ULTRASOUND REVIEW OF OBSTETRICS AND GYNECOLOGY

ULTRASOUND REVIEW OF OBSTETRICS AND GYNECOLOGY

Janice Hickey, RT(R), RDMS
St. Luke's Hospital
Bethlehem, Pennsylvania
Lehigh Valley Hospital
Allentown, Pennsylvania

Franklin Goldberg, MD
Assistant Professor of Radiology
Hotel Dieu Hospital
Kingston General Hospital
Queens University
Kingston, Ontario
Canada

LIPPINCOTT WILLIAMS & WILKINS
A **Wolters Kluwer** Company
Philadelphia • Baltimore • New York • London
Buenos Aires • Hong Kong • Sydney • Tokyo

Lippincott Williams & Wilkins, 530 Walnut Street
Philadelphia, Pennsylvania 19106-3621 USA

Made in the United States of America

Library of Congress Cataloging-in-Publication Data

Hickey, Janice.
The ultrasound review of obstetrics and gynecology / Janice Hickey, Franklin Goldberg.
p. cm.
Includes bibliographical references and index.
ISBN 0-397-51654-1
1. Ultrasonics in obstetrics—Handbooks, manuals, etc. 2. Generative organs, Female—Ultrasonic imaging—handbooks, manuals, etc. I. Title.
[DNLM: 1. Ultrasonography, Prenatal—outlines. 2. Ultrasonography, Prenatal—handbooks. 4. Genitalia, Female—ultrasonography—outlines. WQ 18.2 H628u 1996]
RG527.5.U48H496 1996
618.2'2—dc20
DNLM/DLC
for Library of Congress 95-33416
CIP

The material contained in this volume was submitted as previously unpublished material, except in the instances in which credit has been given to the source from which some of the illustrative material was derived.

Great care has been taken to maintain the accuracy of the information contained in the volume. However, neither Lippincott-Raven Publishers nor the authors can be held responsible for errors or for any consequences arising from the use of the information contained herein.

9 8 7 6 5

Double asterisks (**) denote figures used courtesy of Staff Sonographers and Mr. R. Lappalaine, RDMS, Chief Sonographer at McMaster University Medical Centre, Chedoke-McMaster Hospitals, Hamilton, Ontario, Canada.

To my husband Jim, daughters Julie and Jessica, parents Elizabeth and William Bygrave, and in special memory of my godmother Carol Boyd

JDH

For my mom and dad, sister Sal, and Heidi

FG

CONTENTS

ACKNOWLEDGMENTS

I would like to express my gratitude to a number of wonderful people who deserve my appreciation and thanks:

For content consultation:
Kathleen Foran, R.D.M.S,. R.V.T., Ottawa Civic Hospital, Ottawa, Ontario
Carol Anderson, R.D.M.S., R.D.C.S., Hamilton, Ontario
Janet Markotich, M.D., Radiologist, Kingston Imaging, Kingston, Ontario
Hugh Aldis, M.D., Department of Radiology, Peterborough Civic Hospital, Peterborough, Ontario

For expert computer assistance:
Janet Laubenstein, Associate Professor, Northampton College, Bethlehem, Pennsylvania
Lynn Hudson, Kingston, Ontario, Jim Hickey, my husband

For expert sonographic skills:
Sonographers of McMaster University Medical Centre, Chedoke-McMaster Hospitals, Hamilton, Ontario
Kathleen Foran, R.D.M.S., R.V.T., Ottawa Civic Hospital, Ottawa, Ontario
Angie Henson, R.D.M.S., Hotel Dieu Hospital, Kingston, Ontario
Jan Veenstra, R.D.M.S., Hotel Dieu Hospital, Kingston, Ontario
Anne Joslin, R.D.M.S., Kingston General Hospital, Kingston, Ontario
Tina Cadieux, R.D.M.S., Kingston General Hospital, Kingston, Ontario

For clinical support:
Mike Silver, M.D., Ben Mussari, M.D., Stephanie Young, M.D., Dorothy Lazinski, M.D., Radiology Residents, Queens University, Kingston General Hospital, Kingston, Ontario
Peter Bryson, M.D., and Michael McGrath, M.D., Department of Obstetrics & Gynecology, Queens University, Kingston General Hospital, Kingston, Ontario
Don Sobolesky, M.D., Department of Radiology, Queens University, Kingston General Hospital, Kingston, Ontario
Chris Caco, M.D., and Pat Mohide M.D., McMaster University, Chedoke-McMaster Hospitals, Hamilton, Ontario
Mary Woodman, R.N., R.D.M.S., Fetal Assessment Unit, Kingston General Hospital, Kingston, Ontario

For photography assistance:
Chris Cruise, Kingston General Hospital, Kingston, Ontario
Jack Nochton and the staff at VIP Photographic Lab Services, Bethlehem, Pennsylvania

For graciously lending some sonograms:
Ray Lappalaine, R.D.M.S., Patrick Mohaide, M.D., Christopher Caco, M.D.,' Chedoke-McMaster Hospital, Hamilton, Ontario
Frederick N. Hegge, M.D., Director, Ultrasound Department, Emanuel Hospital, Portland, Oregon
Donald Sobolesky, Eric Sauerbrei, Robert Nolan, Khanh Nguyen, Radiologists, Department of Radiology, Queens University, Kingston General and Hotel Dieu Hospitals, Kingston, Ontario

For assistance with the outline for this project:
Eric Sauerbrei, M.D., Department of Radiology, Queens University, Kingston General Hospital, Kingston, Ontario

And last but not least, especially to Franklin Goldberg, M.D., for assisting me with his invaluable recommendations and comments, expertise, and advice.

Thank you all for your support and encouragement.

PREFACE

This book was to take vast amounts of information and organize it in a format that is:

1. a quick, comprehensive, and convenient source of review for the student or sonographic practitioner;
2. convenient, easy to use, and a quick practical reference for sonographers, radiologists, obstetrician-gynecologists, or residents in these disciplines;
3. a user-friendly text with tables, charts, multiple images, diagrams, and alphabetical listings; and
4. an economical book that keeps in mind students' limited budget.

In preparation for my R.D.M.S. examination, I was unable to find a comprehensive review book that covered all the topics with which I was required to be familiar. I therefore had to accumulate a vast assortment of review articles, handwritten lecture notes, correspondence course material, materials from seminars and conferences, and various textbooks that were informative but too elaborate for review purposes. Valuable time was wasted sorting through and organizing all the material to produce something from which I could review.

Often in textbooks, the sonogram or diagram is not on the same page as the associated text. One is forced to flip pages back and forth or scan the page to match what they were reading to the appropriate image. I drew my own primitive pencil drawings in the margins of my study notes to remind myself what a particular anomaly looked like. Because ultrasound is such a visual modality, I wanted to put into practice the expression, "a picture is worth a thousand words". This was accomplished by placing text next to the multiple sonograms or diagrams. I decided to use tables as a convenient method to sort this information in a clear and concise manner.

The basic core of topics covered in the book are based on the 1994 R.D.M.S. registry examination requirements. Organization of topics is divided into three sections: technical factors, gynecology, and obstetrics. Gynecological anatomy, fetal anatomy, and various anomalies within the chapters are listed alphabetically followed by a complete index. This format will aid in quickly locating information.

Keep in mind that this book is not intended for someone who has never studied ultrasound or who requires a complete and in-depth study of a subject. It presumes a basic knowledge and provides a simple reminder of what we *need* to know, not necessarily what is *nice* to know. I like to think of this book as having the information that you highlight in other texts. If you have located something that needs a more detailed explanation or differential, please refer to one of the excellent sonographic texts I recommend later. This is not an all-inclusive list, as I know there are many other wonderful resource materials as well as periodicals and journals.

I hope this book is a useful addition to your library of sonographic texts. If you have any suggestions or comments, please feel free to contact me at my e-mail address:
JH1361@AOL.com

Janice Hickey

ULTRASOUND REVIEW OF OBSTETRICS AND GYNECOLOGY

CHAPTER 1 - TECHNICAL FACTORS

INDICATIONS FOR ULTRASOUND EXAMINATIONS	
GYNECOLOGY	<u>UTERUS, OVARIES, ADNEXA</u> -abnormal bleeding, pelvic pain and discomfort -IUCD location and complications -pelvic exam reveals mass or enlargement of pelvic organs -evaluation of palpable masses -abnormal laboratory values -ovulation induction therapy and infertility investigation -guidance for abscess drainage, mass biopsy
OBSTETRICS	-"routine" obstetrical ultrasound has varying usefulness according to the literature, but if one was to recommend the best time for a "routine" scan, at 17–18 weeks the fetus is large and developed enough to examine sonographically for most anomalies, yet early enough during the pregnancy when intervention can be considered <u>1ST TRIMESTER</u>: -confirm pregnancy, viability, gestation age -rule out ectopic pregnancy, gestational trophoblastic disease, foreign bodies Large For Dates - fibroids, uterine malformations, multiple gestation, Small For Dates - missed abortion, blighted ovum -ovaries, rule out adnexal lesions, uterine position, rule out uterine anomalies -undetermined etiology of vaginal bleeding -suspected complications, i.e., subchorionic hematoma <u>2ND & 3RD TRIMESTER</u>: -confirm viability, gestational age, fetal number -evaluate fetal growth, anatomy, lie, position, follow-up of anomaly -evaluate placenta, AFV, cord -Biophysical Physical Profile for fetal well being -vaginal bleeding <u>OTHER:</u> -guidance, e.g., amniocentesis, chorionic villi sampling, cordocentesis
ENDOLUMINAL SONOGRAPHY	-better visualization of uterus, ovaries and adnexa -useful in staging endometrial carcinoma
SONO SALPINOGRAPHY/ HYSTEROGRAPHY	-warm fluid is injected via a small catheter to distend lumen of uterus and delineate abnormalities using sonography -used to evaluate tubal patency, uterine anomalies, adhesions, polyps, submucosal fibroids, differentiation between sessile and polypoid fibroids -can explain persistent bleeding in patients with normal endometrial biopsies

TAKING A GOOD HISTORY -recognizing significant clinical information		
GYNECOLOGICAL SONOGRAM	-information such as LNMP, history of unusual bleeding or other significant clinical signs and symptoms, previous surgery, medication, IUCD, Pain-(**P**osition, **Q**uality, **R**adiation, **S**everity, **T**ime), reason for scan, previous scan	
OBSTETRICAL SONOGRAM	-information such as LNMP, pregnancy tests, gravidity (total number of pregnancies), reason for scan, previous scan, unusual clinical signs (eg. bleeding), past abnormal pregnancy history	
DOCUMENTING TOTAL NUMBER OF PREGNANCIES "GPTAL"	**G** - GRAVIDA - number of pregnancies **P** - PARA - number of viable births **T** - TERM - number of term pregnancies **A** - ABORTIONS - number of miscarriages, abortions **L** - LIVING CHILDREN -number of children now living	Multi ...... - has occurred many times Nulli....... - has never occurred Primi ..... - has occurred once

COMPARISON OF TRANSABDOMINAL AND TRANSVAGINAL SCANNING

-techniques are complementary, not mutually exclusive

	TRANSABDOMINAL	ENDO/TRANSVAGINAL
BLADDER VOLUME	<u>Full bladder:</u> 1. provides an acoustic window into the pelvis 2. an anatomic reference point 3. displaces gas-filled bowel loops from pelvis 4. positions uterus more perpendicular to sound beam <u>Amount:</u> -full to point above fundus in non-gravid and early pregnant uterus <u>Volume might need adjusting with:</u> 1. amniocentesis (less full for better pocket of fluid access) 2. over distended bladder presses anterior placenta downward, making it appear previa 3. low lying fetus (a fuller bladder may make BPD more accessible)	-full bladder not required and may limit scan by displacing structures out of view -empty bladder brings pelvic organs into focal zone of transducer
PATIENT POSITION	-supine on comfortable examining table -provided with pillow -patient can be obliqued for a different window	-slight Fowler's position in lithotomy position -transducer must be free to move vertically and horizontally -gynecological table or flat table with large cushion under pelvis
SCANNING TECHNIQUES	-apply gel on area to be scanned -structures imaged in more than one plane: transverse, longitudinal and/or oblique	-insertion of probe into vaginal cavity (gloves worn) -maneuver transducer by in and out rotation and angling motions to visualize pelvic structures
TRANSDUCERS	-careful handling of transducer -cleaning transducer with appropriate solutions between each patient -select frequency for the appropriate penetration with the best resolution: 3.5, 5 MHz sector or convex linear array	-clean techniques are followed with use of condoms and appropriate cleaning solutions after each use -select frequency for the appropriate penetration with the best resolution: 5–7.5 MHz -focal zone 1–5 cm
ADVANTAGES	1. non-invasive 2. greater depth and field of view compared to TV 3. able to scan upper abdomen if required 4. complete sequential and segmental images: can simulanteously image more than one structure at a time (ie. both ovaries)	1. does not require full bladder therefore: i) eases stress with incontinent patients, patients with urinary infections ii) eliminates full bladder discomfort iii) faster medical management 2. higher resolution scanning with more magnification: i) able to better evaluate early pregnancies, ectopic pregnancies, follicular size, small masses, abnormal fallopian tubes, endometrial thickness ii) diagnosis of placenta previa when internal os not well seen with transabdominal approach * iii) better visualization of pelvic organs in obese patients
LIMITATIONS	1. obesity 2. inadequate bladder filling 3. abdominal scarring 4. recent surgery limiting access 5. retroverted or retroflexed uterus 6. fibroids 7. barium or air-filled bowel	1. patients with intact hymens, children 2. smaller field of view 3. requires special probe 4. patient acceptance 5. * placenta previa and incompetent cervix need facilities to deal with possible complications arising from TV scan 6. limited probe mobility due to confines of vagina

GUIDELINES FOR SONOGRAPHIC EVALUATION & DOCUMENTATION

-thorough interrogation, anatomic recognition and demonstration in a systematic pattern using coronal/ transverse and longitudinal planes
-use of appropriate transducer, lowest possible power output settings, correct TGC, field of view, orientation, focus
-each structure labeled on freeze frame with permanent documentation on videotape and/or hard copy
-include images of abnormalities with measurements as necessary

UTERUS, CERVIX & VAGINA	-size, shape, position and echogenicity -endometrial canal
OVARIES	- size, shape, position and echogenicity
OTHER PELVIC STRUCTURES	-musculature, vasculature, anterior and posterior cul-de-sacs, bladder
ANOMALIES & PATHOLOGIES	-location and relationships, size, borders, echotexture, vasculature
OBSTETRICS 1ST TRIMESTER	-ovaries, fetal number, viability, assessment of gestation age (CRL, gestational sac size)
OBSTETRICS 2ND AND 3RD TRIMESTER	-fetal number, viability and lie -placenta location -amniotic fluid volume -assessment of gestation age (BPD, HC, FL, AC) -assessment of fetal anatomy (cerebral ventricles, spine, heart, stomach, urinary bladder, umbilical cord insertion site, renal region, cisterna magna, face, extremities)

TAKING CARE OF THE PATIENT

-staff to adhere to professional code of conduct
-the purpose and procedure should be understood by patient by using verbal explanations, written pamphlets
-explanation of the limitations of diagnostic ultrasound
-put anxious and fearful patients at ease
-protect patient rights, confidentiality and modesty: provide private room for undressing and scanning, use appropriate draping
-check patient ID - ensure the name on the requisition matches the patient's name
-explanation of how and when results will be communicated to patient

GENERAL SONOGRAPHIC CHARACTERISTICS OF MASS TYPE

-correlate sonographic findings with clinical laboratory and clinical results

CYST	COMPLEX	SOLID	BENIGN	MALIGNANT
-anechoic / echo-free even at high gain settings -smooth, well-defined thin wall -distal acoustic enhancement -simple cystic lesion is more likely to be benign	-"mixed" -contains both fluid and solid areas -further subdivided into predominately cystic or predominately solid	-internal echoes -can have irregular, poorly defined margins -distal acoustic shadows caused by increased attenuation -a solid mass can appear anechoic, however, no distal acoustic enhancement will be seen	-anechoic (can have internal echos from blood, septa, dermoid elements) -clear outline, smooth walls, well encapsulated -good sound through transmission -well-defined borders and back wall with prominent echos -mobile	-seen with increasing internal echos, loculations, thick septations -irregular walls, ill-defined borders -no capsule, complex-thickened papillary projections on inner walls -non-mobile

ABSCESS	HEMATOMA
-ovoid masses -anechoic, hypoechoic -thick irregular walls -posterior acoustic enhancement	-appearance depends on time after initial onset and transducer frequency <u>Initially:</u> anechoic <u>After a short interval:</u> highly echogenic due to organization and clot formation <u>After a few more days:</u> becomes more complex due to cellular lysis <u>After several days:</u> after complete lysis the mass becomes anechoic again

DOPPLER

The principle of Doppler is that the frequency of sound reflected from moving objects is related to their speed and direction. Duplex imaging analyzes the difference in frequency between emitted and received signals. An ultrasound beam can be directed at a vessel producing a reflected sound with a Doppler shift. This has a characteristic waveform. The three indices used to evaluate a Doppler Waveform are: resistance index, pulsatility index and the systolic : diastolic ratio. These are arbitrary calculations without a specific unit designation. Blood flow pattern is also analyzed.

Color Doppler is a combination of B-mode, pulsed wave Doppler and a color flow display. It depicts motion. The direction of blood flow is dependent of the direction of flow toward and away from transducer. The color can vary in its hue, brightness and saturation which represent the flows frequency and energy.

As well as evaluating specific vessels, Doppler also has a role in evaluating masses. The velocity and impedance of arterial blood flow in a tumor varies depending on its pathophysiology. There are ongoing studies to measure the velocity and impedance of various types of tumors. Tumor vascularity is often but not always associated with hypervascularity (an increased number of vessels within the mass) and arterial-venous shunting. Tumors often have low resistance to flow due to lack of normal arteriolar smooth muscle. Where the flow is located in a mass can also be significant. For example, in the liver, hemangiomas have no central flow, whereas Focal Nodular Hyperplasia does.

WAVEFORM OF MAXIMUM DOPPLER SHIFT

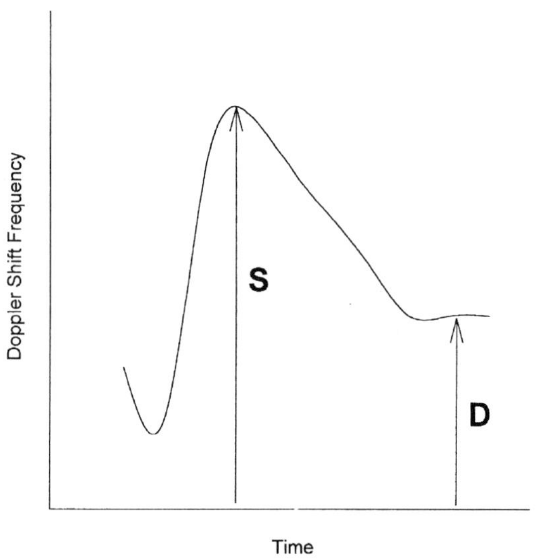

S = peak systolic pressure D = end diastolic pressure

On left side the real time image shows the doppler sample gate through the umbilical artery and shows a normal umbilical arterial waveform

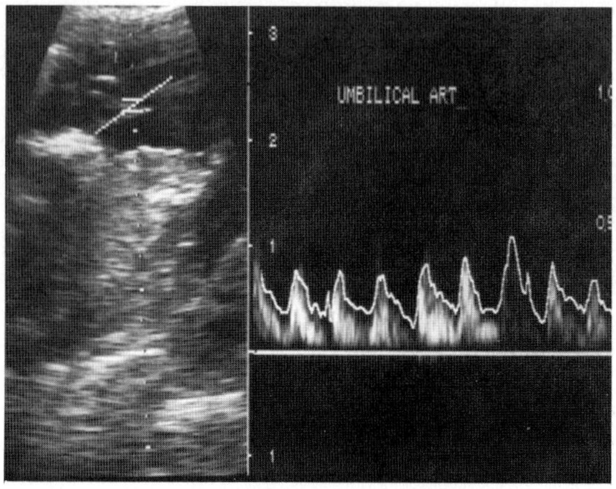

DOPPLER INDICES

Resistive (Pourcelot) Index	Pulsitivity (Impedance) Index	Systolic/Diastolic Ratio
$\frac{S - D}{S}$ -approaches 1 when diastolic velocity approaches zero or is abnormally low and resistance is high	$\frac{S - D}{\text{mean}}$ -ratio of peak to peak height of doppler waveform to mean height -value of PI decreases with increasing resistance -requires precise calculation of mean velocity -will show changes even with no diastolic flow	$\frac{S}{D}$ -simple older indice -value declines as resistance declines -will become infinity when diastolic velocities reach zero

DOPPLER ANALYSIS OF TUMOR CHARACTERIZATION		
HIGH IMPEDANCE	INTERMEDIATE	LOW IMPEDANCE
PI > 1.5 benign RI > 0.7 benign	PI =1.0–1.5 probably benign RI > 0.4 probably benign	PI < 1 suspicious for malignancy RI < 0.4 suspicious for malignancy
-masses such as cystadenomas, hemorrhagic cysts -to avoid false positives due to angiogenesis, avoid scanning between days 3–10 of cycle	-intermediate or variable indices suggest masses such as dermoids and endometriomas	-tumors such as ovarian carcinomas produce neovascularity which can cause a different pattern of low impedance to blood flow -benign tumors such as inflammatory masses, endometriomas, hemorrhagic corpus luteum cysts may show low impedance flow -normal morphology + abn. waveform = suspicious -abn. morphology + normal waveform = suspicious -loss of diastolic notch = suspicious
<u>MASS WITH GREATER PERIPHERAL VASCULARITY</u> + LOW MAXIMUM SYSTOLIC VELOCITY + HIGH IMPEDANCE + DIASTOLIC NOTCH differential includes: simple cyst, dermoid, endometriomas		<u>MASS WITH GREATER CENTRAL VASCULARITY</u> + HIGH MAXIMUM SYSTOLIC VELOCITY + LOW IMPEDANCE + LOSS OF DIASTOLIC NOTCH differential includes: ovarian neoplasms, tubo-ovarian abscess, hemorrhagic masses
<u>ENERGY/ POWER / COLOR POWER ANGIO DOPPLER</u> -this relatively recent type of color doppler shows the perfusion of structures as only flow power is displayed as opposed to flow velocities in the traditional color doppler method. Positive Features: -angle independent, therefore no aliasing, and therefore greater sensitivity -this greater sensitivity is especially useful in small vessels (e.g., testes, and peripheral vessels of organs such as spleen and kidney) -reduced examination time compared to pulsed doppler Negative Features: -prone to flash artifact -no direction or velocity information -not available on all transducers -decreased depth of penetration compared with regular color doppler sonography		

ACRONYMS & ABBREVIATIONS IN OBSTETRICS AND GYNECOLOGY SONOGRAPHY	
AC	abdominal circumference
AFI	amniotic fluid volume index
AFP	alpha-fetoprotein
AFV	amniotic fluid volume
AMA	advanced maternal age
AP	abdominal perimeter
AP	anterior-posterior
APH	ante partum hemorrhage
APKD	adult polycystic kidney disease
ASD	atrial septal defects
BCP	birth control pills
BH	Braxton Hick's contraction
b-hCG	beta- human chorionic gonadotropin
BP	blood pressure
BPD	bi-parietal diameter
BPM	beats per minute
BPP	biophysical profile
BTB	break through bleeding
(C)CAM	(congenital) cystic adenomatoid malformation
CDH	congenital diaphragmatic hernia
CFM	color flow mapping
CI	cephalic index
CMV	Cytomegalovirus
CNS	central nervous system
COC	combined oral contraceptives
COR	coronal
CRL	crown-rump length
CSF	cerebral spinal fluid
CV	cardiovascular
CVS	chorionic villi sampling
CW	continuous wave
CXR	chest x-ray
D+C	dilatation and curettage
DCR	double chorionic ring sign (same as DDS)
DDS	double decidual sac sign (same as DCR)
DDx	differential diagnosis
DES	diethylstilbestrol
DLT	double layer thickness; referring to endometrial measurement
DUB	dysfunctional uterine bleeding
DVT	deep vein thrombosis
DWM	Dandy Walker malformation
EFW	estimated fetal weight
EVS	endovaginal sonography
FDIU	fetal death in utero
FH	fetal heart
FL	femur length
FMC	focal myometrial contraction
FUO	fever of unknown origin
GA	gestational age
GB	gallbladder
GI	gastrointestinal
GIFT	gamete intrafallopian transfer
GTD	gestational trophoblastic disease
GU	genitourinary
HC	head circumference
hCG	human chorionic gonadotropin
HP	head perimeter

ACRONYMS & ABBREVIATIONS IN OBSTETRICS AND GYNECOLOGY SONOGRAPHY cont'd	
HRP	high-risk pregnancy
HRT	hormone replacement therapy
Hx	history
IDDM	insulin dependent diabetitis mellitus
IDM	infant of diabetic mother
IPKD	infantile polycystic kidneys
IUCD	intrauterine contraceptive device
IUD	intrauterine death (also known as intrauterine contraceptive device)
IUG	intrauterine gestation
IUGR	intrauterine growth retardation
IUP	intrauterine pregnancy
IVF	in vitro fertilization
KUB	kidney - ureters - bladder : x-ray of AP abdomen
LBW	low birth weight
LFD	large for dates
LGA	large for gestational age
LH	lutenizing hormone
LKMP	last known menstrual period
LLQ	left lower quadrant
LMP	last menstrual period
LONG	longitudinal
LUQ	left upper quadrant
LVR	lateral ventricular ratio
MA	menstrual age
MCDK	multi-cystic dysplastic kidney(s)
MCK	multi-cystic kidney
MRI	magnetic resonance imaging
MSD	mean sac (gestational) diameter
NIH	non-immune hydrops
NPO	nothing by mouth
NTD	neural tube defect
NYD	not yet diagnosed
OB-US	obstetrical ultrasound
OC	oral contraceptive
OFD	occipital frontal diameter
OHSS	ovarian hyperstimulation syndrome
PCK(D)	polycystic kidney (disease)
PCO	polycystic ovaries
PCOD	polycystic ovarian disease
PDop	power doppler
PE	pleural effusion
PET	pre-eclamptic toxemia
P.I.	pulsatility index
PID	pelvic inflammatory disease
PIH	pregnancy induced hypertension
PMB	post-menopausal bleeding
PMS	pre-menstrual syndrome
PP	post partum
PPV	positive predictive value
PROM	premature rupture of membranes
PUV	posterior urethral valve
PW	pulsed wave
R.I.	resistance index (Pourcelot's Index)
RLQ	right lower quadrant
RUQ	right upper quadrant
SAG	sagittal
SFD	small for dates
SFH	symphysis fundal height

ACRONYMS & ABBREVIATIONS IN OBSTETRICS AND GYNECOLOGY SONOGRAPHY cont'd	
SGA	small for gestational age
SROM	spontaneous rupture of membranes
ST	soft tissue
STD	sexually transmitted diseases
TA	therapeutic abortion
T.A.	transabdominal scan
TAH	total abdominal hysterectomy
TAS	transabdominal sonography
TE	tracheo-esophageal
TIUV	total intrauterine volume
TOA	tubo-ovarian abscess
TORCH	toxoplasmosis, rubella, cytomegalic inclusion disease, herpes simplex virus
TR	transverse
TRAP	twin reversed arterial perfusion syndrome
TTTS	twin-to-twin transfusion syndrome
T.V.	transvaginal scan
TV-CDS	transvaginal color doppler sonography
TVS	transvaginal sonography
TVUS	transvaginal ultrasound
UPJ	uteropelvic junction
UTI	urinary tract infection
UVJ	urethrovesical junction
VBAC	vaginal birth after c-section
VSD	ventricular septal defects
YS	yolk sac
+ve	positive
-ve	negative
<	less than
>	more / greater than

CHAPTER 2 - PELVIC STRUCTURES

BLADDER

-hollow muscular organ located extraperitoneally in pelvis
-discharges urine through the urethra
-contour and size depends on position and size of uterus and volume of bladder

Ureteral Jets:
-flow of urine entering bladder observed with real time scanning and color doppler

Structure:
APEX
-above bladder neck
-most anterior, superior part
-middle umbilical ligament attaches at this point
BLADDER NECK
-lower part, fixed behind symphysis pubis
-portion of bladder surrounding internal urethral orifice
BASE (TRIGONE)
-triangular area between the insertion of the ureters and the urethra
-uretha (bladder neck) opens in apex of trigone
-ureters drain at 2 points of superolateral angle in base of trigone
WALL
-4 layers made up of mucosa, submucosa, Detrusor muscle and serous layer

Relationships:
Anterior -posterior surface of symphysis pubis
-space between is the retropubic space (Retzius)
Posterior -base and trigone of bladder rest on anterior vaginal and uterine wall
Lateral -pelvic diaphragm

transabdominal, transverse view of female pelvis with normal bladder (B) seen anterior to uterus (U) and ovaries (O)

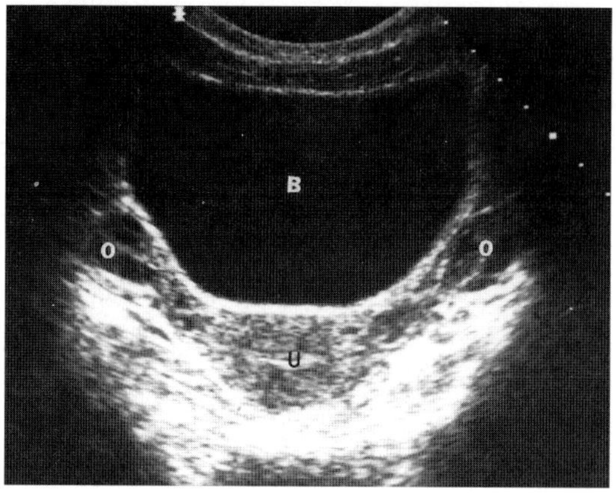

BOWEL

SMALL BOWEL
-when filled with fluid appears a tubular structure in long-axis and as a circular structure in cross section
-normal small bowel wall thickness < 3 mm

LARGE BOWEL
-fusiform structure normally filled with gas and fecal material which can often obscure visualization of pelvic structures during scanning
-changes shape and position due to active peristalsis
-intraluminal fluid will outline projections from bowel wall
-normal colon wall thickness: < / = 4 mm

APPENDIX
-tubular in long axis and circular in cross section
-lies in right iliac fossa
-normal total AP dimension < 6 mm and wall thickness < 2 mm

CLINICAL SIGNIFICANCE
-G.I. disease (eg. appendicitis, inflammatory bowel disease) should be considered in the differential of patients presenting with lower abdominal pain or masses
-normal bowel loops should not be confused as pelvic masses

normal loop of large bowel as seen on transvaginal examination (arrows). Peripheral hypoechoic region represents the muscular layer of the bowel

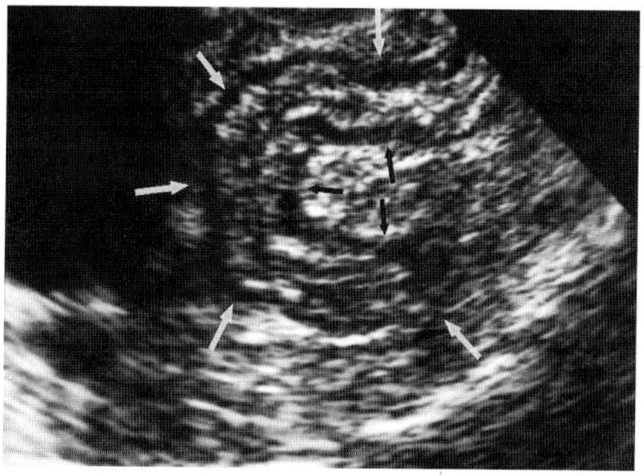

MUSCLES OF PELVIS				
MUSCLE	FUNCTION	ORIGIN	INSERTION	US APPEARANCE
OBTURATOR INTERNUS	rotates thigh outward	pubis, ischium, obturator foramen	inner surface greater trochanter	-can be seen at level of cervix in transverse view
PIRIFORMUS	abducts and rotates thigh outward	anterior sacrum and sacrosciatic notch of ilium	upper margin of greater trochanter	-can be confused with ovary -posterior to rectum, vagina and uterus
ILIO PSOAS	= ILIACUS + PSOAS			-seen sonographically as "bullseye" appearance at level of bony pelvis brim -between true and false pelvis
a) ILIACUS	flexes and rotates thigh	margin of iliac fossa	lesser trochanter	
b) PSOAS MAJOR	flexes thigh, adducts and rotates it medially	thoraco-lumbar spine	lesser trochanter	
c) PSOAS MINOR	tenses iliac fascia	T-12 + L1 vertebrae	iliac fascia, iliopectineal tuberosity	
PELVIC DIAPHRAGM	= LEVATOR ANI + COCCYGEUS -supports pelvic viscera and forms floor of pelvis			-visualized inferiorly on ultrasound near level of vagina on transverse view
a) LEVATOR ANI	anterior portion of pelvic diaphragm supports rectum and pelvic floor	pubis, pelvic fascia, ischial spine	rectum, coccyx, perineum	
b) COCCYGEUS	-posterior portion of pelvic diaphragm supports coccyx, closes pelvic outlet	ishial spine, sacrospinous ligament	coccyx, lower sacrum	

APPEARANCE AND LOCATION OF PELVIC MUSCLES

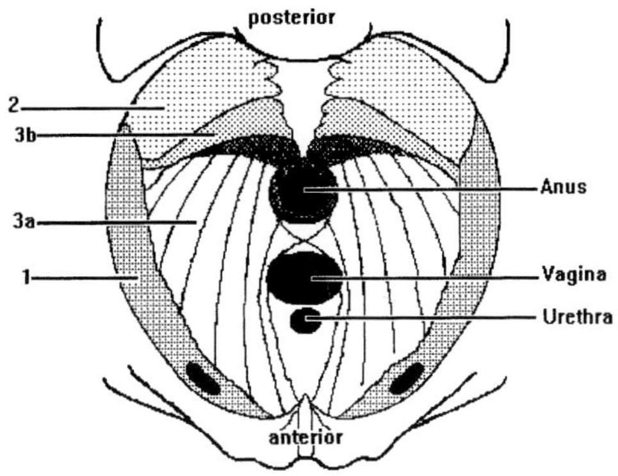

KEY:
1. Obtuartor Internus
2. Piriformus
3a. Levator Ani
3b. Coccygeus

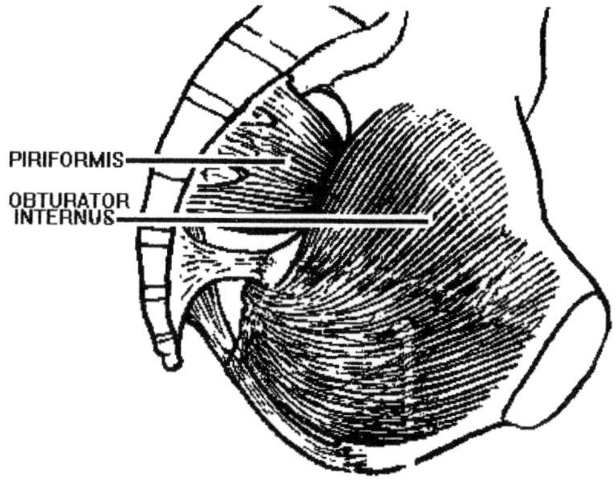

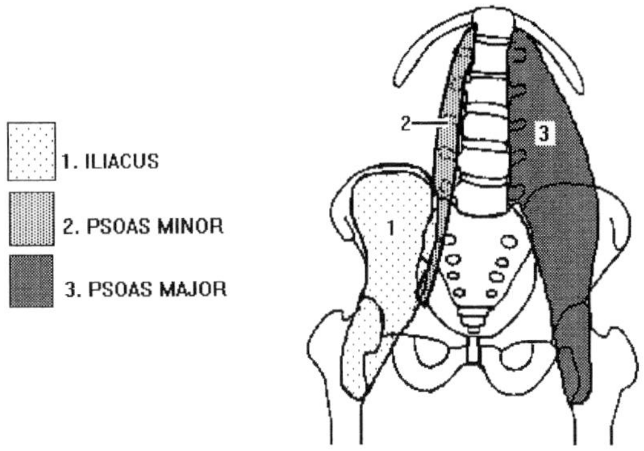

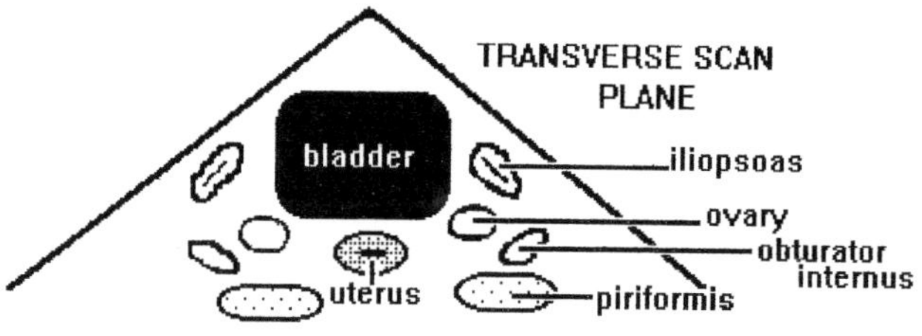

transabdominal longitudinal scan of right pelvic side wall which visualizes the bladder (B) external iliac vessels (EI), psoas major (P) and iliacus (I) in their long axes

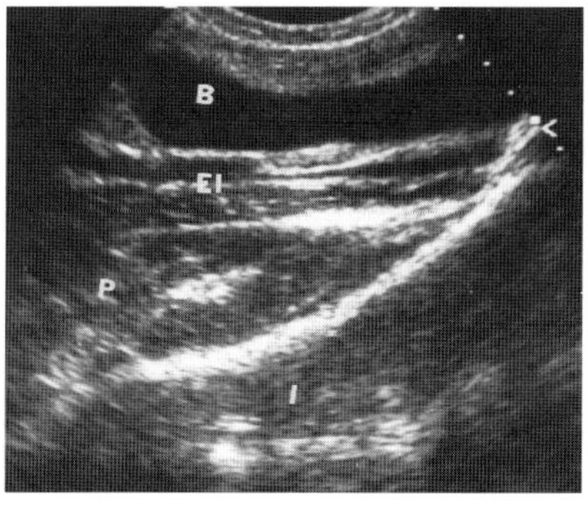

transabdominal transverse scan of female pelvis; uterus (U) and ovaries (O) are seen above the piriformus muscle (white arrows)

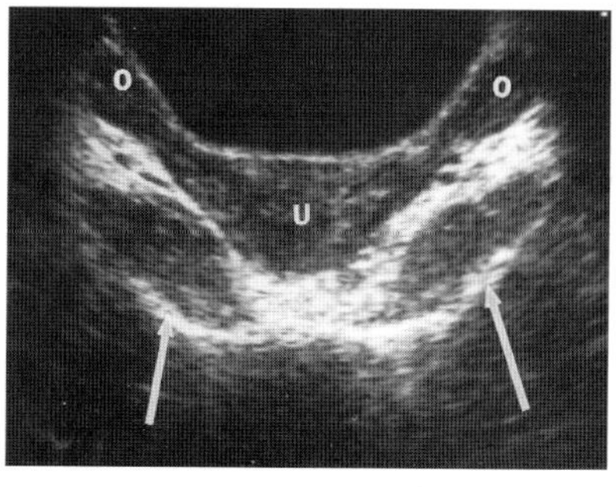

PELVIS - BONY

-consists of
1. paired innominate bones which are a fusion of 3 bones
   a) Ischium
   b) Pubis
   c) Ilium
2. sacrum
3. coccyx
4. ligaments uniting them

-functions as support for vertebrae and articulation for femurs
-separated into true (inferior) and false (superior) by iliopectineal line and upper margin of symphysis pubis

<u>True (minor) pelvis:</u>
-lies below linea terminalis (bony ridge on inner surface of ilum which continues onto pubis)
-lower border formed by coccyx, ishial protuberances, ishial rami

<u>False (major) pelvis:</u>
-above the linea terminalis and represents the lower portion of the abdomen

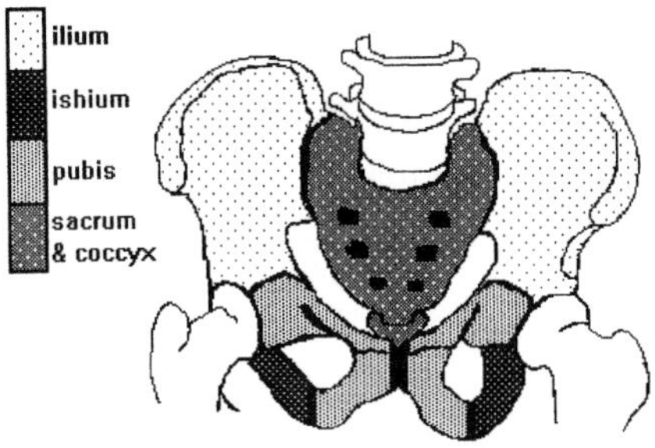

PELVIC FREE FLUID

POSTERIOR ABDOMINAL WALL DIVIDES

-free fluid runs off heights created by these structures and accumulates in dependent areas called the paravertebral, paracolic gutters and pelvic cavity (anterior and posterior cul-de-sacs)

<u>1. LONGITUDINAL DIVIDE</u>
-an elevation of the posterior abdominal wall formed by the lumbar spine, psoas muscles, aorta, IVC, crus of diaphragm, quadratus lumborum
<u>2. OBLIQUE DIVIDE</u>
-consists of bony pelvic brim, iliopsoas muscle and common and external iliac vessels

culdocentesis:
-transvaginal needle aspiration of fluid from the posterior peritoneal cul-de-sac
-useful technique for evaluating the type of fluid pooled there

NORMAL FINDINGS	ABNORMAL FINDINGS
-posterior cul-de-sac is frequently the first site for intraperitoneal fluid to collect—small amount of fluid is normal finding during menstrual cycle in asymptomatic patients	-ascites -blood due to rupture of ectopic pregnancy, cyst -infected collections: pus, abscess -hematomas
transvaginal sagittal scan of posterior cul de sac showing a small collection of free fluid (arrows) 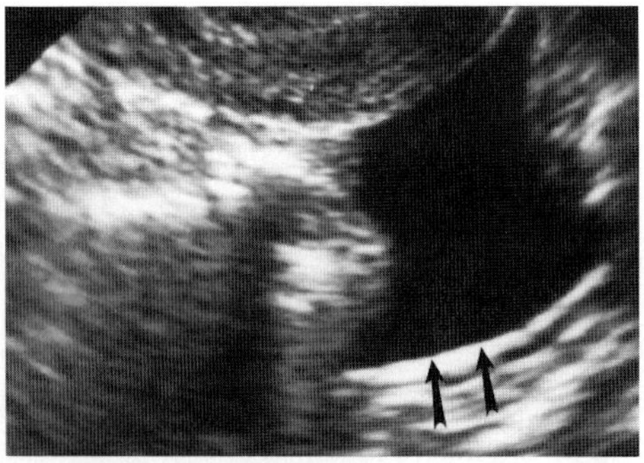	transvaginal scan of hematoperitoneum (arrows) surrounding a hemorrhagic cyst (C) in the posterior cul de sac 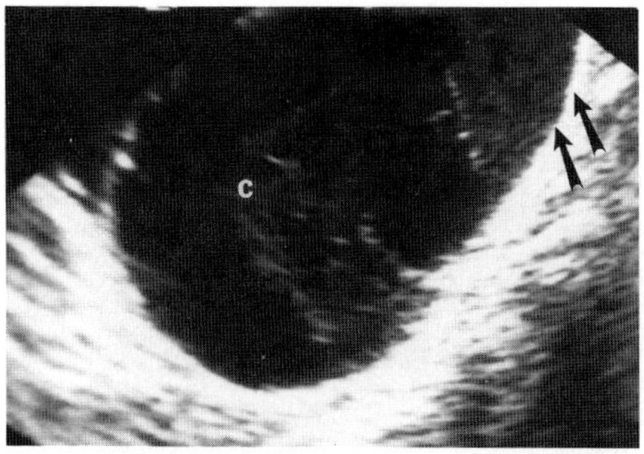

PERINEUM - female	
-diamond-shaped area consisting of skin and several layers of muscle, overlying pelvic outlet between thighs and buttocks -divided into two sections: 1. Anterior Urogenital Triangle -contains orifice for urethra and vagina 2. Posterior Anal Triangle -contains anus boundaries of perineum: <u>Lateral Boundaries:</u> -sacrotuberous ligament, ischial tuberosity, pubic arch -transverse line across divides perineum into anterior/posterior <u>Anterior Boundary</u>: -symphysis pubis, pubic arch <u>Posterior Boundary</u>: -coccyx	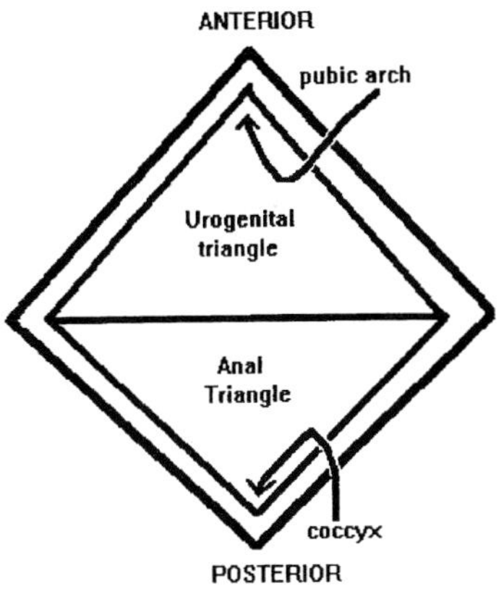

ANOMALIES THAT CAN MIMIC GYNECOLOGICAL PATHOLOGY	
PELVIC MASSES	bladder diverticuli bladder masses bowel disease: appendicitis, diverticulitis, Crohns disease, colitis, bowel cancer duplication cysts ectopic kidneys fluid/fecal filled bowel loops lymphoma mesenteric cysts urachal cysts
COMPLICATIONS OF TRAUMA, SURGERY	abscess hematoma hemorrhage lymphocele seroma thrombosis urinoma

Superior - towards head
Anterior - close to transducer
Posterior - towards back
Inferior - towards feet

CHAPTER 3 - UTERUS

A) NORMAL ANATOMY

UTERUS	-thick-walled, hollow, muscular organ-shaped like an inverted pear -located in lesser pelvis between urinary bladder and rectum -consists of two main parts: body and cervix
FUNCTION	-menstruation, pregnancy, labor
STRUCTURE	-wall of uterus contains 3 layers: <u>1. ENDOMETRIUM</u>- MUCOSAL LAYER -inner layer of uterus divided into two sublayers A. DECIDUAL LAYER (STRATUM FUNCTIONALIS) -functional layer closer to uterine cavity -thickens and changes appearance throughout cycle and is shed during menstration B. BASAL LAYER (STRATUM BASALIS) -permanent layer that produces a new decidual layer following menstruation -contains numerous glands <u>2. MYOMETRIUM</u>- MUSCULAR LAYER -forms bulk of uterine wall. Contains 3 layers of smooth muscle <u>3. PERIMETRIUM</u>- SEROUS LAYER -outer layer of uterus. Part of visceral peritoneum. Laterally it becomes broad ligament. Anteriorly it wraps over the urinary bladder and forms the anterior cul-de-sac, posteriorly if it reflected onto the rectum and forms the posterior cul-de-sac
BODY (CORPUS)	-fundus (dome-shaped portion of uterus above fallopian tubes) to cervix -corpus to cervix ration 2:1
SIZE	-length 7.5–9 cm x width 4.5–6 cm x thickness 2.5–4 cm -multiparity may increase size by 1–2 cm in all directions
LOCATION	-superior and posterior to empty bladder and anterior cul-de-sac -anterior to rectum and posterior cul-de-sac (Pouch of Douglas)
RELATIONSHIPS	<u>Anterior Surface</u>: flat surface, covered by peritoneum which is reflected onto the bladder to form the ANTERIOR CUL-DE-SAC <u>Posterior Surface</u>: convex surface covered by peritoneum which continues downward over the cervix and upper vagina and then reflected onto the anterior portion of the rectum to form the POSTERIOR CUL-DE-SAC (lowest point in peritoneal cavity)
CERVIX	-neck of the uterus which is rounded and conical in shape opening into the vagina at 90° -cavity called the endocervical canal -made up of two parts, supra-vaginal and vaginal
SIZE	-length 2.5 cm x diameter 2.5 cm
LOCATION	-the lower part of the uterus below the level of the isthmus which protrudes into vagina
RELATIONSHIPS	<u>Anterior Surface</u> - bladder <u>Posterior Surface</u> - uterosacral ligament, posterior cul-de-sac <u>Lateral Aspect</u> - uterine artery in connective tissue -ureters pass downward and forward about 2 cm lateral <u>Proximal Aspect - Supra-Vaginal part -</u> communicates with body at isthmus <u>Distal Aspect - Vaginal part</u> - projects into vagina forming vaginal fornices creating 4 recesses (anterior, posterior and two lateral fornices)
VAGINA	-fibromuscular tube extending from vestibule of vulva externally to cavity of uterus internally <u>Fornices:</u> recess that surrounds vaginal attachment to cervix -divided into four segments: ANTERIOR, POSTERIOR, and two LATERAL
SIZE	-length 9 cm (posterior wall) 7.5 cm (anterior wall)
LOCATION	-directed posterosuperiorly at 45° angle in relation to pelvic inlet -its axis forms approximately at a 90° angle to cervix
RELATIONSHIPS	<u>Anterior Surface</u> - cervix, base of bladder, distal ureters, urethra <u>Posterior Surface</u> - posterior cul-de-sac, rectum, anal canal, urogenital diaphragm <u>Lateral Aspect</u> - root of broad ligament, ends of ureters, levator ani muscle <u>Proximal Aspect</u> - surrounds vaginal part of cervix extending higher posteriorly and forming four continuous recesses

UTERUS Longitudinal View

1. CUL-DE-SACS:
   A. ANTERIOR CUL-DE-SAC (VESICOUTERINE POUCH)
   B. POSTERIOR CUL-DE-SAC (RECTO-UTERINE POUCH/POUCH OF DOUGLAS)
2. BLADDER
3. ANTERIOR FORNIX OF VAGINA
4. POSTERIOR FORNIX OF VAGINA
5. SPACE OF RETZIUS (PREVESICAL / RETROPUBIC SPACE)
-space between bladder and pubis filled with extraperitoneal adipose tissue

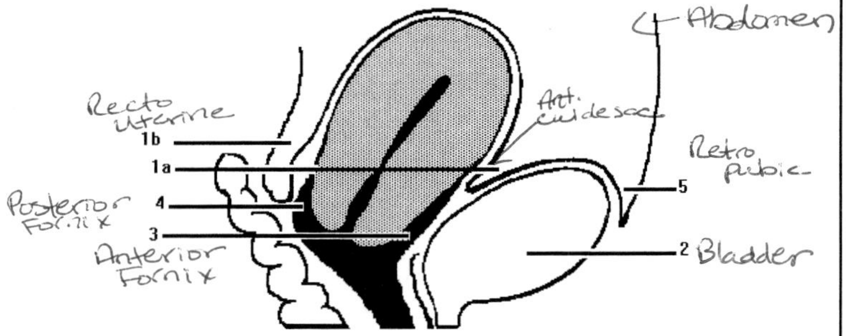

UTERUS Frontal / Coronal View

1. FUNDUS
2. BODY (CORPUS)
   a. CORNUA-LATERAL ANGLES
   -superolateral aspect of body where fallopian tubes enter
3. ISTHMUS
   -constricted area represents lowest part of body of uterus, known as lower uterine segment during pregnancy
4. CERVIX
   a. VAGINAL CERVIX
   b. SUPRAVAGINAL CERVIX
5. LATERAL FORNICES OF VAGINA
6. INTERNAL OS
7. EXTERNAL OS
8. ENDOCERVICAL CANAL
9. UTERINE CAVITY
   -interior of the uterine body is a potential space
10. VAGINA
11. PERIMETRIUM
12. MYOMETRIUM
13. ENDOMETRIUM
14. FALLOPIAN TUBE

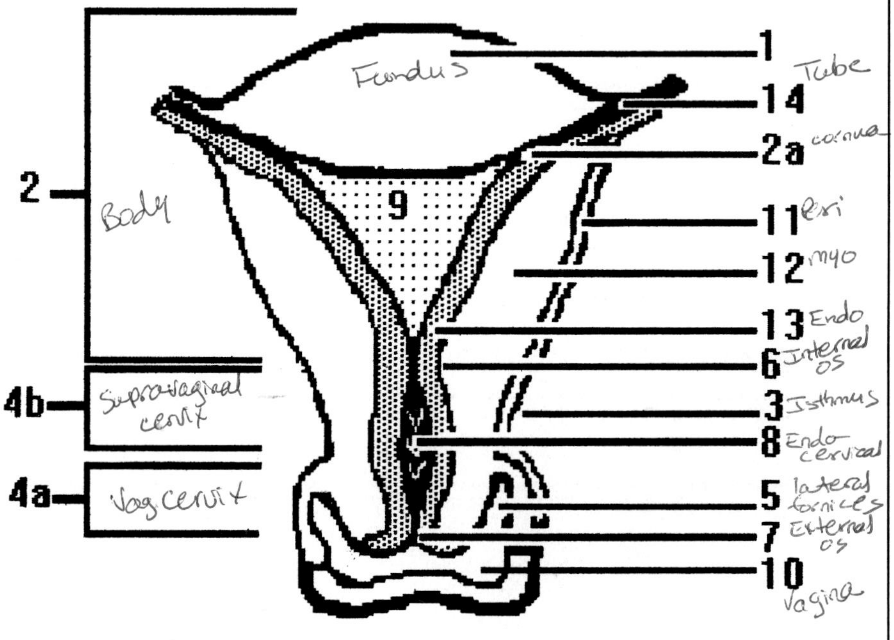

Anterior-cul-de-sac (vesicouterine)
between bladder + uterus

Posterior-cul-de-sac (rectouterine) / Pouch of Douglas
between rectum + uterus

Space of Retzius (Retropubic)
between bladder + pubis

UTERINE SUPPORTS - many ligaments attach to uterus but main supports are bony pelvis and muscles of pelvic floor

1. UTERO-SACRAL LIGAMENT
-posterior support
-maintain the anteverted position of the uterus
-deep to peritoneum, pair of ligaments that lie on either side of the rectum and connect the cervix to the sacrum

2. CARDINAL LIGAMENT (MACKENRODT/TRANSVERSE CERVICAL)
-principle lateral support, especially for cervix
-extend laterally in bottom of anterior part of broad ligament
-passes over ureters
-lying below the broad ligament, they position the uterus above vagina by extending between the pelvic wall and the cervix and vagina
-path for uterine blood vessels and nerves

3. BROAD LIGAMENT
-lateral support
-double fold of parietal peritoneum that drapes over the uterus and divides pelvic cavity into anterior and posterior portions
-stretches from the uterus to the lateral side walls and floor of the pelvis
-helps support the structures it encloses

Contains:
-uterine blood vessels, nerves, round ligament and ligament of ovary
-free edge contains fallopian tube
-at its posterosuperior surface it gives attachment to ovary through the mesovarium

4. ROUND LIGAMENT
-anterior support
-runs anteriorly and inferiorly from junction of fallopian tube and uterus between layers of broad ligament

5. SUSPENSORY LIGAMENT OF OVARY

6. OVARIAN LIGAMENT

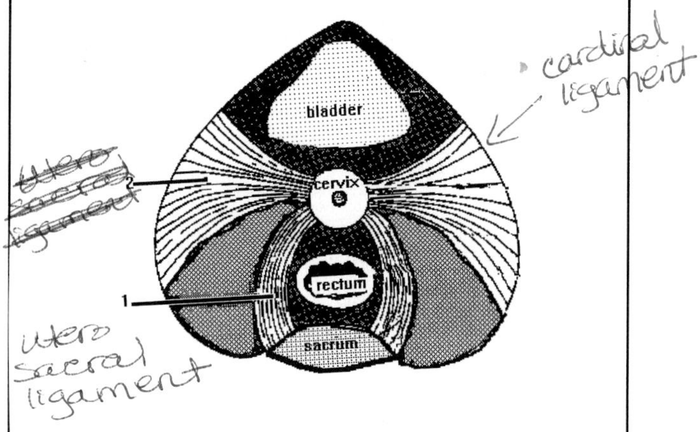

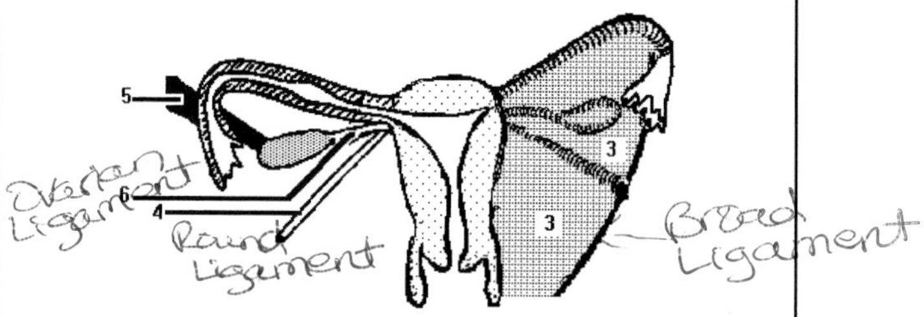

POSITIONS OF UTERUS

ANTEFLEXION - a thrust forward of the uterine body on the cervix resulting in a sharp angle where it bends

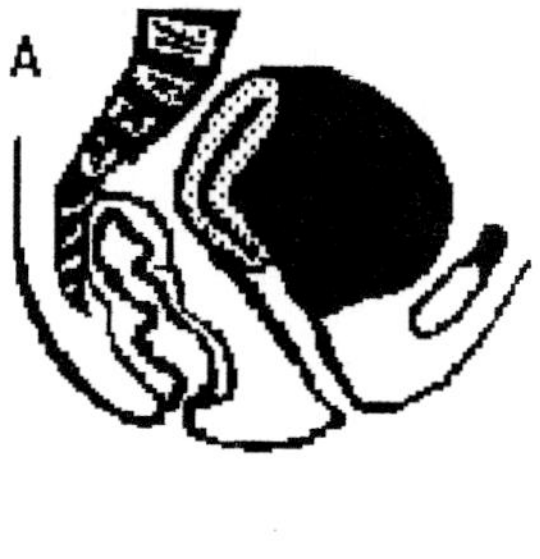

ANTEVERSION - a tipping forward of the uterus without a sharp angle between the body and the cervix

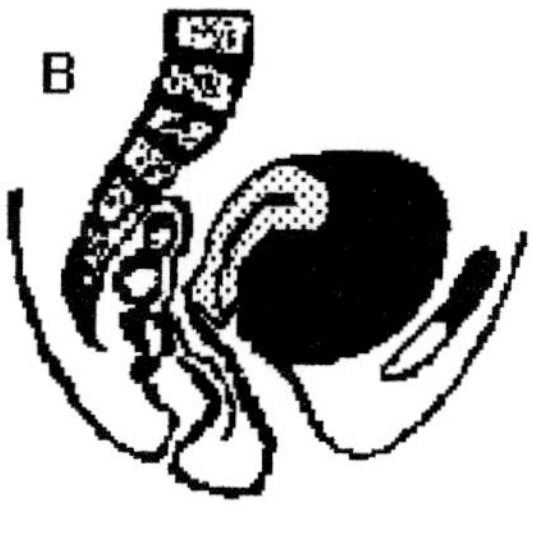

RETROVERSION - a tipping backward of the uterus without a bend between the cervix and body

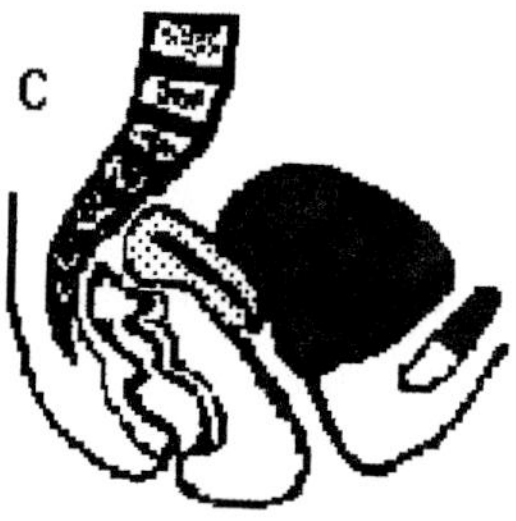

RETROFLEXION - a bending backward of the uterine body on the cervix resulting in a sharp angle where it bends

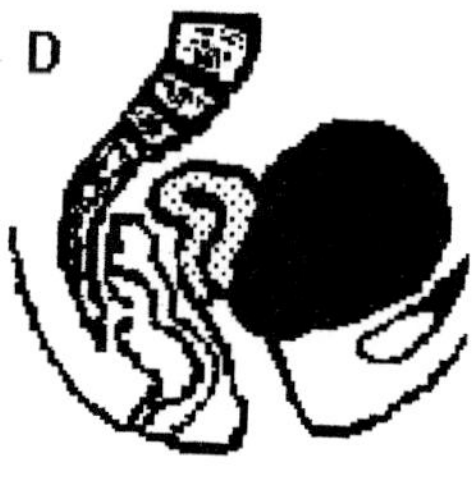

VASCULATURE OF UTERUS

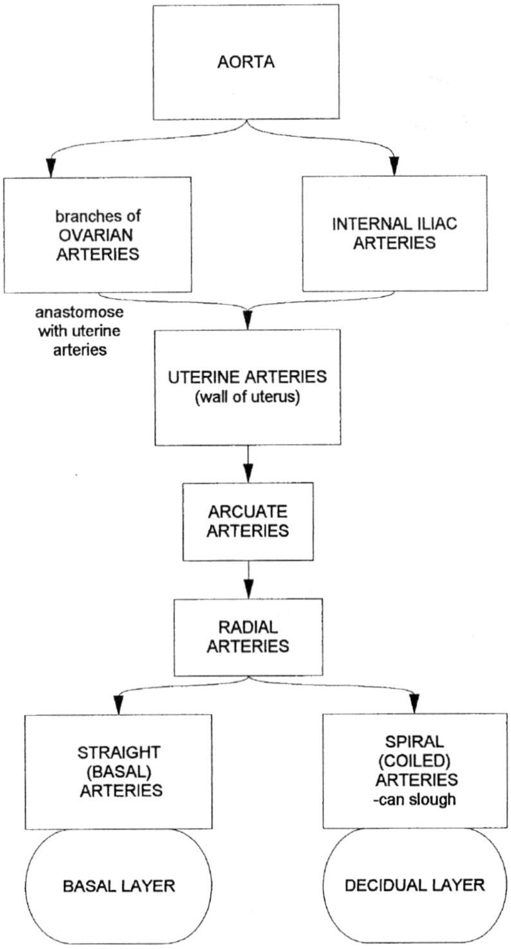

ARTERIAL CIRCULATION

-uterine artery runs medially off the internal iliac artery toward the cervix where it then ascends lateral to uterus in the broad ligament to cornua

-there it coarses laterally toward the ovary to where it astomoses with a branch of the ovarian artery

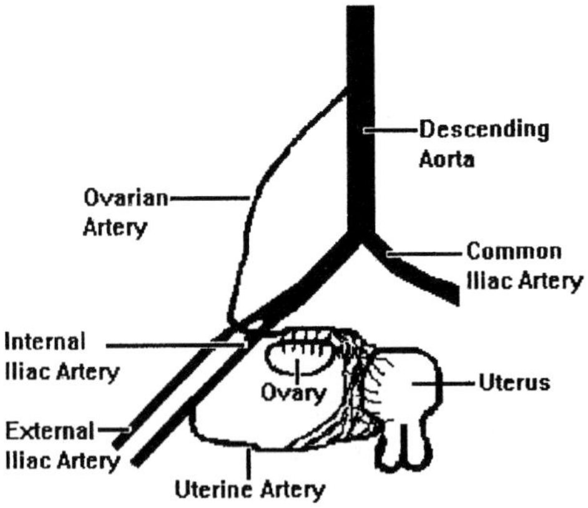

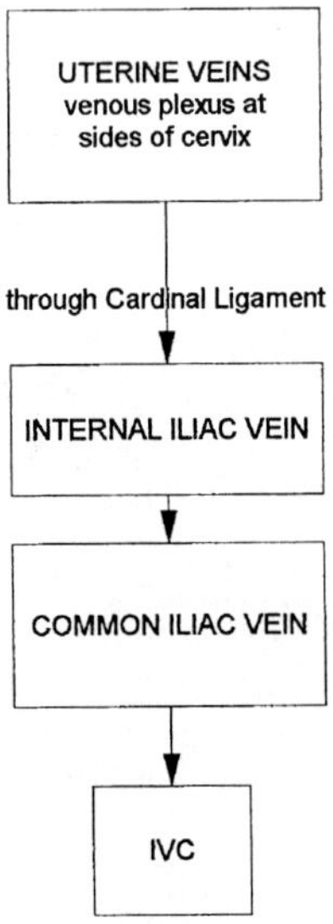

VENOUS CIRCULATION

Uterine Plexus

-situated along sides and cornua of uterus

-veins composing this plexus anastomose with each other and the ovarian veins

-are not tortuous like the arteries

Common Iliac Veins

-are formed by the union of the external and internal iliac veins

-ascend to join and form the inferior vena cava posterior and lateral to their corresponding artery

-right common iliac vein shorter and more vertical than left

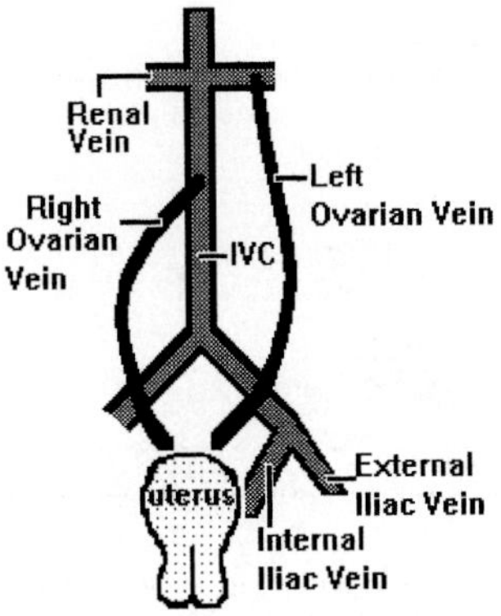

URETER AND VESSEL RELATIONSHIP

ILIAC ARTERY AND VEINS AND URETER

Common Iliac Artery:
-anterior and medial to psoas muscle
-posterior to ureters, ovaries and fallopian tubes
Common Iliac Vein:
-medial and posterior to Common Iliac artery
Internal Iliac Artery:
-supplies pelvic viscera, walls, perineum
-posterior to ureter
Internal Iliac Vein:
-posterior to internal iliac artery
External Iliac Artery:
-travels through false pelvis and femoral canals to supply lower limbs

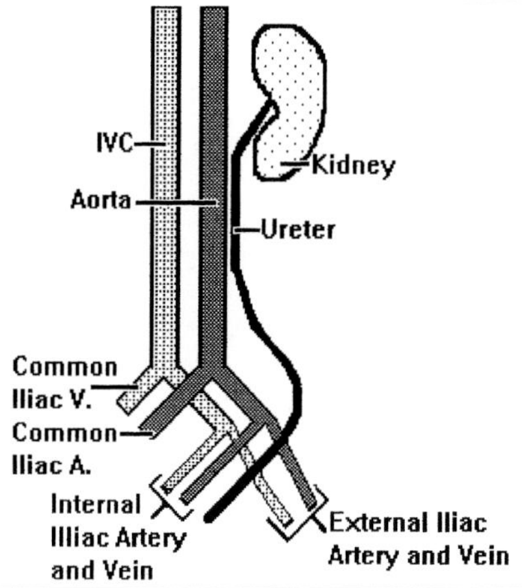

UTERINE ARTERY AND URETER

Ureters:
-cross either the common iliac or external artery to enter the pelvis medially to the ovarian vessels beneath the peritoneum
-descend into pelvis antero-medial to internal iliac vessels
-assumes anterior direction at the level of the ischial spine to pass about 2 cm lateral to cervix under uterine artery
-then it travels medially to enter the bladder anterior to the upper vagina

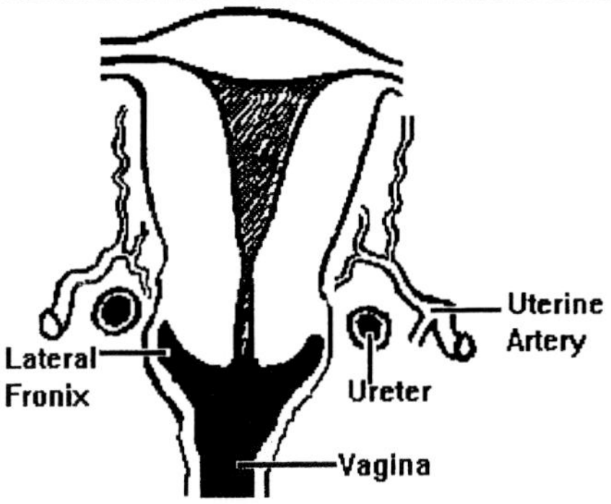

ENDOMETRIAL BLOOD SUPPLY

1. ENDOMETRIUM
2. MYOMETRIUM
3. ARCUATE ARTERIES
-arranged in circular fashion in myometrium
-appear as tortuous tubular anechoic structures in outer myometrium
4. RADIAL ARTERIES
-penetrate myometrium
5. SPIRAL ARTERIOLES
-coiled vessels which penetrate and supply the functional layer of endometrial
-change markedly during cycle
-during menstruation are sloughed off
-during pregnancy become the uteroplacental arteries in decidua
6. STRAIGHT (BASAL) ARTERIOLES
-supply continual nourishment to basal layer
-not affected by cyclical hormone changes and are therefore not sloughed off
7. UTERINE ARTERY
-branch of internal iliac artery
-along with uterine veins seen as hypoechoic linear structures near lateral border of cervix

CROSS SECTION OF UTERUS

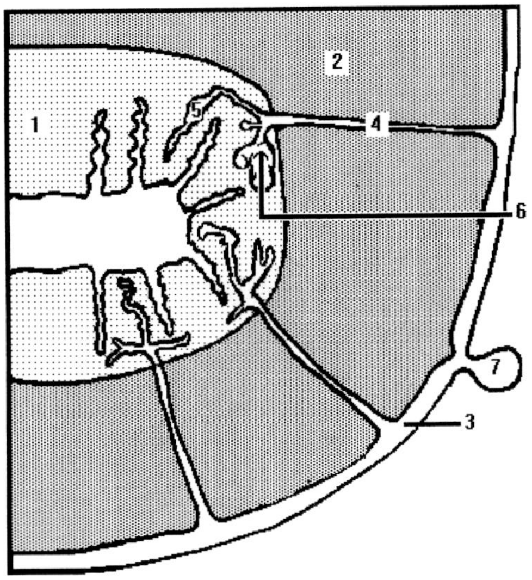

LYMPHATIC DRAINAGE OF FEMALE GENITAL SYSTEM

UPPER BODY & FUNDUS, FALLOPIAN TUBES, OVARIES	-drain into lumbar lymph/para aortic nodes -accompany ovarian vessels
LOWER PART OF BODY	-drain into external iliac nodes
CERVIX	-drains posterolaterally into external iliac nodes -drains posteriorly into sacral and common iliac noes
VAGINA	-drains into superficial inguinal nodes

NORMAL SONOGRAPHIC APPEARANCES OF UTERUS

-apart from normal growth, the appearances of the genital tract depend entirely on the supply of estrogens

DESCRIPTION and SIZE L= length W= width D= AP diameter	ULTRASOUND APPEARANCE
NEONATAL (birth - 6 weeks) -can be slightly enlarged, secondary to residual maternal hormonal stimulation -no isthmus -1/2–1 cm larger than infantile INFANTILE (6 weeks - 2 years) -the cervix is longer than (comprising 2/3 total length) the uterine body, and there is no flexion between the cervix and the uterus L: 2–3.3 cm D: 0.5–1.0 cm CHILDHOOD (2 years - menarche) -tubular or inverse pear-shaped uterus which persists in this appearance until puberty -cervix twice AP diameter of uterine fundus -uterus continues to grow slowly until just before puberty L: 3.5 cm PUBERTY (8–12 years) -growth is rapid for short time -uterus becomes pear shaped -with the gradual increase in estrogen, the body of the uterus grows in relation to the cervix L: 6 cm D: 3 cm	sagittal scan of infant uterus (arrows), (B) bladder 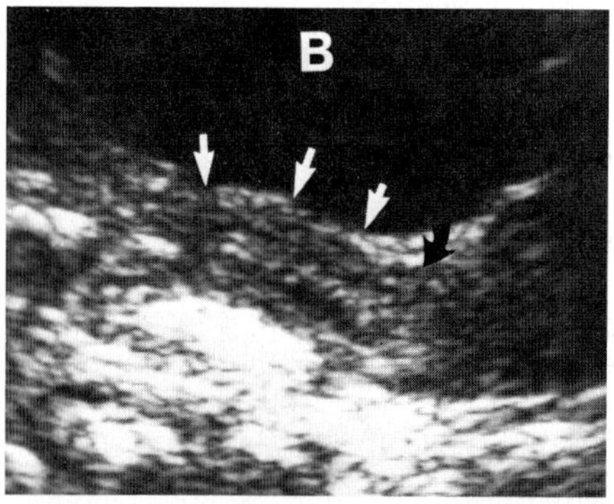 transabdominal sagittal scan of 10-year-old uterus 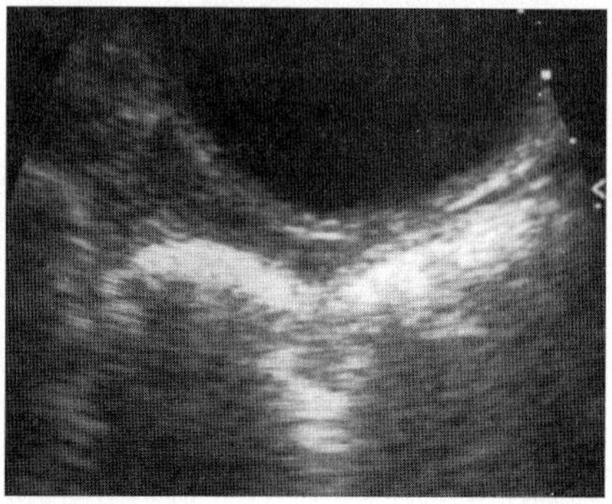
ADULTHOOD -under hormonal influence the fundus now becomes twice the depth of the cervix Uterus Endometrium: -measured at thickest point in AP diameter in a long axis view and includes all layers -DLT: double layer thickness measured on mid sagittal scan -thickness and echogenicity varies throughout menstrual cycle Myometrium: -sonographically is normally homogenous with low to moderate echogenicity -3 layers can be differentiated into a hypoechoic inner zone, slightly more echogenic thicker middle zone and vessels between the middle and outer zone Cervix -cervical canal appears as echogenic stripe continuous with uterine canal -cervix is that portion of the uterus which lies behind the posterior angle of the bladder on the sagittal scan plane Vagina -hypoechoic tubular structure -echogenic lumen	**TRANSABDOMINAL UTERUS** transabdominal transverse scan of adult uterus 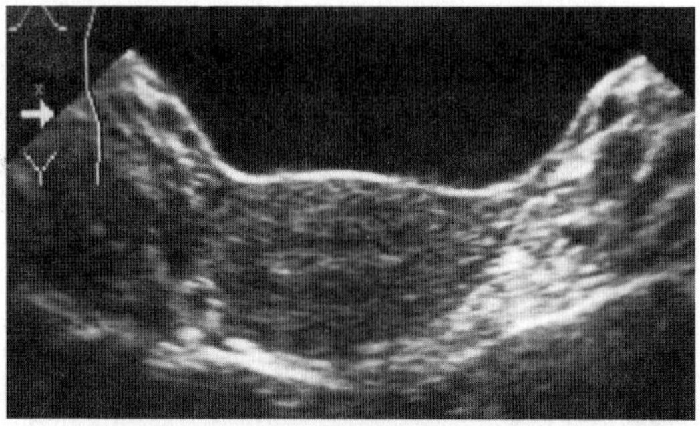 transabdominal sagittal scan of adult uterus 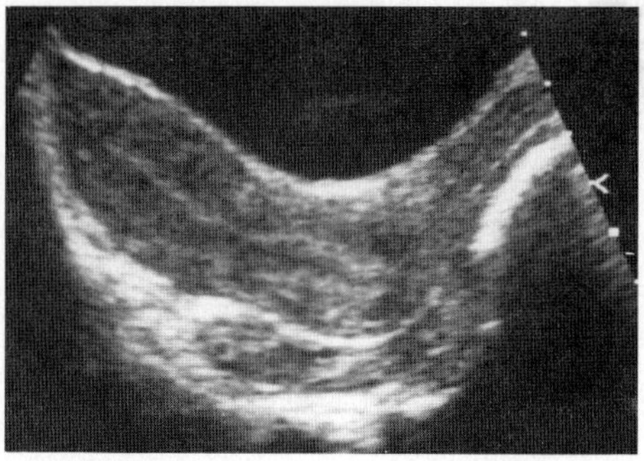

ADULTHOOD UTERUS cont'd

NULLIPAROUS

-woman who has not produced viable offspring

-the body reaches twice the size as the cervix and the permanent degree of flexion is achieved

-position varies depending on bladder and rectum volume

L: 5.0–8.0 cm

W: 3.0 cm

D: 3.0 cm

MULTIPAROUS

-after childbirth uterus remains slightly larger than a nulliparous uterus by about 1–2 cm in all dimensions

L: 8.0–9.0 cm

W: 5.0–6.0 cm

D: 5.0 cm

TRANSVAGINAL UTERUS

transvaginal transverse scan of adult uterus

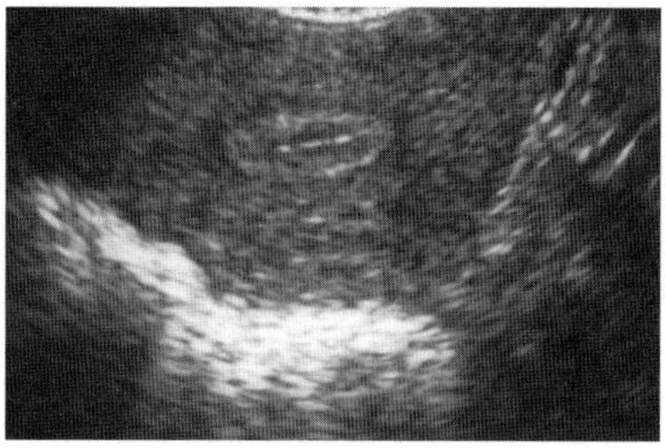

transvaginal sagittal scan of adult uterus

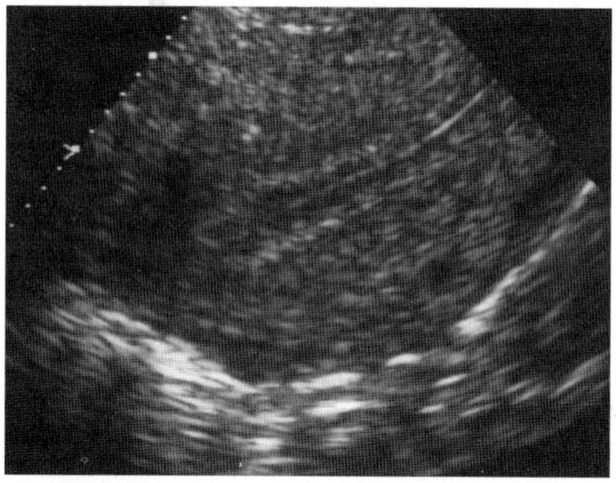

RETROVERTED AND RETROFLEXED ADULT UTERUS

-variants of normal uterine position

Retroversion:

-posterior tilting of the uterus with no bend between the uterine body and the cervix

Retroflexion:

-posterior tilting of uterine body on the cervix creating an angle at the point where it bends

-a uterus tilted to the right or left are variations of normal

transabdominal sagittal scan of retroflexed uterus; calipers measuring endometrial thickness

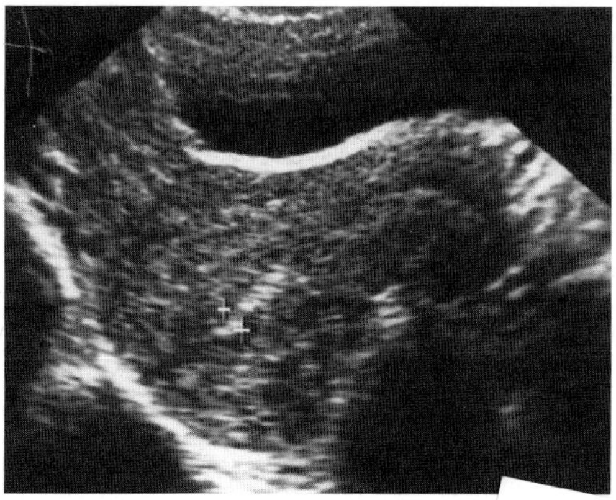

ADULTHOOD UTERUS cont'd

PREGNANCY

-in first trimester, careful scanning to rule out any uterine malformations should be made as these anomalies may be difficult to detect later in pregnancy
-fundus of uterus is palpable and the documentation of symphysis fundal height is charted by obstetricians
-fundal height increases until about 36 weeks when baby "drops"

transabdominal sagittal scan of cervix during pregnancy; endometrial canal (black arrows), internal os (white arrow)

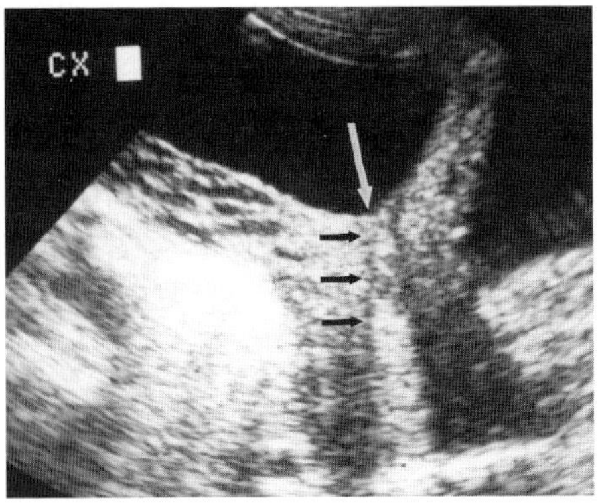

transabdominal sagittal scan of gravid uterus in first trimester

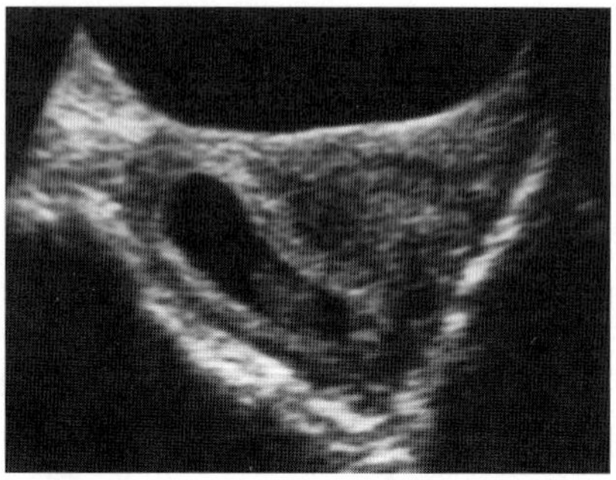

POST- PARTUM

-uterus contracts after delivery
-many times larger than resting uterus
-inhomogenous endometrium
-postpartum uterus remains enlarged 1–2 months following delivery

transabdominal sagittal scan of enlarged post-partum uterus (within 24 hours of delivery) (note bladder flap hematoma and fluid within an irregular endometrium)

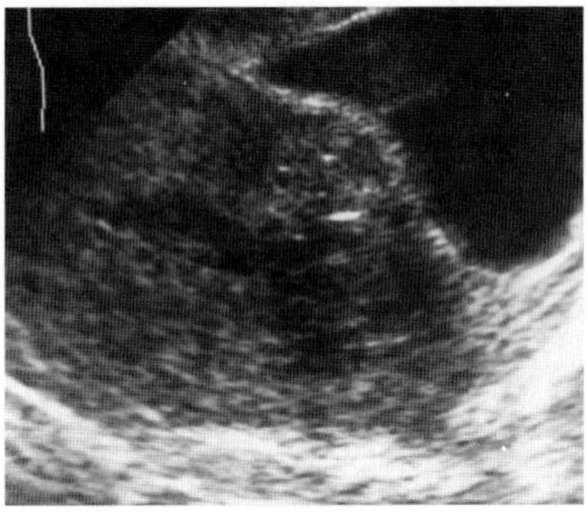

transabdominal transverse of post-partum uterus within 24 hours of delivery showing a normal amount of endometrial fluid within an enlarged uterus

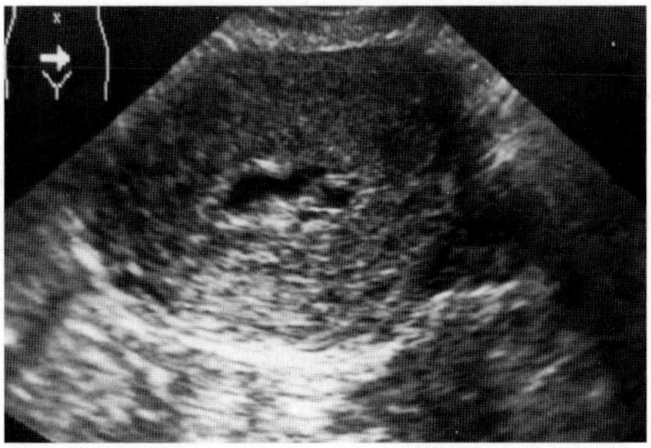

ADULTHOOD UTERUS cont'd	
POST-MENOPAUSE -menstrual cycles become less frequent due to failure of ovaries to respond to stimulation of gonadotrophic hormones from anterior pituitary -causes a decrease in production of follicles and subsequent reduction of estrogen -atrophy of reproductive organs -the uterus gradually atrophies over time and becomes similar in appearance to infantile proportions, with a relatively large cervix and small body L: 3.5–6.5 W: 1.0–2.0 D: 2.0 Post-Menopausal Bleeding Differential: -hormone replacement therapy -vaginitis -endometrial carcinoma, polyp, hyperplasia -cervical carcinoma, polyp -ovarian tumor -bleeding from urinary tract	transabdominal sagittal scan of a 70-year-old's uterus 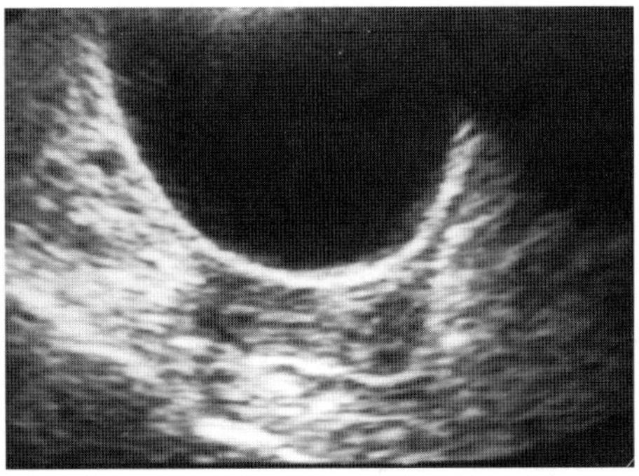 transabdominal transverse scan of a 65-year-old's uterus 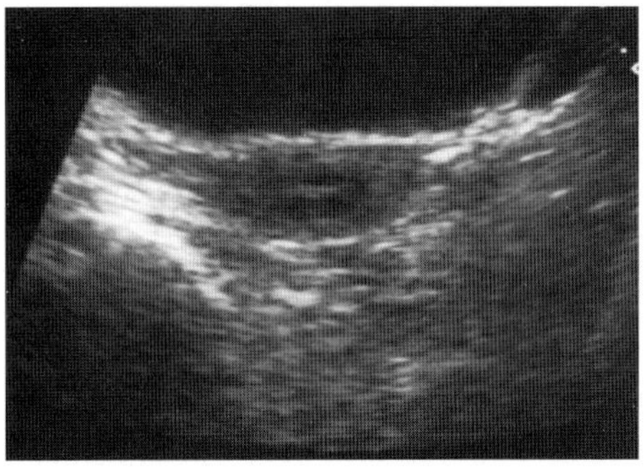 transvaginal sagittal scan of a normal post-menopausal uterus 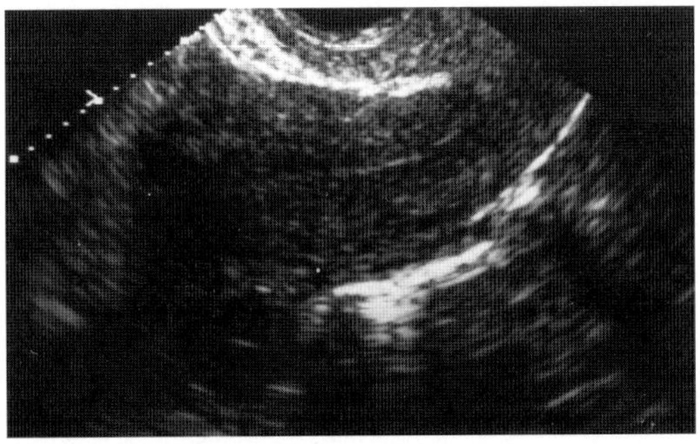
HORMONE REPLACEMENT THERAPY -therapy of replacing estrogen and progesterone in post-menopausal women -relieves symptoms associated with menopause, prevents severe osteoporosis, improves cardiovascular risks -DUB: Dysfunctional Uterine Bleeding or cyclic bleeding can be a side effect of hormonal stimulation of endometrium -uterus is similar in size to nulliparous	transabdominal sagittal scan of a 65-year-old's uterus on hormone replacement therapy (note the prominent echogenic endometrial echo) 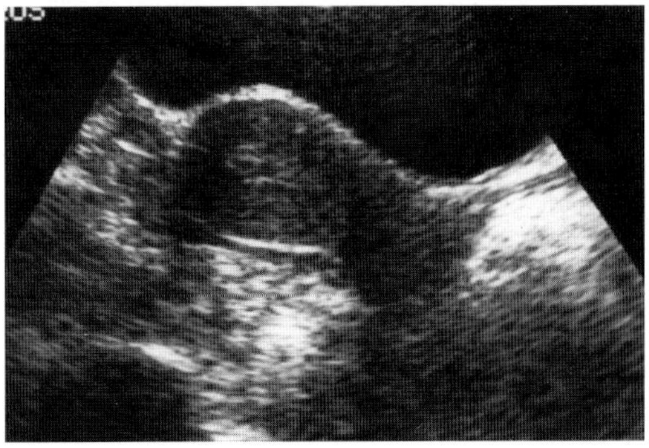

NORMAL SONOGRAPHIC APPEARANCE OF ENDOMETRIUM

-visualization of a normal endometrial stripe can almost certainly rule out endometrial disease
-consists of 2 layers:
1. Functional layer (Decidual)
-appearance changes constantly throughout all phases of menstrual cycle
-innermost layer of endometrium
-endometrial cavity is a potential space between apposed functional layers and can generate a bright linear echo
2. Basal layer
-thin and hyperechoic
-outermost layer of endometrium

PSEUDOTHICKENING
-a normal endometrium can appear too thick when there is echogenic material within the lumen or if endometrium is imaged with an oblique scan plane

MEASURING THE ENDOMETRIUM
-measure in midline sagittal plane in the widest area of the fundus and include all layers of endometrium
-thickness depends on phase of menstrual cycle
-if possible, scan when endometrium should be its thinnest, ie.,
a) pre-menopausal women—near end of menstruation
b) post menopausal women with hormone replacement therapy—after completion of progesterone or near end of withdrawal bleeding

SINGLE (SLT) OR DOUBLE LAYER THICKNESS (DLT)
-endometrial thickness can be reported as single layer thickness (total width divided in half) but it is more commonly accepted to report it as a double layer thickness

transvaginal sagittal uterus with calipers placed to measure the endometrium

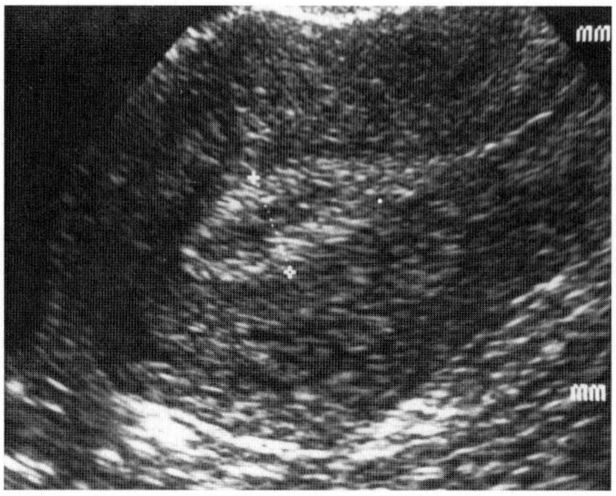

measure endometrium between black arrows

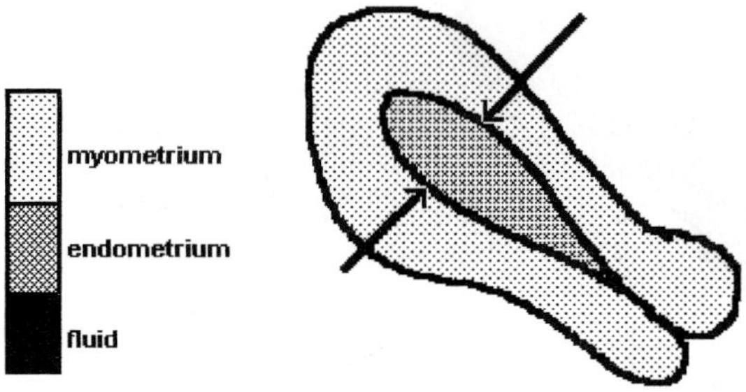

uterus with fluid in endometrium: endometrium between each black and white arrow pair and add values together

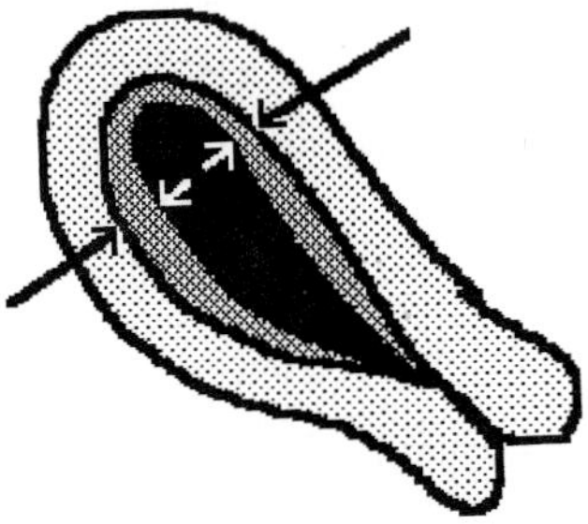

MENSTRUAL PHASE	SIZE–DLT	US APPEARANCE
<u>MENSTRUATING PHASE</u> -variable appearance depending on the amount of clot or blood present -thin broken echogenic central interface -uterine artery has a higher impedance	2–4 mm	transvaginal sagittal scan of uterus; first day of menstrual cycle 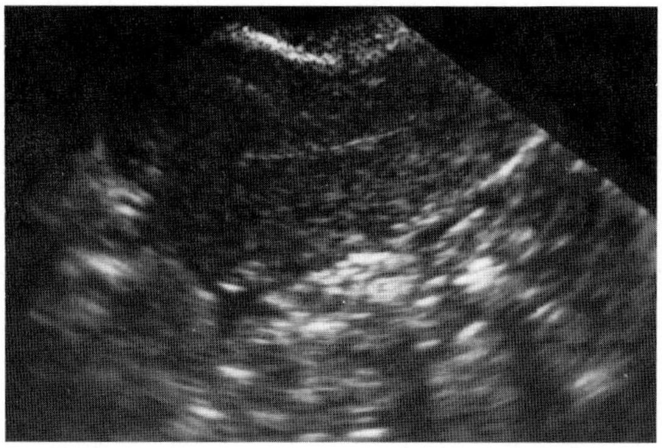
<u>PROLIFERATIVE PHASE</u> EARLY -relatively thin echogenic line composed of echogenic basal layer next to the central endometrial interface LATE -becomes more hypoechoic during the late proliferative phase with a multilayered triple layer or "halo" appearance 3 layers; 1. central thin echogenic line of the endometrial interface 2. hypoechoic functional layer 3. echogenic basal layer -trace amount of fluid can be found within endometrium	4–8 mm	transvaginal sagittal scan of uterus; late proliferative stage 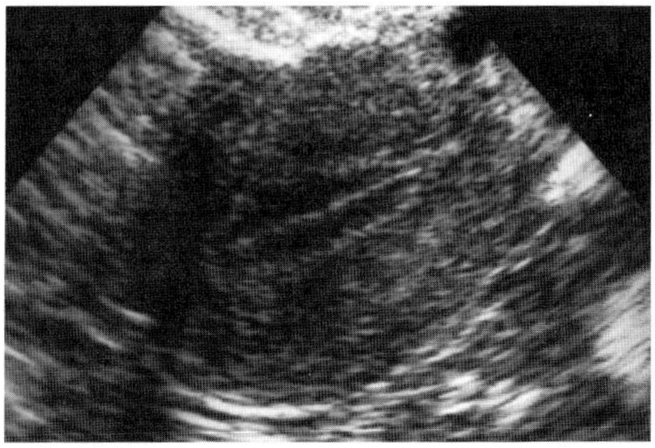
<u>SECRETORY PHASE</u> -thick uniformly echogenic central band as all three layers mentioned in late proliferative are all echogenic and merge together to form one region -endometrial glands become tortuous and filled with glycogen and mucin -uterine artery has lower pulsativity index	at maximum thickness of 7–16 mm	transvaginal sagittal scan of uterus in secretory phase 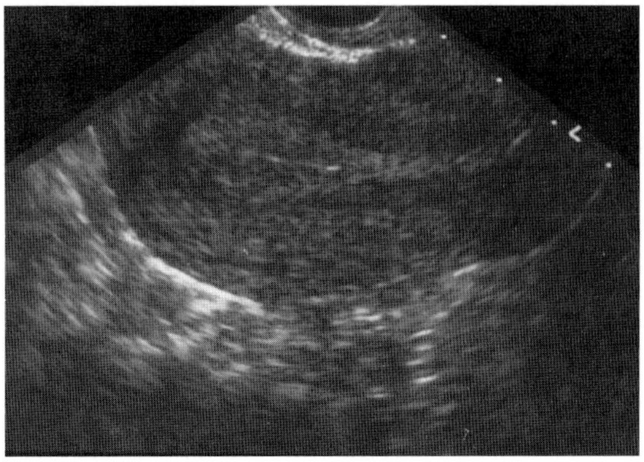

MENSTRUAL PHASE	SIZE–DLT		US APPEARANCE
<u>POST-MENOPAUSAL</u> -thin echogenic line due to atrophy -myometrium may be seen as a subendometrial hypoechoic halo	NO BLEEDING </= 8 mm acceptable >8 mm unacceptable, needs further investigation >15 mm urgent attention	BLEEDING </= 4 mm atrophy 6-8 mm equivocal > 8 mm further investigation (biopsy)	abnormal transvaginal sagittal scan of post-menopausal uterus; patient has bleeding, but not on hormone replacement: Endometrium = 2.4 mm 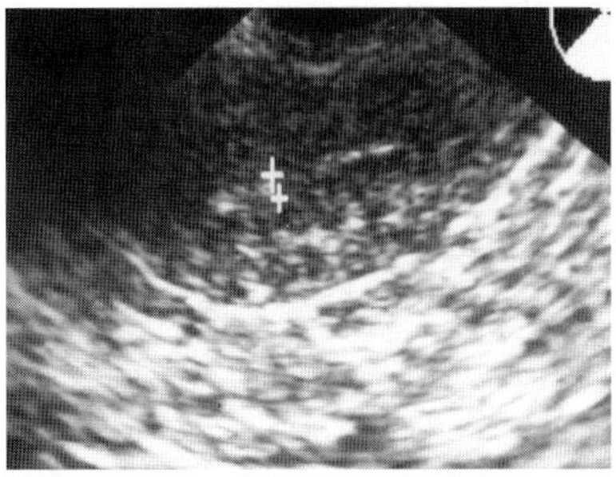
<u>POST-MENOPAUSAL + HORMONE REPLACEMENT THERAPY</u> Estrogen + Progesterone: typically seen as thin echogenic interface Unopposed Estrogen: thicker endometrium due to cellular proliferation which is induced by the estrogen	NO BLEEDING </= 8 mm acceptable > 8 mm unacceptable, needs further investigation (biopsy, D&C)	BLEEDING </= 4 mm acceptable 5–8 mm equivocal > 8 mm unacceptable, needs further investigation, treatment	transvaginal scan of a 70-year-old female's uterus showing a very enlarged heterogeneous endometrium measuring 26 mm (between arrows) 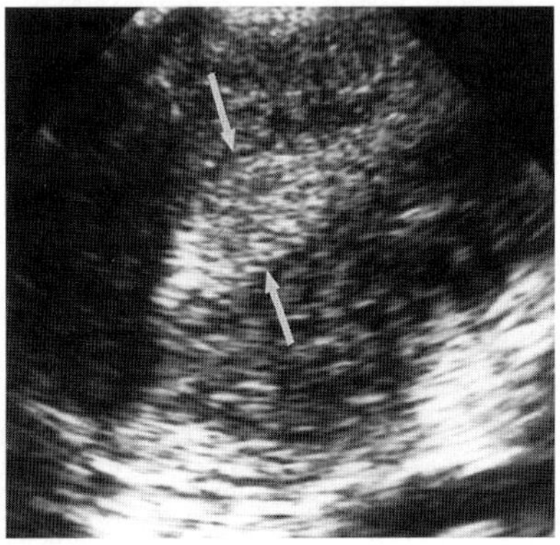 transabdominal sagittal uterine scan with hormone replacement–endometrium measures 10 mm, but transvaginal measurements should be done, especially if measurement is equivocal 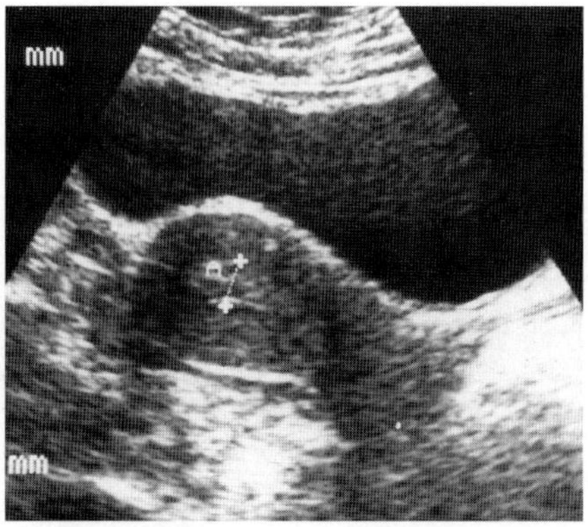

B) ABNORMALITIES

ABNORMALITY SS= signs and symptoms US= ultrasound findings	**US APPEARANCE**
ADENOMYOSIS AND ENDOMETRIOSIS -although pathologically different, these diseases are both abnormal growths of endometrial tissue outside endometrium therefore are considered for simplicity's sake together <u>ADENOMYOSIS</u> -benign invasion of the myometrium by ectopic deposits of endometrium SS -if severe, can cause menorrhagia, dysmenorrhea, and pelvic pain prior to menstruation US -normal scan / or diffusely enlarged uterus -can show increase in low echo area of myometrium around endometrium -scattered cysts within myometrium <u>ENDOMETRIOSIS</u> -ectopic deposits of endometrium on the peritoneum and pelvic organs SS -depends on location of lesion -discomfort can occur if ovaries and tubes involved (can also lead to sterility) -pain in defecation, urination if rectal wall or and bladder involvement -dyspareunia if uterine involvement -almost always dysmenorrhea and pelvic pain due to pelvic bleeding and or adhesions US -can have normal scan /or present with endometriomas	transvaginal scans of a large, thick-walled (arrows mark walls) "chocolate cyst" 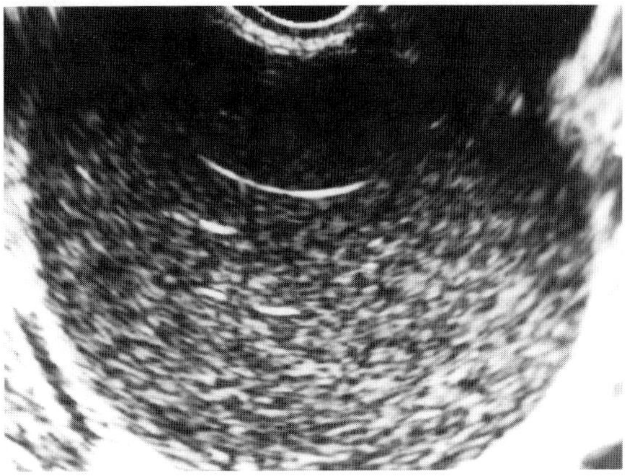 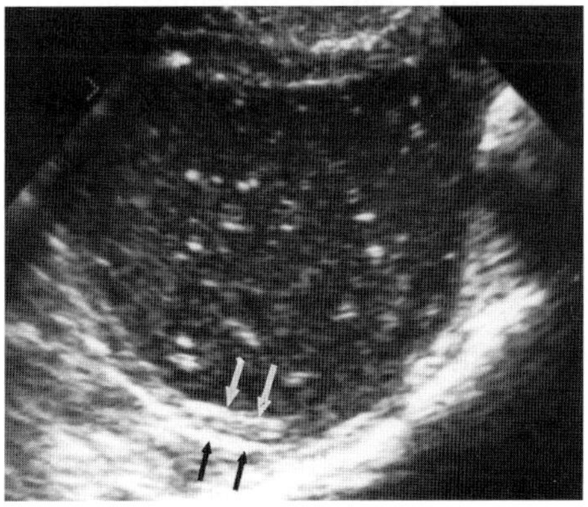

ABNORMALITY	US APPEARANCE
ENDOMETRIOMAS CONTINUED. ENDOMETRIOMAS (ENDOMETRIAL CYSTS, CHOCOLATE CYSTS): -localized blood collections caused by endometrial foci which respond to hormonal changes and bleeding during the menstrual cycle -variety of sonographic appearances -fairly round and discrete adnexal and/or cul-de-sac masses with enhanced through transmission -low level echos within the dependent portion, sometimes with a fluid-debris level -can be echolucent, complex or echogenic with septations -thick, irregular and/or shaggy walls	-transvaginal scan of endometrioma 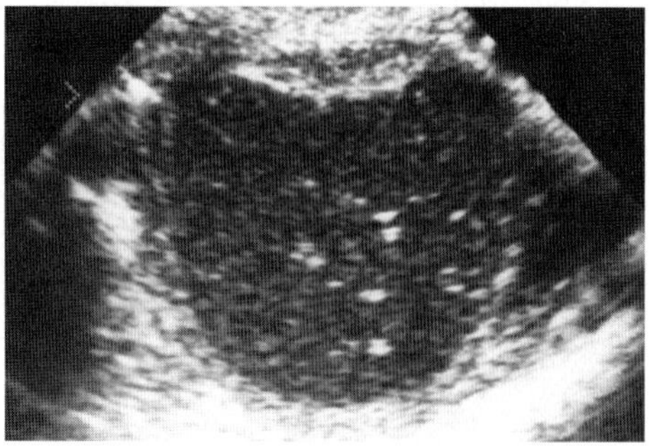
CERVICAL CARCINOMA (CIN : cervical intra-epithelial neoplasia) -diagnosis is made by examining smears of cells from the surface of the ectocervix -cytology can be normal, show dysplasia, carcinoma in situ or invasive carcinoma -increased incidence with peri-menopausal women SS -early: none -advanced: bleeding, pain, weight loss US -without local invasion: none or irregular cervical mass, enlargement of cervix -with local invasion can cause ureteral obstruction, hematometria	-transabdominal scan of transverse cervix: small isoechoic mass (M) projecting posteriorly from cervix 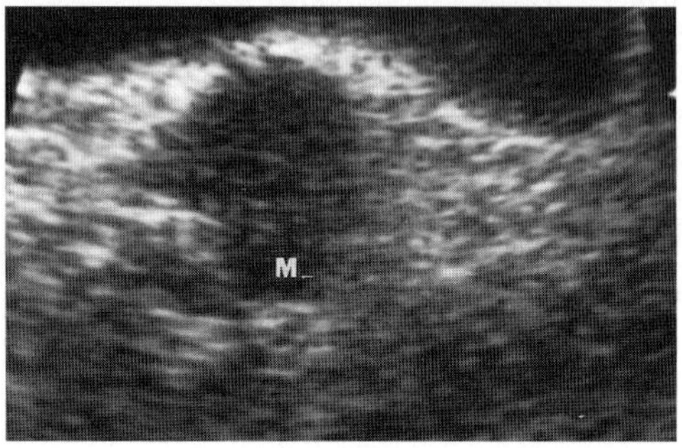

Septate- medium septum
Bicornate- uterus
Bicollis/unicolis- cervix

ABNORMALITY

CONGENITAL UTERINE MALFORMATIONS

-can occur as a sporadic event or as an adverse effect of diethylstilbestrol (DES) which has been noted in female offspring exposed before birth

(A) failure of fusion of the Mullerian ducts
- i-total failure—uterus didelphys: 2 uteruses, 2 cervices, 2 vagina
- ii-partial failure
  - -uterus bicornis bicollis: 2 uteruses, 2 cervices, 1 vagina
  - -uterus bicornic unicolis: 2 uteruses, 1 cervix, 1 vagina

(B) Failure of resorption of median septum
- i-complete failure—septate uterus
- ii-partial failure—subseptate uterus

(C) Failure of development of Mullerian ducts
- i-complete unilateral failure—unicornate uterus (uterus unicornis unicollis)
- ii-partial unilateral failure—uterus with 1 normal horn + 1 rudimentary horn
- iii-complete bilateral failure—uterine aplasia—total agenesis, ovaries present

(D) Uterus Arcuatus

-most common anomaly but not depicted on US
-saddle-shaped uterine fundus that increases transverse diameter of uterine cavity
-not associated with reproductive failure

SS FOR ALL ABOVE UTERINE MALFORMATIONS
-none, infertility, miscarriages, endometriosis, dysmenorrhoea
-associated with renal tract anomalies

US
-didelphys & bicornate uterus—deep fundal notch, 2 widely separate endometria
-septate uterus—shallow notch/smoother fundal contour, 2 separate endometria
-unicornate uterus—difficult to recognize

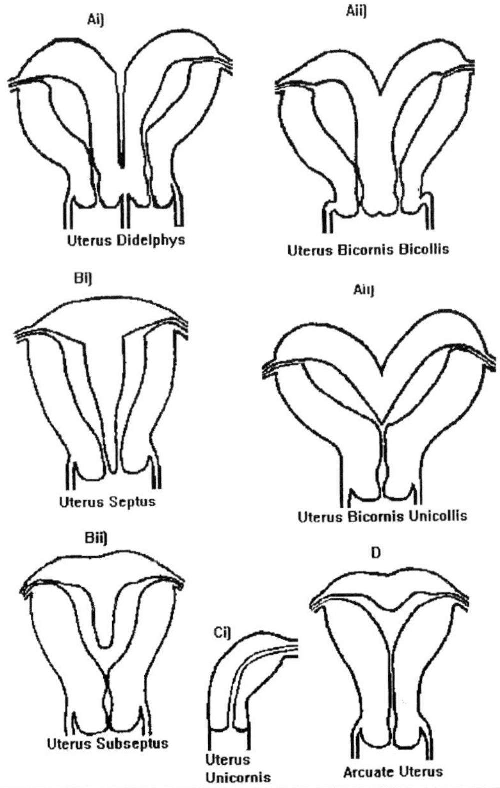

US APPEARANCE

Granvid Bicornate Uterus: transvaginal, transverse scan of bicornate gravid uterus with gestational sac in one horn and echogenic endometrium in other horn

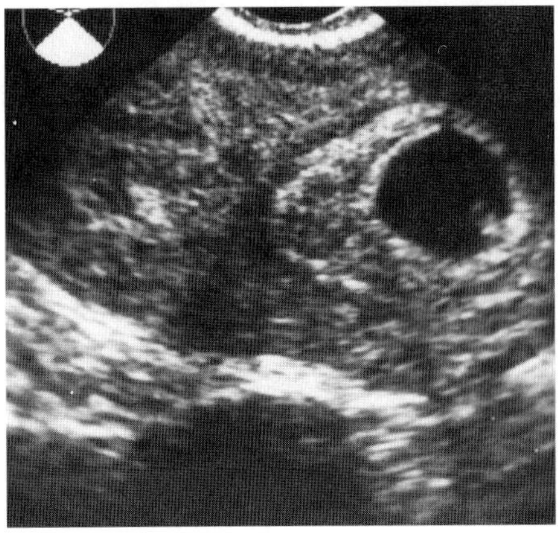

Uterus Didelphys: transabdominal transverse scan through fundi showing uterus didelphys; separate endometrial cavities

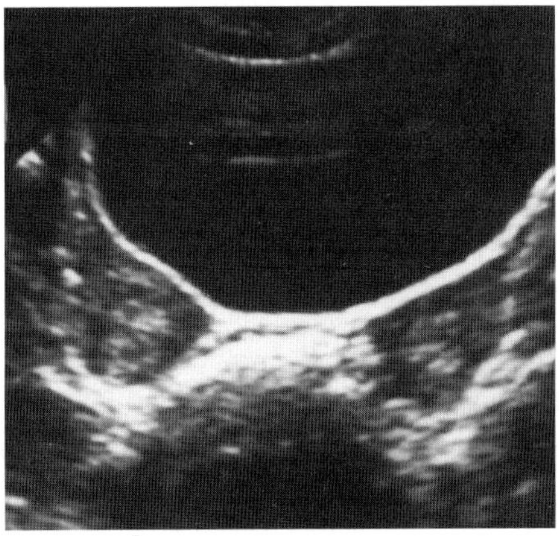

Bicornate Uterus: transvaginal transverse view of uterus depicting two separate endometrial canals

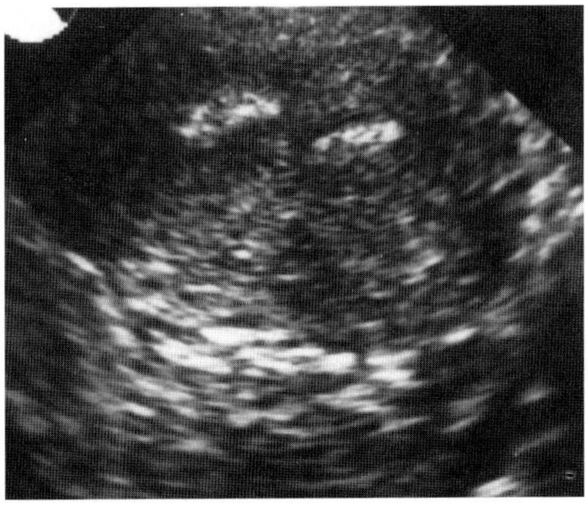

ABNORMALITY	US APPEARANCE
ENDOMETRIAL DISEASE ASHERMANS SYNDROME -normal endometrial lining is replaced by fibrous adhesions -secondary to previous D+C, multiple abortions, infections -sonographically can have varying appearances from normal, thin to thick endometrium SS -can cause loss of menstruation.	endometrial carcinoma-transabdominal sagittal scan of post-menopausal uterus with calipers measuring enlarged, inhomogenous endometrial canal 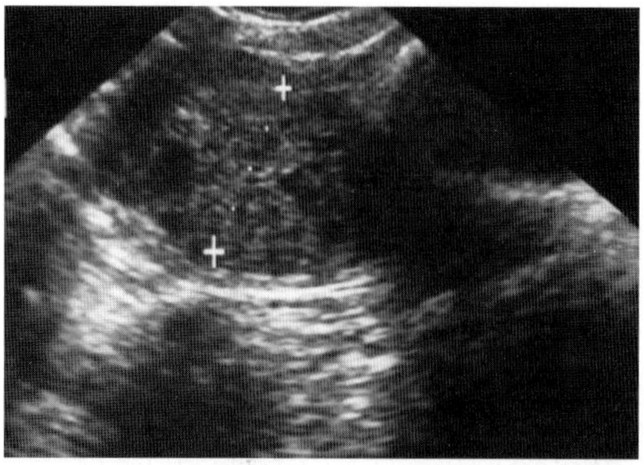
ENDOMETRIAL CARCINOMA -usually found in post-menopausal women, >50 years -increased risk associated with unopposed estrogen stimulation -linked with obesity, diabetes mellitus, hypertension, nulliparity, late menopause, polycystic ovaries, exogenous hormones SS -post-menopausal bleeding, normal sized or enlarged uterus	endometrial hyperplasia: transvaginal sagittal scan of perimenopausal uterus with thickened echogenic endometrium 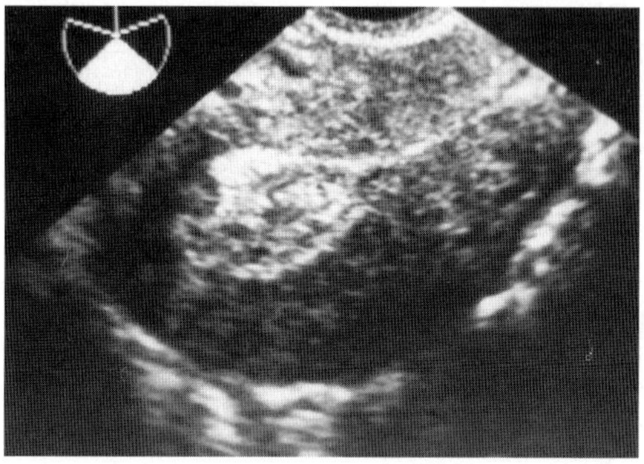
ENDOMETRIAL HYPERPLASIA -non-specific thickening of the endometrial lining -can be caused by estrogen over stimulation -common cause of uterine bleeding -irregular thickening of endometrium with cystic changes has been reported related to tamoxifen therapy for breast cancer SS -abnormal bleeding in women of any age	endometrial hyperplasia-transvaginal sagittal scan of uterus with calipers measuring a 2 cm enlarged endometrium 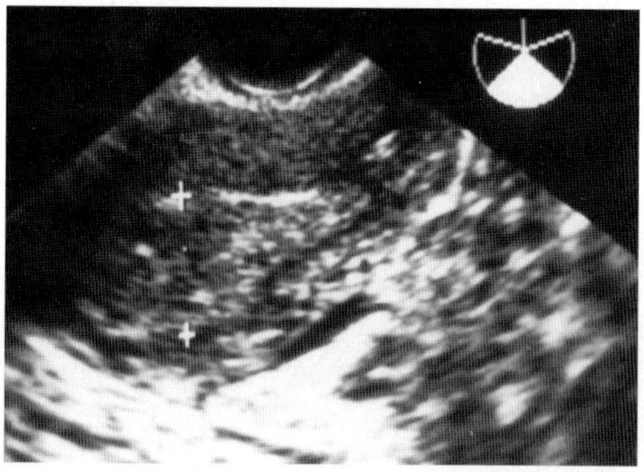

ABNORMALITY	US APPEARANCE
ENDOMETRIAL DISEASE CONTINUED <u>ENDOMETRIAL POLYPS</u> -types 1. hyperplastic or adenomatous endometrial tissue 2. some endometrial cancers are polypoid 3. some submucosal leiomyomas are pedunculated SS -asymptomatic or abnormal uterine bleeding <u>ENDOMETRITIS</u> -infection of endometrium following abortion, delivery or as a result of PID US FINDINGS IN ENDOMETRIAL DISEASE -usually non specific with prominent enlarged, inhomogenous echo complex -polyps may be large enough to produce a discrete mass within endometrial cavity -tiny cysts within the thickened endometrium can be a benign indication -clinical correlation can be helpful	endometrial polyp (arrow) surrounded by a small amount of fluid within the endometrial canal 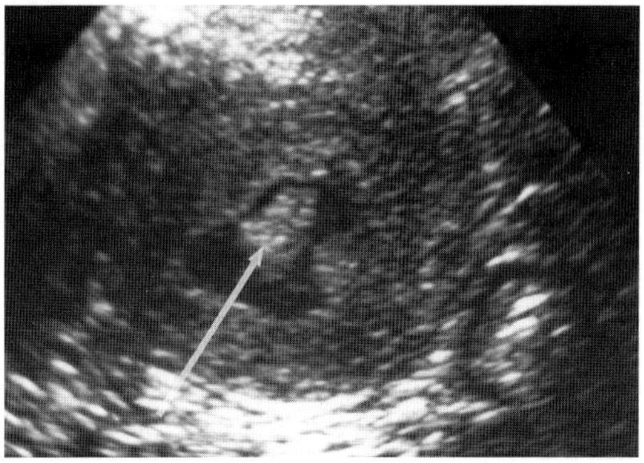 endometritis: transvaginal sagittal scan of uterus with complex collection within endometrial canal (arrows) 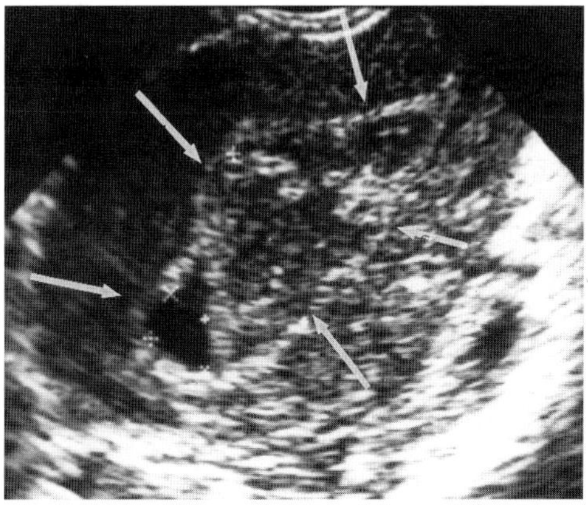

ABNORMALITY

INTRAUTERINE AND VAGINAL FLUID COLLECTIONS:

-abnormal fluid collections within uterus (metria)
-abnormal fluid collections within vagina (colpos)
Hydro - aqueous fluid collection
Pyo - infectious fluid collection
Hemato -bloody fluid collection

three types: depending where fluid has pooled
<u>Hematocolpos</u>
-only the vagina is distended with fluid
<u>Hematometracolpos</u>
-the uterus is also distended
<u>Hematometracolpossalpinx</u>
-in long-standing cases the tubes are also involved

Causes
1) Congenital Obstruction
-imperforate hymen, vaginal septum or atresia
2) Acquired Obstruction
uterine malignancy, radiotherapy, scarring, foreign body, surgery
-endometrial fluid in post-menopausal women can be associated with a benign process (eg. cervical stenosis) or malignancies (eg. endometrial or cervical carcinoma)

SS
-none, amenorrhea, enlarged uterus, pelvic pain or discomfort, pain on voiding or with bowel movements

US
-distention of involved anatomy with fluid which can appear anechoic (hydro), with echos or have a fluid–fluid level (pyo/hemato)
-occasionally echogenic fluid may be indistinguishable from an endometrial polyp or cancer

US APPEARANCE

transabdominal sagittal scan of uterus containing large fluid collection

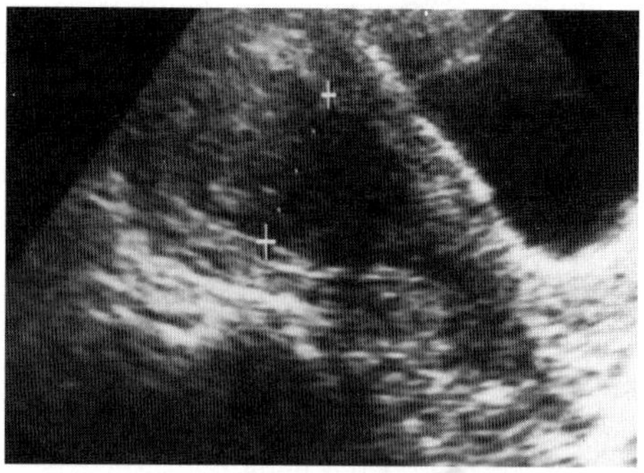

transabdominal sagittal scan uterus showing a normal amount of fluid

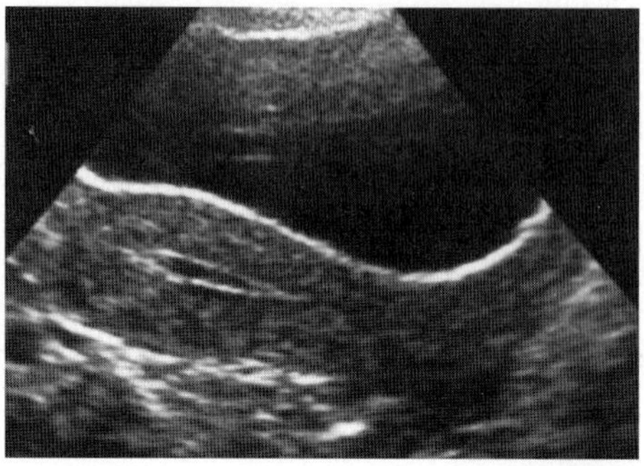

transabdominal sagittal scan of uterus enlarged with echogenic collection representing either an infectious or bloody accumulation

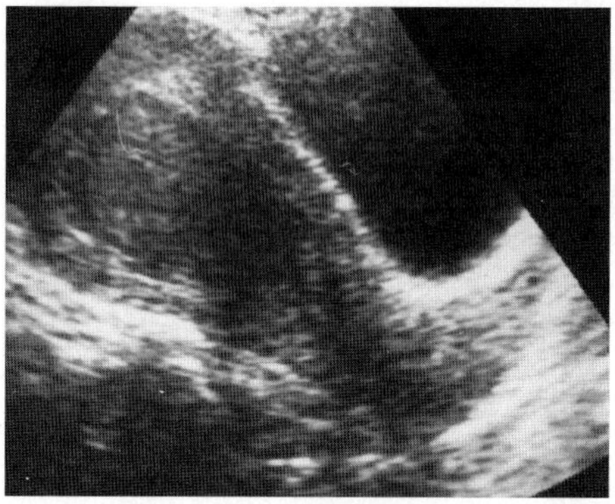

hematocolpos: transabdominal sagittal scan of blood filled vaginal (black arrows) inferior to the cervix (C) and posterior to bladder (white arrows) indicating an imperforate hymen

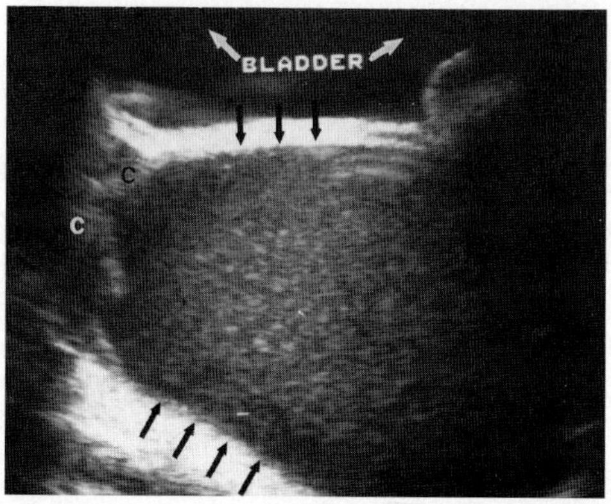

ABNORMALITY	US APPEARANCE
IUCD - INTRAUTERINE CONTRACEPTIVE DEVICE -variety of devices inserted into the uterus to prevent pregnancy by creating an unfavorable environment for implantation of the fertilized ovum common types—Copper 7, Copper T, Lippes Loope, saf-T-Coil US -hyperechoic linear echos in the endometrial canal, distal acoustic shadowing, 65% have entrance–exit artifact which are multiple double parallel interrupted echos -type specific echos (eg. Lippes Loop - 5 interrupted echos) -pitfalls that make visualization difficult include fibroids, retroverted uterus, pregnancy CLINICAL SIGNIFICANCE <u>EXPULSION / LOST IUCD</u> -"lost" occurs when the locator threads at the proximal end of the IUCD cannot be felt on physical exam -possible reasons: detachment of thread, expulsion of IUCD, uterine perforation by IUCD, migration of thread -ultrasound is often ordered to ensure the correct location and position of the IUCD <u>MALPOSITION / INCOMPLETE EXPULSION</u> -can hinder effectiveness and cause pain <u>PERFORATION</u> -occurs when an ectopic IUCD penetrates through the myometrium -causes pain and cramping <u>PID</u> -IUCD users may have increased risk for PID <u>PREGNANCY</u> -pregnancies that occur with IUCD are at an increased risk for spontaneous abortion, ectopic location	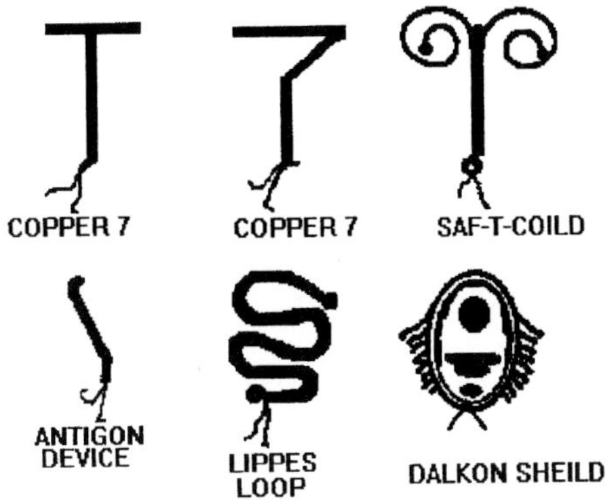 transabdominal, sagittal scan of uterus with hyperechoic linear area (IUCD) within endometrial cavity 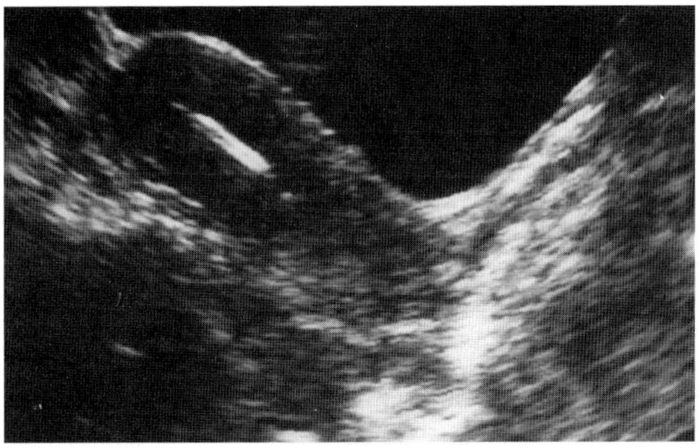 early pregnancy (fetal head = H) with IUCD indicated by entry–exit echos (parallel lines indicated by arrow) 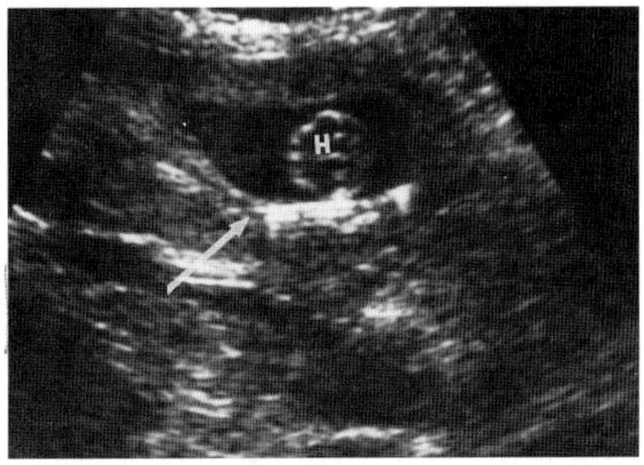
LEIOMYOLIPOMAS -rare fatty tumor of the uterus -usually found in postmenopausal women SS -asymptomatic or similar to those caused by fibroids US -hyperechoic mass which can be surrounded by a hypoechoic ring of myometrium	transvaginal transverse scan of uterus with hyperechoic mass within the myometrium 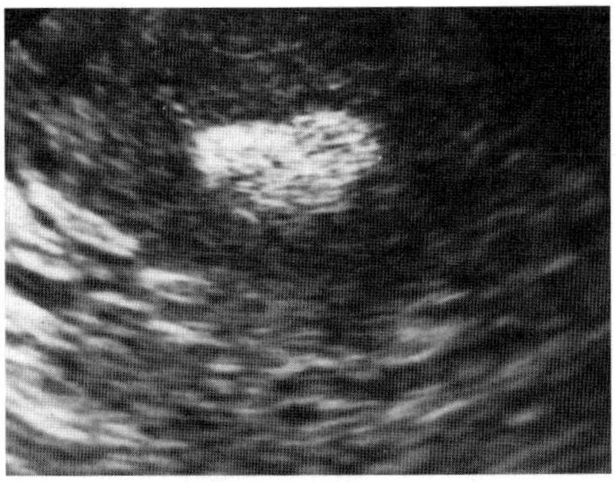

ABNORMALITY	US APPEARANCE

LEIOMYOMAS (FIBROIDS)

-most common benign gynecological tumor with increased incidence in women > 35 years
-circumscribed, spherical mass arising from the smooth muscle of the myometrium
-not encapsulated, but develops a false capsule of compressed myometrial tissue
-atrophy and vascular changes cause the fibroid to undergo degeneration which can cause fibrotic changes, hemorrhage, necrosis and calcification
-respond to estrogen and may enlarge rapidly in pregnancy and shrink during menopause

the location of the fibroid describes the type:

<u>Broad Ligament Myomas</u>
-simulate adnexal masses

<u>Cervical Myomas</u>
-rare, can cause dystocia

<u>Intramural (Interstitial)</u>
-most common within myometrium

<u>Submucosal</u>
-grow inward beneath the endometrial
-least common but cause the most symptoms
-can be pedunculated and extend out of cervix

<u>Subserosal (Subperitoneal)</u>
-grow outward and are covered by peritoneum; can be pedunculated which can simulate adnexal mass

<u>LEIOMYOSARCOMA:</u>
-uncommon rapidly growing, aggressive malignancy arises from pre-existing benign leiomyomas

SS
-depends on location and size of fibroid
-bulky uterus, palpable abdominal mass, heavy menstruation, infertility, nulliparity, urinary frequency, dysuria, constipation, low back pain

US
-large range of appearances
Classic appearance-discrete masses that are homogenous, hypoechoic with poor sound through transmission and drop out
Multiple Fibroids can appear with a large inhomogenous, bulky, nodular uterus with lobulated contour
-smaller fibroids: more attenuating with increased shadow
-larger fibroids: easier to penetrate
-upon degeneration they can calcify, become more cystic or undergo fatty degeneration
Doppler - high impedance, low-flow

transvaginal sagittal scan with an attenuating fibroid (arrows) on the posterior aspect of uterus

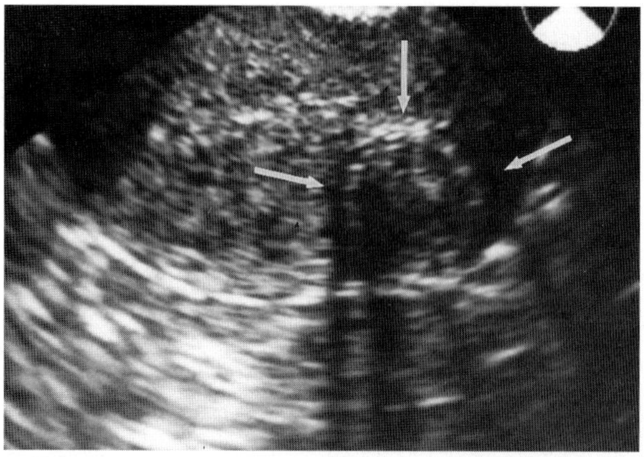

transvaginal sagittal scan with a well circumscribed leiomyoma (arrows) within the myometrium (note also small amount of fluid within endometrial canal)

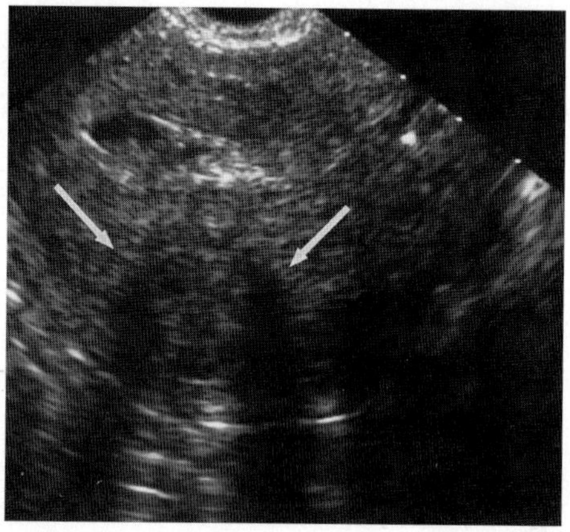

transabdominal transverse scan of a pedunculated fibroid (calipers) to the right of the uterus

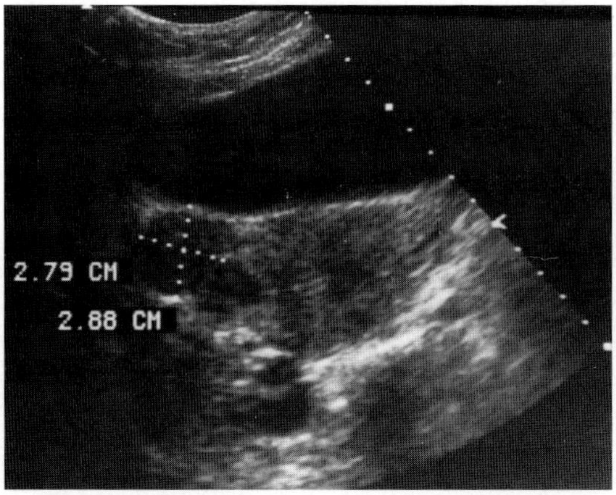

ABNORMALITY	US APPEARANCE
<u>LEIOMYOMAS CONTINUED</u> SS -depends on location and size of fibroid -bulky uterus, palpable abdominal mass, heavy menstruation, infertility, nulliparity, urinary frequency, dysuria, constipation, low back pain US -large range of appearance -classic appearance: discrete masses that are homogenous, hypoechoic with poor sound through transmission and drop out -multiple fibroids can appear with a large inhomogenous, bulky, nodular uterus with lobulated contour -smaller fibroids: more attenuating with increased shadow -larger fibroids: easier to penetrate -upon degeneration they can calcify, become more cystic or undergo fatty degeneration Doppler - high impedance, low-flow	transabdominal sagittal scan of calcified fibroid (bright echos-arrows) within the uterus 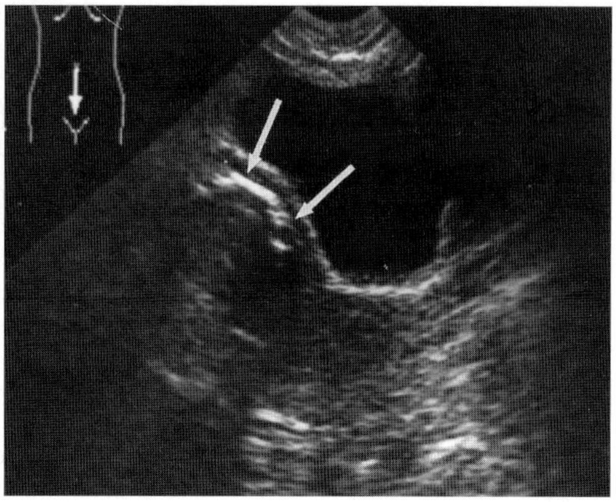 transvaginal scan of polypoid fibroid (arrows) within endometrial canal 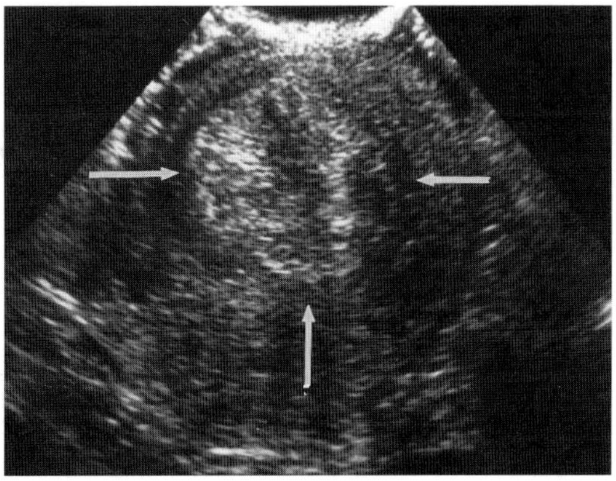

ABNORMALITY	US APPEARANCE
NABOTHIAN CYSTS -entrapped cervical secretions forming retention cysts in cervix -a feature of chronic cervixitis -no clinical significance SS -asymptomatic US -small simple cysts found along margin of cervix or within cervical canal	transvaginal sagittal scan of cervical nabothian cyst (arrow) with posterior acoustic enhancement 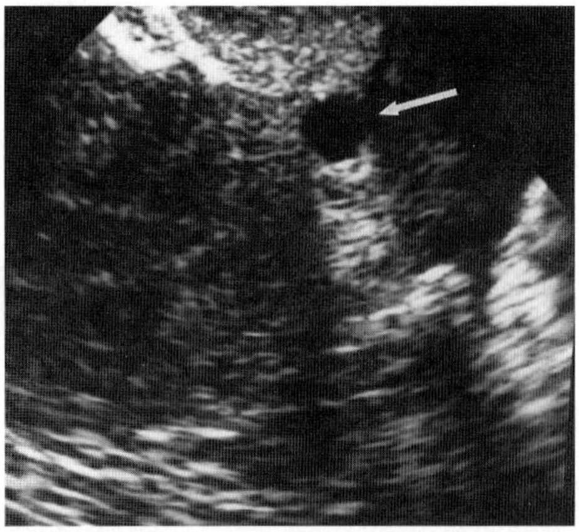 transabdominal sagittal scan of cervix with two small nabothian cysts (arrows) 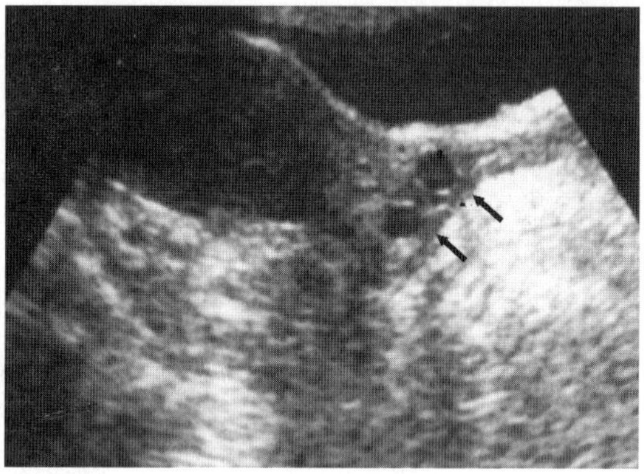

UTERINE ANOMALIES AND CHANGES WITH PREGNANCY

FOCAL MYOMETRIAL CONTRACTURES

-painless, localized contractures of myometrium
-occur throughout pregnancy and are not always clinically apparent
-not to be confused with Braxton Hicks contractions

<u>Braxton Hicks contractions:</u>
-entire uterus contracts
-similar to contractions in labor except these do not dilate cervix
-not commonly seen on ultrasound

US
-focal thickening of uterine wall that may last up to 45 minutes
-can create pitfalls:
1. may mimic hematomas or fibroids
-contractures change over time and do not attenuate like fibroids
-usually only distort endometrial surface, whereas fibroids tend to distort serosal and endometrial contour
2. may mimic placenta previa by altering the relationship of the placenta and cervix

transabdominal sagittal scan of gravid uterus with posterior placenta (P) being "pushed" anteriorly by contracture (C) beneath it

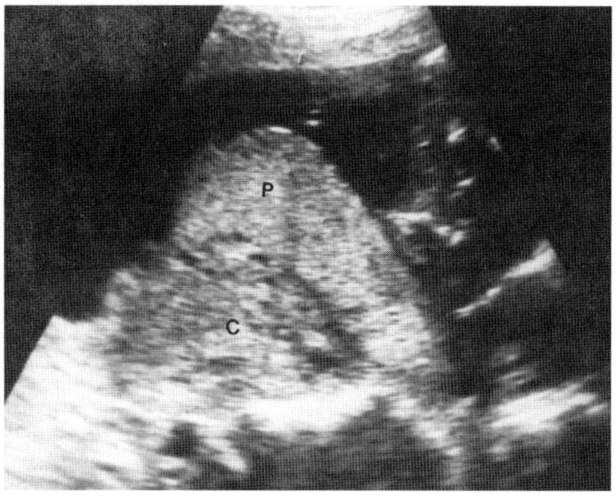

INCOMPETENT CERVIX

-an incompetent cervix is unable to retain an intrauterine pregnancy
-functional condition with many etiological factors; congenital, trauma, hormones

SS
-history of recurrent, painless second-trimester abortions
-treatment: cervical cerclage

US
-competent cervix length < 3 cm
-width of cervix > 2 cm in second trimester
-width of cervical canal > 8 mm
-open internal os
-protrusion of membranes into endocervical canal

PITFALL
-overdistension of bladder causes distortion, giving an open cervix a closed appearance therefore ensure bladder volume is appropriate
-transvaginal scanning allows for better resolution and results that are easily reproduced

transabdominal sagittal scan of cervix: fetal head (H), maternal bladder (B), amniotic fluid in widened endocervical canal (arrows), calipers measuring distal competent shortened cervix (**)

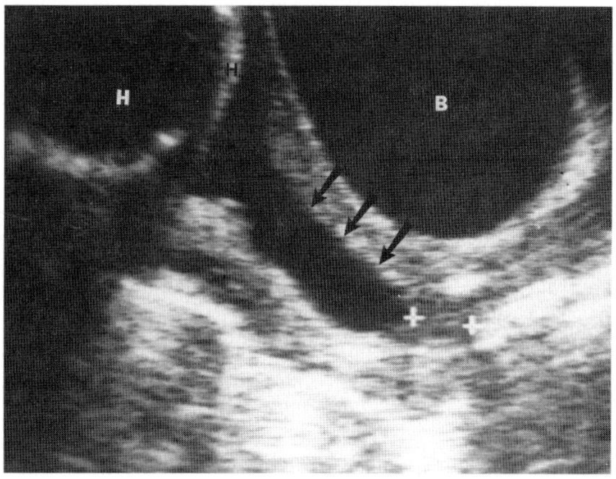

UTERINE ANOMALIES AND CHANGES WITH PREGNANCY cont'd

LEIOMYOMAS

-most common solid mass encountered with pregnancy
-increased hormone levels during pregnancy enlarge pre-existing fibroids

Clinical Significance
-can be misinterpreted as a contraction
-may cause dystocia and can prevent vaginal delivery
-can be misinterpreted as placental tissue

US
-different echogenicity from placental tissue
-has discrete borders
-fibroid remains static over time compared to uterine contractions
-usually bulges uterine margin

-sagittal scan of endocervical canal (C)
-maternal bladder (B), fetal abdomen (A), fibroid on anterior wall of uterus (F)
-if this fibroid continues to increase in size, it could cause obstruction of vaginal delivery

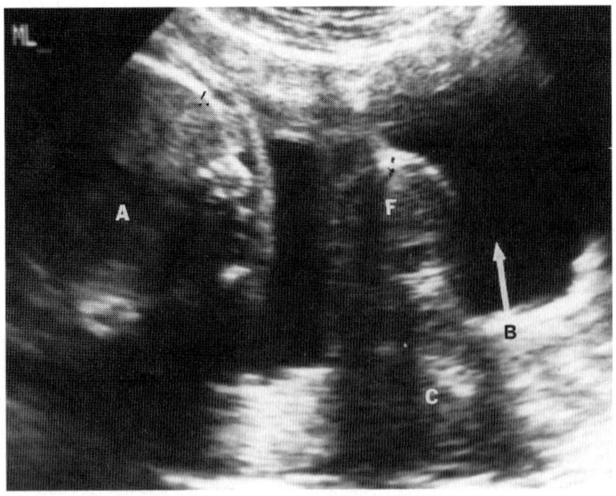

MENORRHEA - TERMINOLOGY OF ABNORMAL MENSTRUATION	
AMENORRHEA	absence of menstrual flow when expected A - non
CRYPTOMENORRHEA	monthly symptoms of menstruation without bleeding
DYSMENORRHEA	painful menstruation Dys - pain
HYPERMENORRHEA	abnormal increase in duration and amount of flow Hyper - ↑
HYPOMENORRHEA	deficient amount of flow, but regular Hypo - ↓
MENARCHE	the start of the first menstrual cycle
MENORRHAGIA	excessive bleeding at time of menstrual period in amount or duration
MENSES	monthly flow of bloody fluid from uterus
METRORRHAGIA	bleeding from uterus at anytime, spotting between periods
MITTELSCHMERZ	pain midway between periods, occurring at ovulation
OLIGOMENORRHEA	scant, infrequent menstrual flow
POLYMENORRHEA	menstrual periods with abnormal, increased frequency
PSEUDOCYESIS	false pregnancy

PELVIC PAIN DIFFERENTIAL	
TYPE & LOCATION	**DIFFERENTIAL**
ACUTE, LOCALIZED	-ovarian/pedunculated fibroid torsion -ruptured ovarian cysts -ectopic pregnancy -appendicitis or other gastrointestinal disease
CHRONIC	-pelvic infection / PID -adhesions
POST MENOPAUSAL	-infections -uterine/ovarian neoplasms
PREPUBERTAL	-pelvic mass -urinary infection -masked menstration -cryptomenorrhea
DYSMENORRHEA	-endometriosis, salpingoophoritis, pelvic venous congestion, acute uterine retroversion
DYSPAREUNIA (PAIN WITH INTERCOURSE)	-endometriosis -PID

COMMON ULTRASOUND FINDINGS AND DIFFERENTIALS	
THICKENED ENDOMETRIUM	-endometrial hyperplasia, polyps -endometrial carcinoma -ashermans syndrome -retained products ; ~~Ashermans syndrome~~
THIN ENDOMETRIUM	-hormonal imbalances (eg. pituitary, ovarian abnormalities) -post menopausal uterus -Ashermans syndrome
ECHOGENIC ENDOMETRIUM	-PID -secretory phase of menstral cycle -post D+C -endometritis -post iUCD removal -decidual proliferation in ectopic pregnancy -endometrial carcinoma, hyperplasia
FLUID IN ENDOMETRIAL CANAL	-pregnancy -malignancy -obstructive process -small amount is normal
SMALL HYPOPLASTIC UTERUS	-hypofunction: pituitary/hypothalmus -Turners 45XO syndrome -primary ovarian failure -mother with exposure to DES (female offspring with path.)
UTERINE ENLARGEMENT	-fibroids -polyps -adenomyosis -Trophoblastic disease -endometrial cancer -hematometra -pyometra

CHAPTER 4 - OVARIES

A) NORMAL ANATOMY

OVARY	-paired almond-shaped glands -variable shape, but of equal size -not surrounded by peritoneum; lies directly exposed to peritoneal cavity
FUNCTION	-ovulation -hormone production
STRUCTURE	-composed mainly of fibroareolar tissue called stroma -two major parts: 1. CORTEX- outer glandular section that contains follicles 2. MEDULLA- deeper connective tissue and smooth muscle that contains blood vessels
SIZE volume = $\frac{\text{height X width X length}}{2}$	Child < 5 years volume < 1 cc Menstruating volume 6-10 cc; maximum volume 14–16 cc (3 x 2 x 2 cm) Peri -Menopausal -3–5 years post cessation of menses, ovary retains ovoid shape Post–Menopausal (volume decease with age) Volume 3-6 cc.; maximum volume <7 cc. (2 x 1.5 x 0.5 cm.) ** **normal size depends on investigator Post Menopausal with Hormone Replacement Therapy -ovarian volume does not decrease
LOCATION	-posterior lateral wall of pelvic cavity in a shallow depression called Waldeyer's fossa -can be extremely variable as ovaries are mobile -posterior to broad ligament
RELATIONSHIPS	Medial Surface- faces pelvic cavity, may be largely covered by fallopian tube which drapes over it Lateral Surface- lies against pelvic wall in ovarian fossa (Fossa of Waldyer) Posterior Border - convex, anterior to ureter, internal iliac artery and vein, free border Anterior Border- mesovarian (broad ligament) -also known as the hilum or the ovary as vessels and nerves enter here Antero Medial - uterus
SONOGRAPHIC APPEARANCE	-hypoechoic ovoid structures with homogenous echotexture -more echogenic central medulla -reproductive age: follicles help to identify -menopausal age: difficult to identify due to small size and lack of follicles

OVARIAN BLOOD SUPPLY

ARTERIAL SUPPLY

AORTA
(below level of renal artery)

⇓

OVARIAN ARTERY
(in suspensory ligament)

⇓

through anterior border of ovary to anastomose with

⇓

UTERINE ARTERIES

⇓

ovarian divisions of uterine arteries anastomose with ipsilateral ovarian arteries creating dual blood supply

VENOUS DRAINAGE -follows course close to that of ovarian artery

OVARIAN HILUM
- ➡ LEFT OVARIAN VENOUS PLEXUS ⇒ LEFT OVARIAN VEIN ⇒ LT RENAL VEIN ⇒ IVC
- ➡ RIGHT OVARIAN VENOUS PLEXUS ⇒ RIGHT OVARIAN VEIN ⇒ IVC

DOPPLER OF ARTERIAL VESSELS IN OVARY

-resting state: high impedance waveform pattern
-corpus luteum phase: (day 8–21) low impedance waveform pattern

OVARIAN SUPPORTS

1. OVARIAN LIGAMENT
-band of fibrous tissue which runs in the broad ligament connecting the uterine extremity of the ovary to the lateral wall of the uterus
-becomes round ligament at the anterior surface of uterus

2. MESOVARIAN
-ovary's own mesentery; double fold of peritoneum which attaches ovary to broad ligament

3. SUSPENSORY LIGAMENT
(INFUNDIBULOPELVIC LIGAMENT)
-part of the broad ligament between the infundibulum and ovary and pelvic wall; contains ovarian vessels and nerves
-passes over external iliac vessels and psoas major muscle

<u>OTHER</u>
4. OVARIAN / WALDYER'S FOSSA
-shallow "V"-shaped fossa formed by the crossover of ureter and iliac vessels on pelvic side wall

5. UTERINE EXTREMITY
-lower, more pointed end closer to uterus
-connected to lateral angle to uterus behind and below level of fallopian tube by ovarian ligament

6. TUBAL EXTREMITY
-upper, larger, rounder end closer to fallopian tube
-suspended from pelvic brim by suspensory ligament

SAGITTAL CROSS SECTION:
lateral to midline

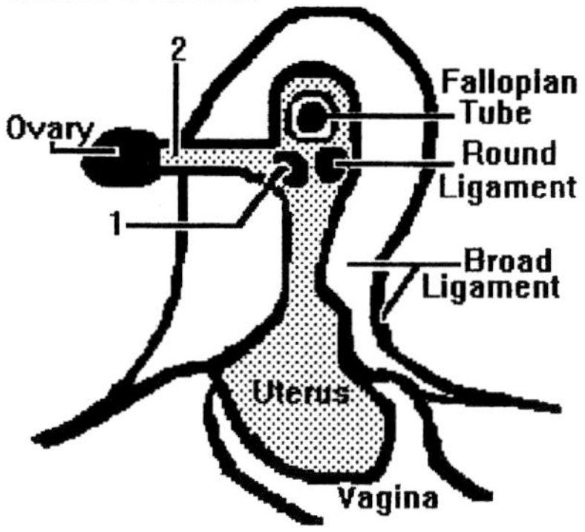

CORONAL RIGHT ADNEXA

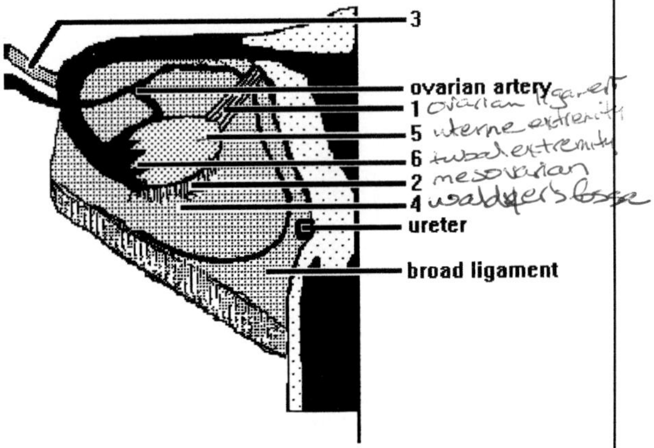

NORMAL SONOGRAPHIC APPEARANCE OF OVARIES

	TRANSABDOMINAL	TRANSVAGINAL
MATURE OVARY -demonstration of follicular cysts surrounded by ovarian parenchyma	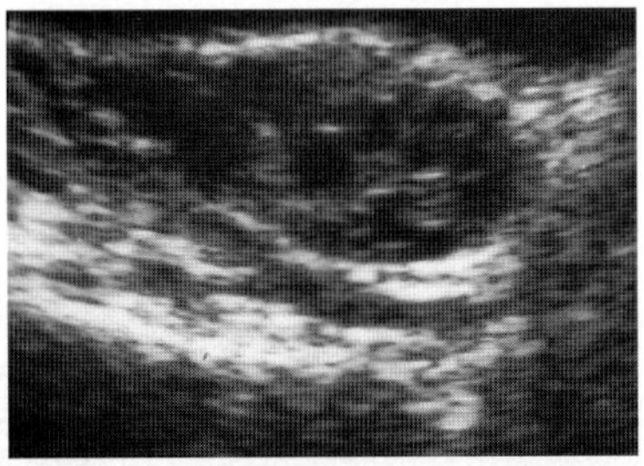	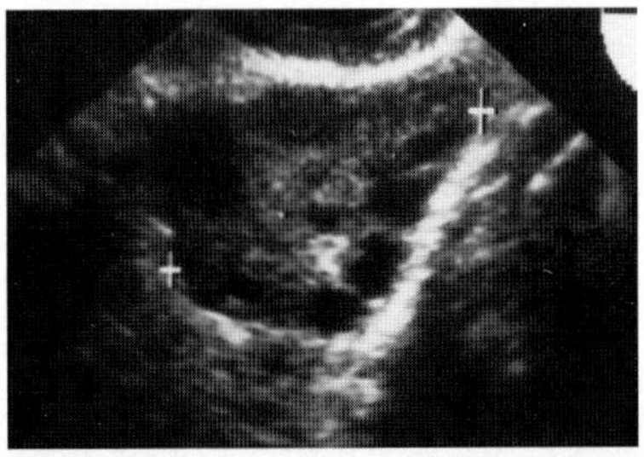
POST-MENOPAUSAL OVARY -becomes thinner, smaller and elongated with decreased or absence of folliculogenesis which makes sonographic delineation difficult	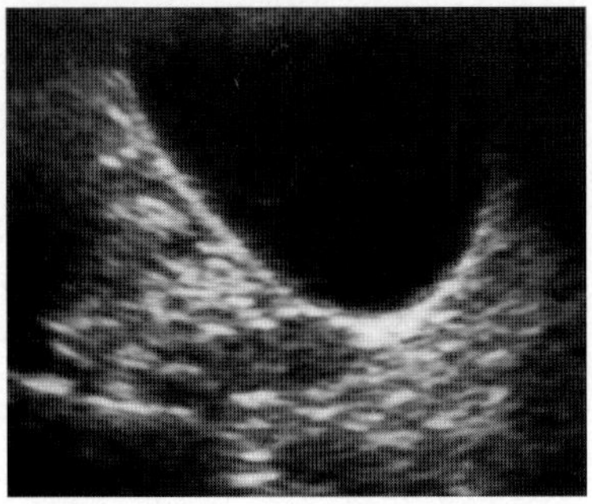	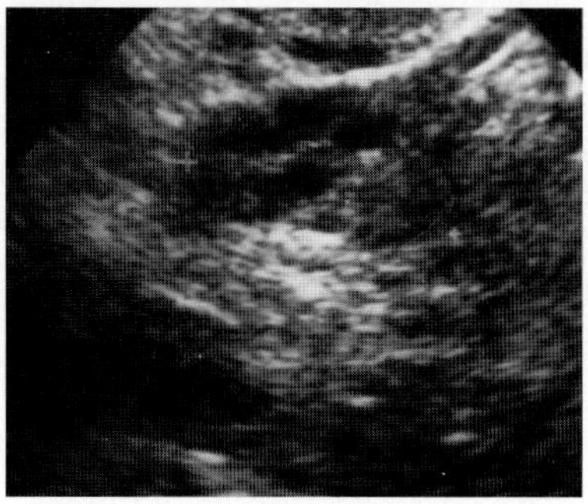

B) ABNORMALITIES

OVARIAN CYSTS	US APPEARANCE
CORPUS LUTEAL -functional post ovulatory cysts-graffian follicle ruptures, seals off and may hemorrhage; usually 12–17 mm in size -most common cystic mass with pregnancy; usually regresses after first trimester SS -asymptomatic or may present with pain if cyst hemorrhages US -simple cysts: anechoic, thin walled, round/oval with sharp margins, increased sound through transmission, usually unilateral -larger ones can have internal low level echos	transvaginal scan of a corpus luteal cyst (arrows) within an ovary 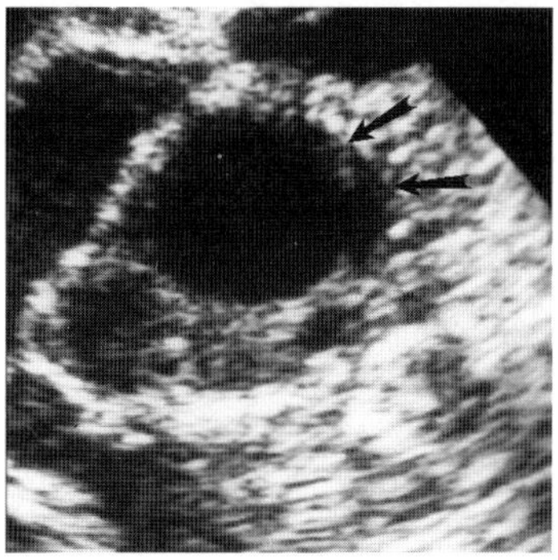
FOLLICULAR -functional/physiological cysts form when a mature follicle fails to ovulate or involute -resolve spontaneously SS -asymptomatic US -simple cysts: anechoic, thin walled, round/oval with sharp margins, increased sound through transmission -usually 1.5– 2.5 cm at time of ovulation, may increase up to 6 cm	transabdominal scan of ovary with small follicular cyst 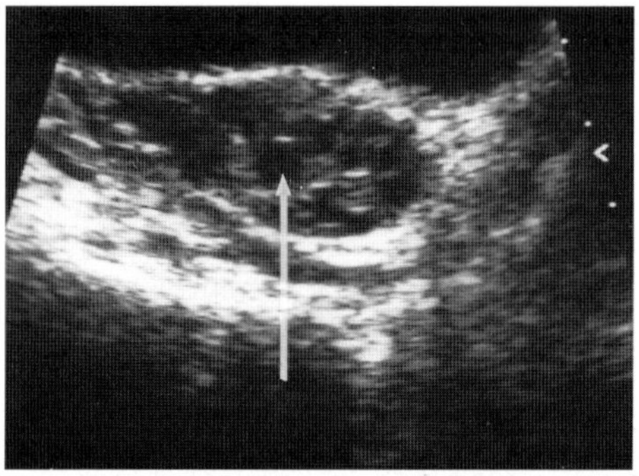
HEMORRHAGIC -bleeding into a cyst SS -pelvic pain US -variable characteristics because of clot formation, lysis and retraction can mimic other adnexal masses -can appear solid, or show a fluid–fluid level or focal wall thickening -increased sound through transmission	transvaginal scan of a hemorrhagic ovarian cyst 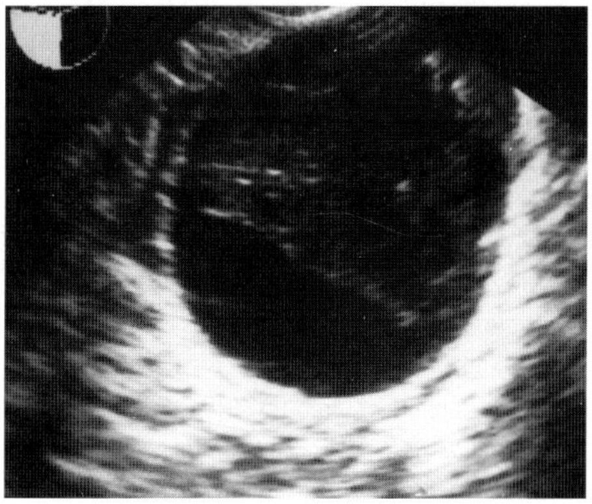

OVARIAN CYSTS	US APPEARANCE
PARAOVARIAN (TYPES: GARTNER'S DUCT, PAROOPHORON, EPOOPHORON, HYDATID OF MORGAGNI) -arise in broad ligament as remnants of Wolffian body paralleling vagina and fallopian tubes SS -asymptomatic unless hemorrhage US -simple, thin walled unilocular cysts up to 18 cm	transabdominal scan of uterus with a Gartner's duct cyst along the wall of the vagina (calipers) 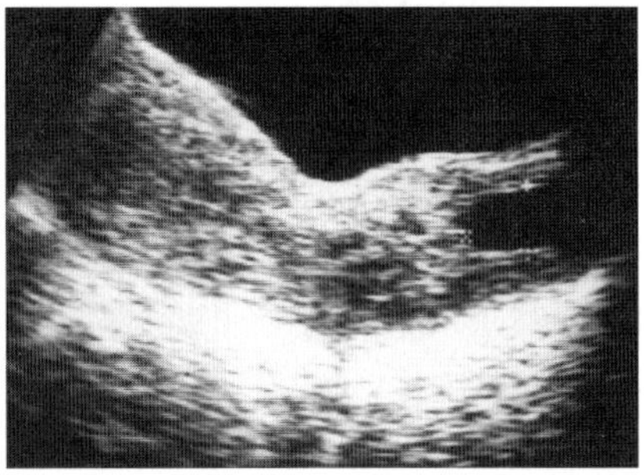
POLYCYSTIC OVARIES (PCO) -no mid-cycle peak of estrogen and a low steady-state of estrogen causes a complex imbalance of the ovarian cycle -can cause chronic anovulation -occurs in reproductive age group -associated with endometrial carcinoma due to chronic unopposed estrogen stimulation -diagnosed with blood work (normal/decreased FSH levels, increased androstenedione/testosterone, LH, estrone/estradiol levels) SS <u>STEIN–LEVENTHAL SYNDROME</u>: hirsutism, amenorrhea, obesity, infertility US -normal or bilaterally enlarged echogenic ovaries (vol. > 10 cc) -multiple, small (2–6 mm) varying sized cysts located in the periphery of the ovary resembling a "string of pearls"	transvaginal scan of enlarged polycystic ovary; multiple follicles around periphery of a 5 cm ovary 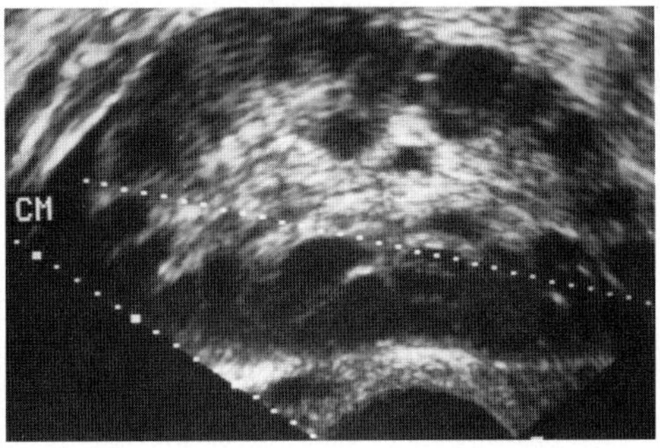
THECA LUTEAL OVARIAN HYPERSTIMULATION SYNDROME -hyperstimulated follicles formed in response to gonadotrophic hormones -functional cysts associated with abnormally high levels of hCG levels -associated with gestational trophoblastic disease, ovarian hyperstimulation, multiple pregnancy, choriocarcinoma SS -pain due to pressure caused by size, abdominal distention, nausea, vomiting US -bilateral enlarged ovaries with multiple, multifollicular, septated cysts	transvaginal scan of enlarged, multicystic ovaries; they are so enlarged that they appear as one continuous mass 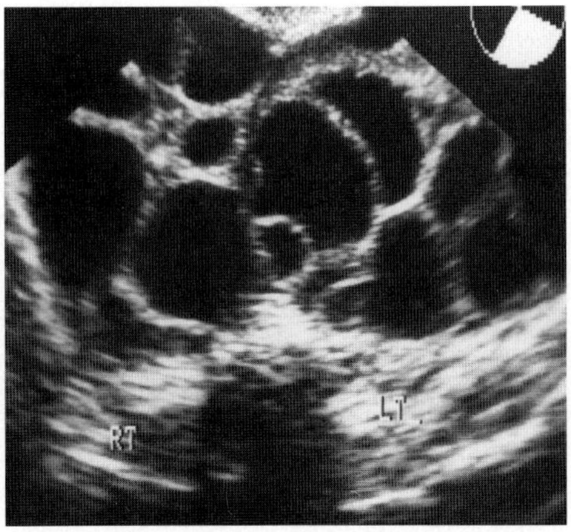

NON NEOPLASTIC ADNEXAL MASSES				
MASS	**SIZE**	**BILATERAL OR UNILATERAL**	**SIGNS AND SYMPTOMS**	**OUTCOME OR FOLLOW-UP**
CORPUS LUTEUM CYST	1.5-2.5 cm	unilateral	amenorrhea, pain, abnormal bleeding	resolves if persists called corpus albicans cyst
ECTOPIC PREGNANCY	approximate 1-3 cm.	unilateral	pain, bleeding, positve pregnancy test	clinical intervention
ENDOMETRIOMA	up to 15-20 cm.	uni or bilateral	symptoms of endometriosis	depends on clinical information.
FOLLICULAR CYST	0.5-2 cm.	unilateral sometimes bi	none	resolve
HEMORRHAGIC CYSTS	2 mm./day 3-10 cm	unilateral sometimes bi	none or pain, pressure	resolve 3 months, rupture, torsion
OVARIAN TORSION	enlarged ovary	unilateral	acute, severe pain	clinical intervention
PARAOVARIAN CYST	tiny to several cm.	uni or bilateral	none	incidental finding
POLYCYSTIC OVARIES STEIN-LEVENTHAL SYNDROME	tiny cysts but large ovary	bilateral	hirtsuitism amenorrhea obesity infertility hypertension	clinical intervention (associated with increased incidence of endometrial carcinoma)
THECA LUTEAL CYSTS	large	bilateral	pain, pressure	associated with gestational trophoblastic disease, ovarian hyperstimulation

OVARIAN PATHOLOGIES

EPITHELIAL TUMORS

BRENNER TUMOR
-mainly benign solid tumor, most common in the 6th decade
-primarily unilateral (96%)
-can be associated with Meigs' Syndrome
MEIGS' SYNDROME: unknown etiology
-condition in which a solid benign ovarian tumor is associated with ascites and right hydrothorax

US
-well-defined solid mass, usually hypoechoic
-up to 10 cm in diameter

ENDOMETROID CARCINOMA
-20% of ovarian malignancies
-bilateral 50%
-30% accompanied by endometrial carcinoma

US
-mixed; solid and cystic components
-papillary projection common into cystic spaces

MUCINOUS TUMORS
-mucin containing tumors comprise 20–25% of ovarian tumors
-less common than the serous type and more likely to be benign

MUCINOUS CYSTADENOMA
-can occur at any age (mainly seen in 20–40 age group)
-unilateral (95%)

US
-multi-septated, smooth walled +/- a few small papillary projections
-large to massive in size, often filling pelvic cavity up to 30 cm in size

MUCINOUS CYSTADENOCARCINOMA
-rarer than its benign counterpart
-bilateral (20%)
-usually found in 4th–6th decade
-10% of all ovarian malignancies

US
-large multiloculated cystic neoplasms, solid and papillary areas projecting from walls are common
-can measure up to 50 cm

PSEUDOMYXOMA PERITONEI
- rare condition caused by metastasis of a mucin producing tumor
-epithelial cells implant on peritoneum and continue to secrete a gelatinous material which is not absorbed well
-the abdominal cavity can eventually fill with the mucinous jelly

US APPEARANCE

Brenner–transvaginal scan of ovary with small solid mass (arrow) that on pathology was determined to be a Brenner Tumor

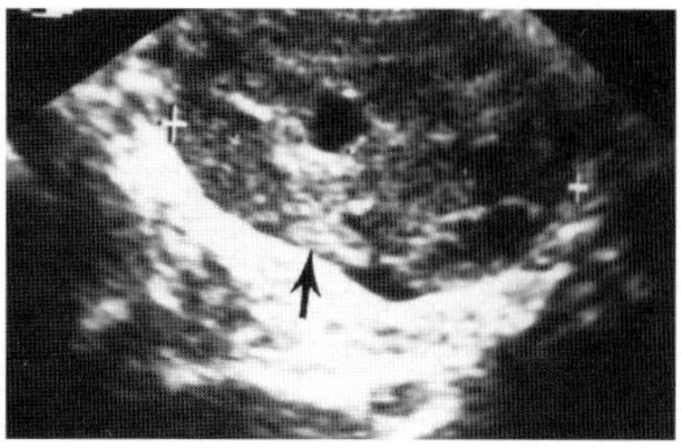

mucinous cystadenocarcinoma—transabdominal sagittal scan of early mucinous cystadenocarcinoma; note thickened central septum

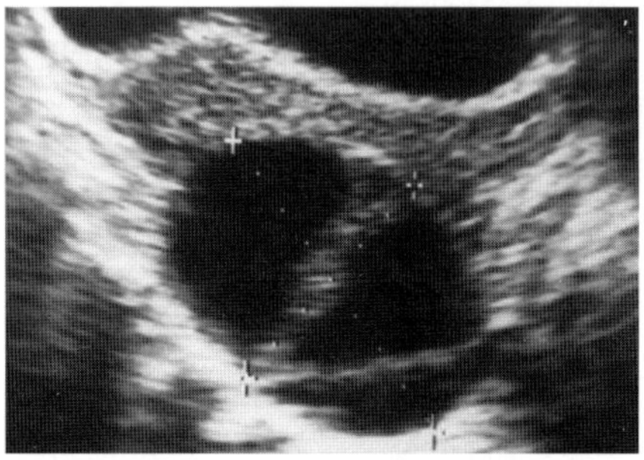

mucinous cystadenocarcinoma-transabdominal scan of large mucinous cystadenocarcinoma

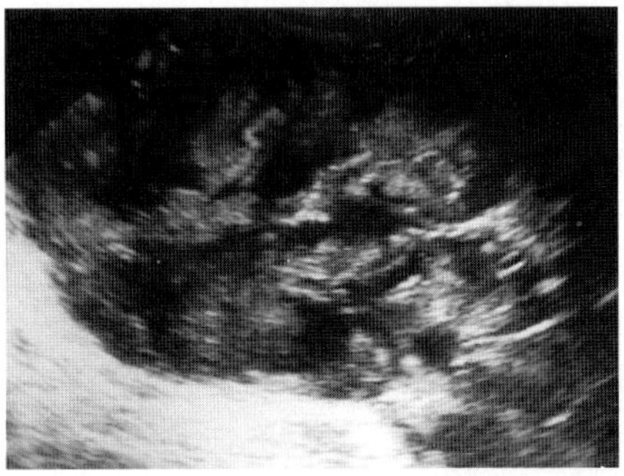

Meig's - epitheleal tumor; ascites + right hydrothorax

ABNORMALITY	**US APPEARANCE**
EPITHELIAL TUMORS CONTINUED SEROUS TUMORS SEROUS CYSTADENOMA -benign, bilateral 20% -occur peri-menopausal age -can be quite large US -cystic lesions, most are unilocular -septa if present are thin -few, if any, papillary projections from wall SEROUS CYSTADENOCARCINOMA -most common primary carcinoma of ovary (40%) -50% bilateral -50% are greater than 15 cm in size US -multiloculated and multiple papillary projection from walls which can be irregularly thickened	transabdominal scans of a serous cystadenocarcinoma. Notice thickened septum and papillary projections 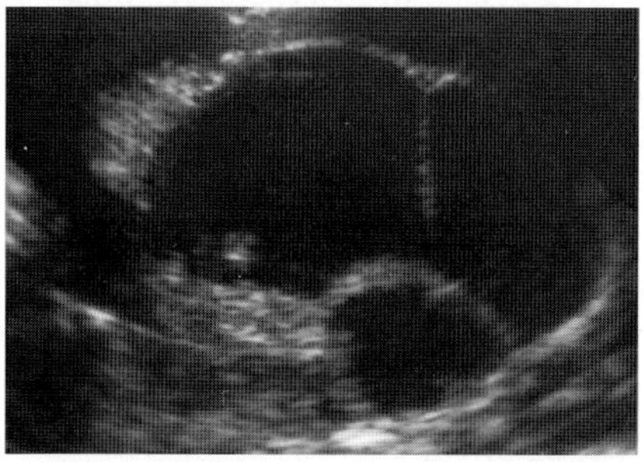 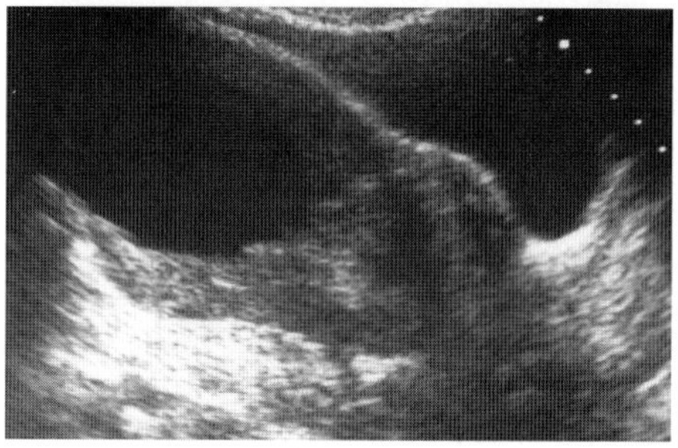

ABNORMALITY	US APPEARANCE

ABNORMALITY

GERM CELL TUMORS

DYSGERMINOMA
-rare, usually found in younger groups (under 30)
-can be bilateral, usually unilateral and moderate size
-most malignant germ cell tumor
-in children tend to be more malignant
-homologue of testicular seminomas

SS
-localized pain, pressure

US
-hyperechoic solid mass, may have areas of hemorrhage and necrosis

TERATOMAS
-used to be divided into cystic and solid, but more recently are classified according to the type of tissue found within

IMMATURE
-contains elements from all 3 embryonic layers; endoderm, mesoderm and ectoderm
-highly malignant
-occurs at an early age than mature teratomas, usually in childhood

US
-usually solid but may contain cystic areas

MATURE
-contains well-differentiated fetal to adult-type tissues
-cells are totipotential, i.e., able to form any type of tissue mass; typically hair, teeth, bone, fat
-most common of mature teratomas are cystic, usually a dermoid cyst which accounts for > 20% of all ovarian neoplams

US
-vary in size and sonographic appearance depending on composition
-cystic/fat fluid levels/echogenic mural nodules/thick septations/solid/ calcifications/mixed solid & cystic
-"Tip of Iceberg Sign"- echogenic portion of poorly-defined mass due to high attenuation

MONODERMAL
- predominance of a single of tissue, e.g., thyroid in the struma ovarii tumor

US APPEARANCE

transvaginal scan of cystic teratoma

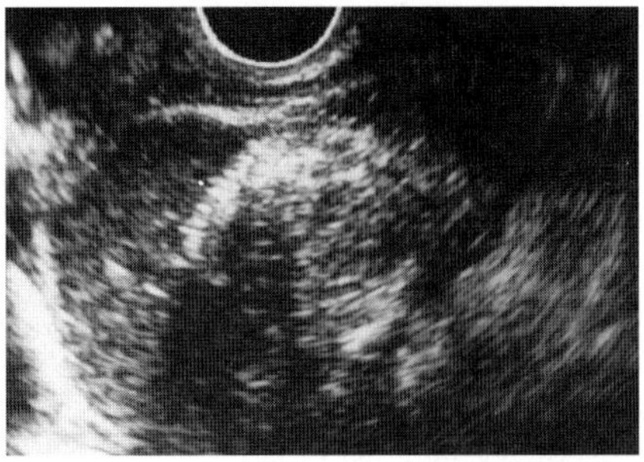

transvaginal scan small teratoma within an ovary

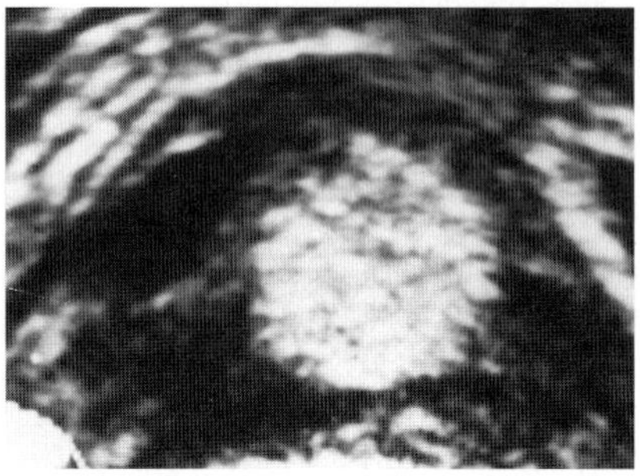

transabdominal transverse scan of mature teratoma (arrows) in left adnexa

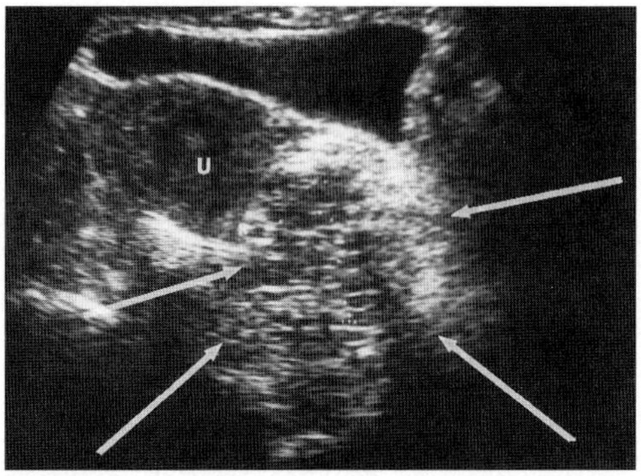

transvaginal scan of a large mature teratoma (arrows) adjacent to uterus (U)

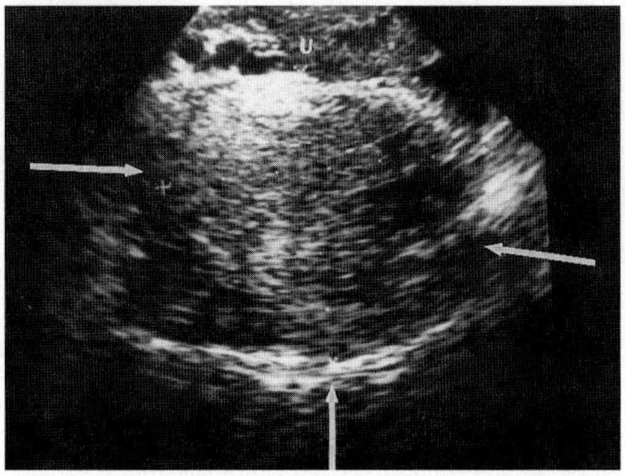

<table>
<tr><th>ABNORMALITY</th><th>US APPEARANCE</th></tr>
<tr><td>
METASTASES TO OVARY
-relatively uncommon
-primaries include: breast, stomach, large intestine
-owing to their rapid growth they tend to be friable and hemorrhage which gives blood-stained ascites

<u>KRUCKENBERG TUMOR</u>
-secondary tumor of the ovary from a G.I. primary (classically from stomach carcinoma)
-can be bilateral, equal-sized solid masses
-may be accompanied by ascites

US
-complex mass
</td><td>
Kruckenberg Tumor: two large complex masses; bowel mass (B) and ovarian mass (O)
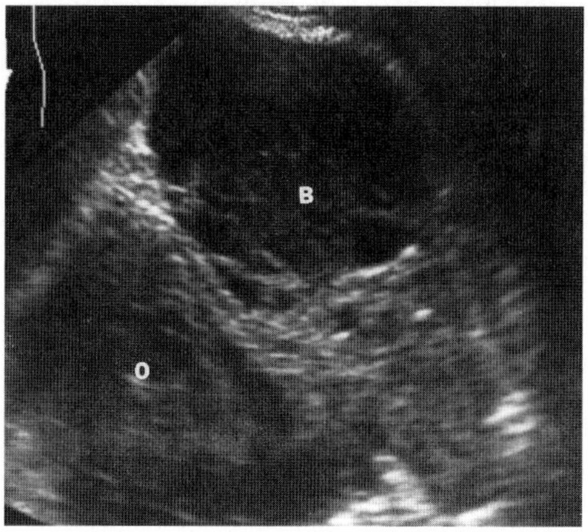

same patient as above with fluid in the left upper quadrant; spleen (S) and left pleural effusion (P)
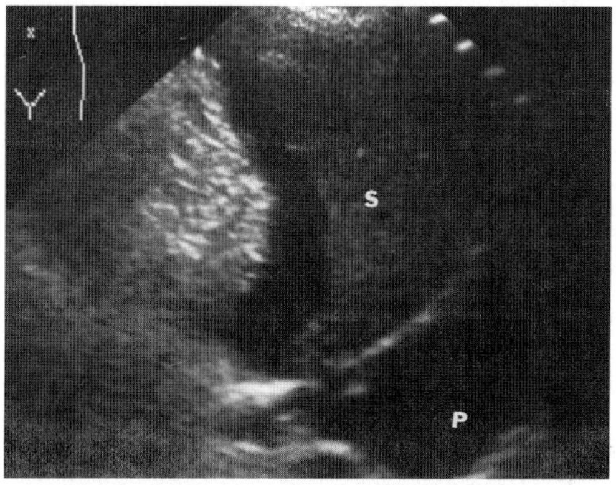

</td></tr>
<tr><td>
OVARIAN TORSION
-twisting or rotation of ovary
-can be seen secondary to ovarian masses which can be pedunculated

SS
-acute, severe pain, nausea, vomiting

US
-enlarged, mixed echogenic mass, irregular cystic/solid areas of hemorrhage classically showing multiple anechoic peripheral follicles
-differential includes ectopic pregnancy, appendicitis, pelvic inflammatory disease, endometrioma, hemorrhagic cyst

<u>Doppler</u>
-absent vascular flow within enlarged ovary
-high resistance flow in hilar vessels and possible venous flow in capsular vessels
-differential diagnoses include ectopic, appendicitis, PID, endometrioma, hemorrhagic cyst
</td><td>
transabdominal scan of enlarged torted ovary; note multiple anechoic peripherally placed follicles
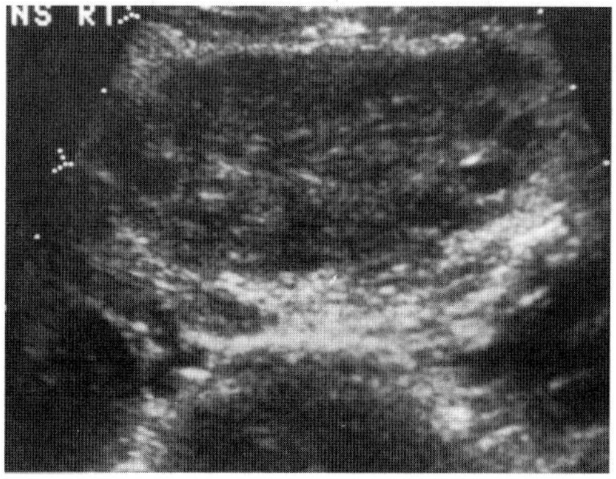

</td></tr>
</table>

ABNORMALITY	US APPEARANCE

ABNORMALITY

SEX CORD-STROMAL TUMORS
-hormone producing tumors
-least common ovarian tumors

ESTROGEN PRODUCING
(feminizing)
FIBROMA
-usually small, unilateral solid, benign
-occurs most commonly in peri- and post-menopausal women
-> 5 cm can sometimes be associated with Meigs' Syndrome

GRANULOSA CELL TUMOR
-post-menopausal and reproductive age group (5% occur before puberty)
-estrogenically active ovarian tumor
-low grade malignancy, unilateral
-can be solid or cystic

THECOMA (THECA CELL TUMOR)
-older population, primarily post-menopausal
-unilateral, benign
-estrogenically active ovarian tumor

SS
-excessive estrogen causes: enlarged uterus, irregular bleeding, occasional amenorrhea, enlargement and tenderness of breasts, post-menopausal bleeding, precocious puberty

ANDROGEN PRODUCING
(masculinizing)
SERTOLI–LEYDIG CELL / ARRHENOBLASTOMA /ANDROBLASTOMA
-rare <1% of ovarian neoplasms, occurs in young adult females

SS
-period of defeminization followed by a period of masculinization: (atrophy of breasts and female genital organs, oligomenorrhea, amenorrhea, facial and abdominal hair etc.)

US FOR BOTH TYPES
-unilateral (95%) solid mass with cystic components
-no real distinctive gross or ultrasound appearance

US APPEARANCE

transabdominal scans of a Sertoli–Leydig tumor

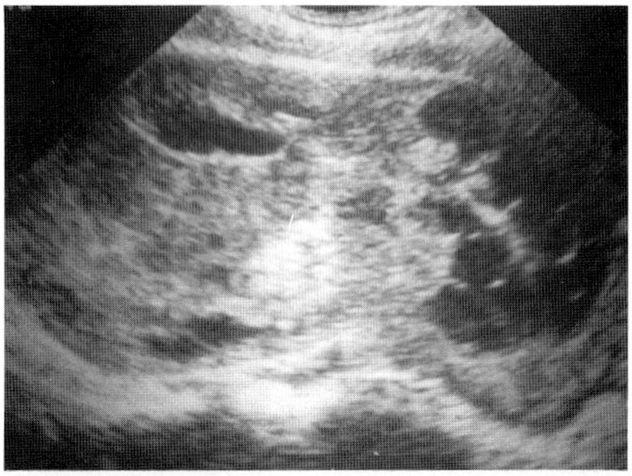

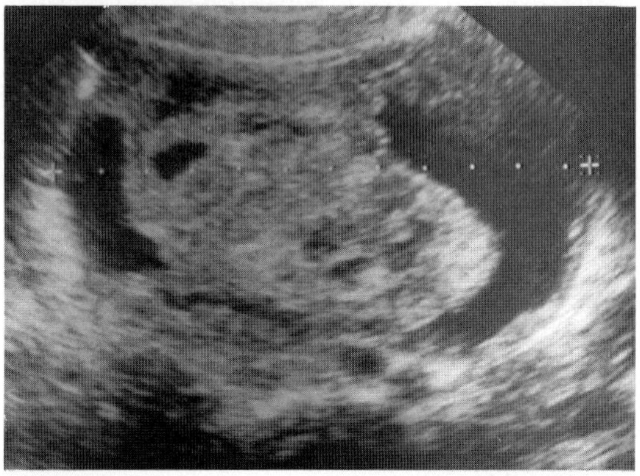

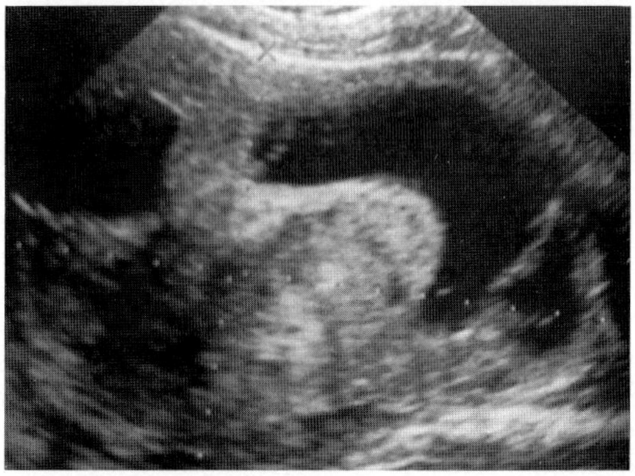

OVARIAN CANCER		
STAGING OF CARCINOMA OF OVARY		
STAGE I	- growth limited to ovaries	Ia. one ovary - no ascites Ib. both ovaries - no ascites Ic. ascites or +ve peritoneal washings
STAGE II	- pelvic extension	IIa. spread to uterus/tubes IIb. spread to other pelvic tissues IIc. IIb. with ascites
STAGE III:	- extrapelvic intraperitoneal spread and/or retroperitoneal positive nodes -limited to true pelvis with involvement of small bowel or omentum	Spread can be via several routes - -Direct - peritoneum, uterus, bladder, bowel, omentum -Transcolonic: - along paracolonic gutters by serous fluid -Lymphatics - para-aortic drainage
STAGE IV	- invasion beyond the true pelvis -distant metastases -pleural effusion with +ve cytology	-blood stream spread - to liver, lungs, lymph nodes

HISTOLOGY: EPITHELIAL (90%), GERM CELL (15%), METASTASES (10%), STROMAL (5%)

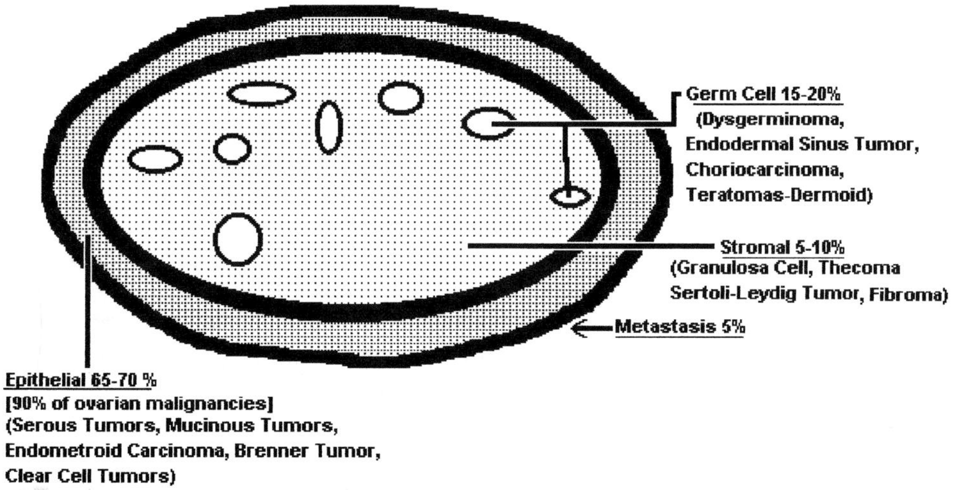

OVARIAN NEOPLASMS: incidence of types

TUMOR BIOMARKERS:
-serum CA-125: increased values are associated with carcinomas, but are also associated with other benign and malignant conditions such as PID, breast cancer

CHAPTER 5 - FALLOPIAN TUBES

A) NORMAL ANATOMY

FALLOPIAN TUBES (UTERINE TUBES, SALPINGES, OVIDUCTS)	
SIZE	-approximately 10 cm in length
LOCATION	-extend laterally and horizontally from cornua of uterus into peritoneal cavity -ascend along mesovarian border to tubal extremity of ovary
FUNCTION	-provide passage for ovum into uterus -assist ovum onward by peristalsis -be long enough to allow ovum time to mature after it has been fertilized in ampulla
BLOOD SUPPLY	-vessels from anastomosis between uterine and ovarian arteries
US APPEARANCE	-not normally seen on transabdominal ultrasound examination but can occasionally be seen using transvaginal scanning

TUBE ANATOMY	
1. INFUNDIBULUM -2 cm—terminal expansion of tube a. TUBAL FOLDS 2. FIMBRIA -processes at end of tube which help attract the ovum 3. AMPULLA -5 cm 2/3 of tube—thin-walled and convoluted -variable diameter -usual site of fertilization 4. ISTHMUS -2 cm 1/3 of tube—straight and cord-like -continuous with ampulla 5. INTRAMURAL SEGMENT OF TUBE (interstitial/uterine part of tube) -1 length x < 1 mm width -embedded in uterine wall -cornual pregnancies would occur here but they are rare	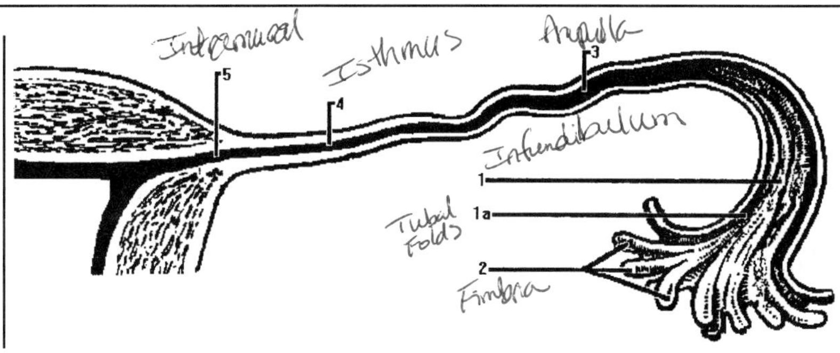

B) ABNORMALITIES

ABNORMALITY
PELVIC INFLAMMATORY DISEASE (PID) -infection of the fallopian tubes with ovaries and peritoneum caused by a variety of organisms (gonococcal, pyogenic, tuberculosis) -gonorrhea can be the most common and destructive depending on the area infected -acute PID may occur following surgery but usually is a result of ascending infection and associated with IUCDs -chronic PID can involve adhesions, edema, hydrosalpinx, pyosalpinx, ovarian abscess SS acute: pain, fever, vaginal discharge US -nonspecific, enlarged uterus with ill-defined margins, mild adnexal enlargement with loss of tissue definition -obstructed tubes: appear as funnel or tube-shaped kinked cystic adnexal structures (hydro or pyosalpinx) -free fluid in pelvis -abscess has variable appearance: unilocular or multilocular complex masses with irregular borders and thickened walls -differential should include appendicitis, diverticulitis, ovarian torsion, ectopic pregnancy -endometritis-thickening of endometrium +/- fluid within the endometrial cavity -hydro/pyosalpinx-see below
MANIFESTATIONS OF PELVIC INFLAMMATORY DISEASE HYDROSALPINX -distention of fallopian tube by clear fluid seen in nonvenereal salpingitis or with long-standing, resolved gonococcal infection -complex mass on abdominal scanning, on transvaginal scanning appear as anechoic tubular structure -when moderately enlarged the tubes continuity with the uterine cornua can help to identify it sonographically as a tube, although when a tube is maximally distended, it is difficult to distinguish it from an ovarian mass PYOSALPINX -distention of fallopian tube by pus usually secondary to a gonococcal infection -results from blockage of the lumen of the tube at the fimbriated and one or more points along the tube -usually bilateral -with transabdominal scanning will appear as complex adnexal mass -with transvaginal scanning will appear as tubular-shaped structure with echogenic walls -can contain low level echos that represent pus -can progress to tubo-ovarian abscess which can appear as a multicystic and solid complex mass TUBO-OVARIAN ABSCESS (T.O.A.) -tubal abscess that extends beyond the confines of the fallopian tube -caused by pelvic inflammatory disease -ovary may be seen as part of abscess mass [Differential for fluid filled fallopian tubes: Hematosalpinx - usually as a result of an ectopic tubal pregnancy or can rarely be part of a hematometracolposalpinx that is caused by obstruction of menstrual fluids]
TUBAL CARCINOMA -rare neoplasm -most primary carcinomas are adenocarcinomas -secondaries are more common and usually originate in adjacent pelvic organs US -ill-defined complex / solid fusiform mass adjacent to the uterus and ovary which can mimic intraligamentary or peduculated fibroids

SONOGRAPHIC APPEARANCES OF TUBAL MASSES

transvaginal scan of hydrosalpinx (arrows), right ovary (R OV), uterus (UT)

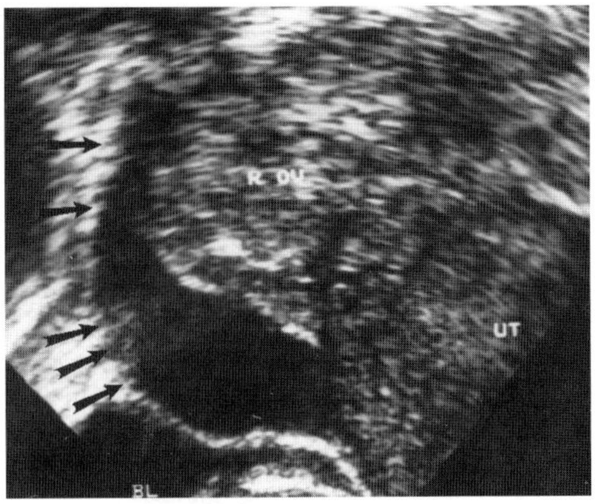

transvaginal scan of hematosalpinx; echogenic fluid within fallopian tube (arrows)

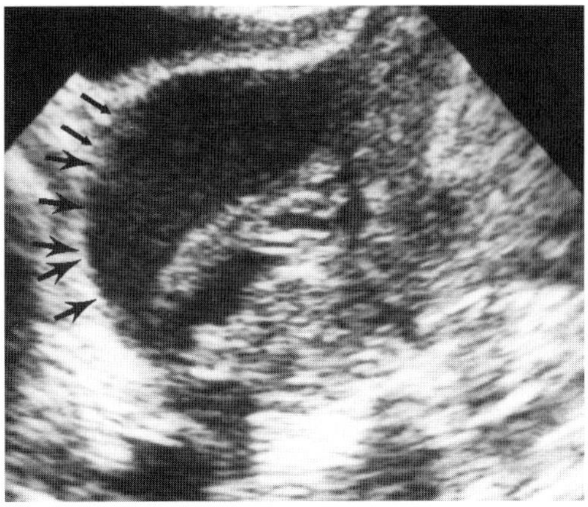

transvaginal scan of a large tubo-ovarian abscess

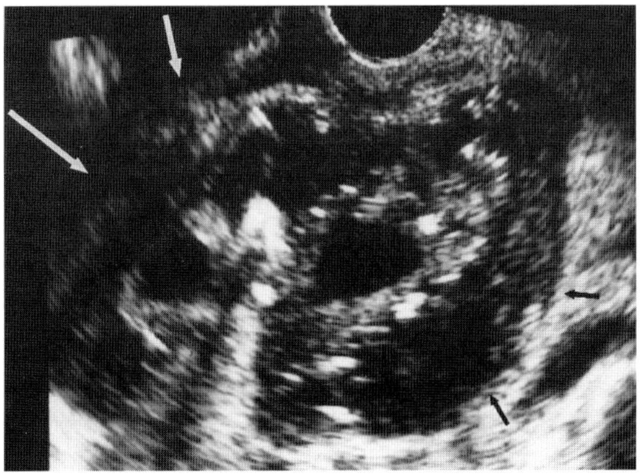

transabdominal scan of a pelvic abscess

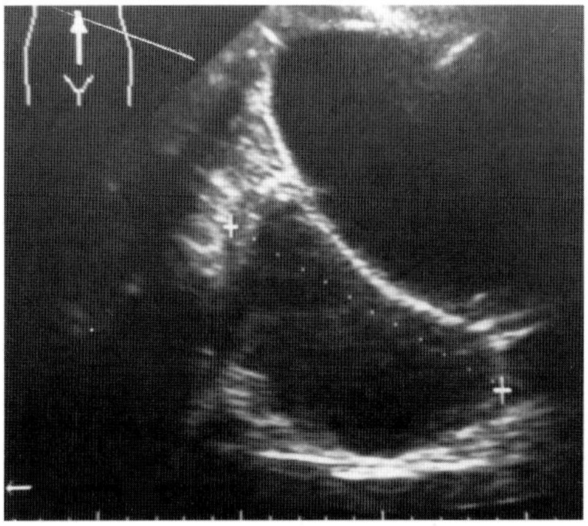

OVARIAN AND UTERINE CHANGES WITH MENSTRUAL CYCLE

HORMONE LEVELS DURING MENSTRUAL CYCLE

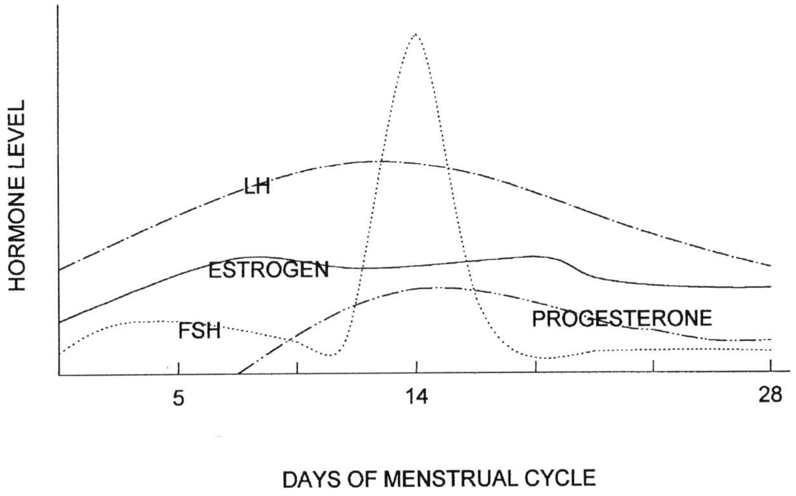

DAYS	1-5	5-14	10-14	14-22	22-28	
HORMONE LEVELS	LOW ESTROGEN LOW PROGEST LOW LH ↑ FSH	↑ ESTROGEN ↑ LH ↓ FSH excretion tapers off dips due to rising ESTROGEN then FSH peaks just before ovulation	↓ ESTROGEN ↑↑ LH surge before then drops FSH drops	↑ EST: 2nd peak at maximum corpus luteum activity ↑ PROG peaks day 20-22	**NO Fertilization** ↓↓ PROG & ESTROGEN	**+ Fertilization** corpus luteum secretes EST & PROG
OVARIAN CYCLE	**FOLLICULAR / PRE-OVULATORY PHASE**		**OVULATION**	**LUTEAL / POST-OVULATORY PHASE**		
OVARIAN CYCLE PHASES	-primary follicles start to produce estrogen -zona pellucida develops around potential ovum - secondary follicles develop which elevate EST level	↑EST by developing follicle graafian/dominant follicle ready for ovulation -mean diameter about 2 cm	rupture of graafian follicle with release of immature ovum into pelvic cavity	LH stimulates development of corpus luteum which secretes PROG & EST	corpus luteum degenerates into corpus albicans which decreases EST & PROG levels	corpus luteum is maintained 3-4 months by placental HCG -both secrete EST & PROG
UTERINE CYCLE	**MENSTRUAL/ BLEEDING PHASE**	**PROLIFERATIVE PHASE**	**PERI-OVULATORY**	**SECRETORY PHASE**		
UTERINE CYCLE PHASES	-endometrium degenerates, shrinks and then is shed -menstruation -caused by sudden ↓ in EST & PROG	-decidual layer regenerates from basal layer causing endometrium to thicken	-glands develop and arterioles coil and lengthen	-prepatory changes in glands and vascularature -edema, rich blood supply	-contraction of tissue, resorption of fluid, spiral arteries kink & buckle	-endometrium maintained for implantation of fertilized ovum

MENSTRUAL CYCLE

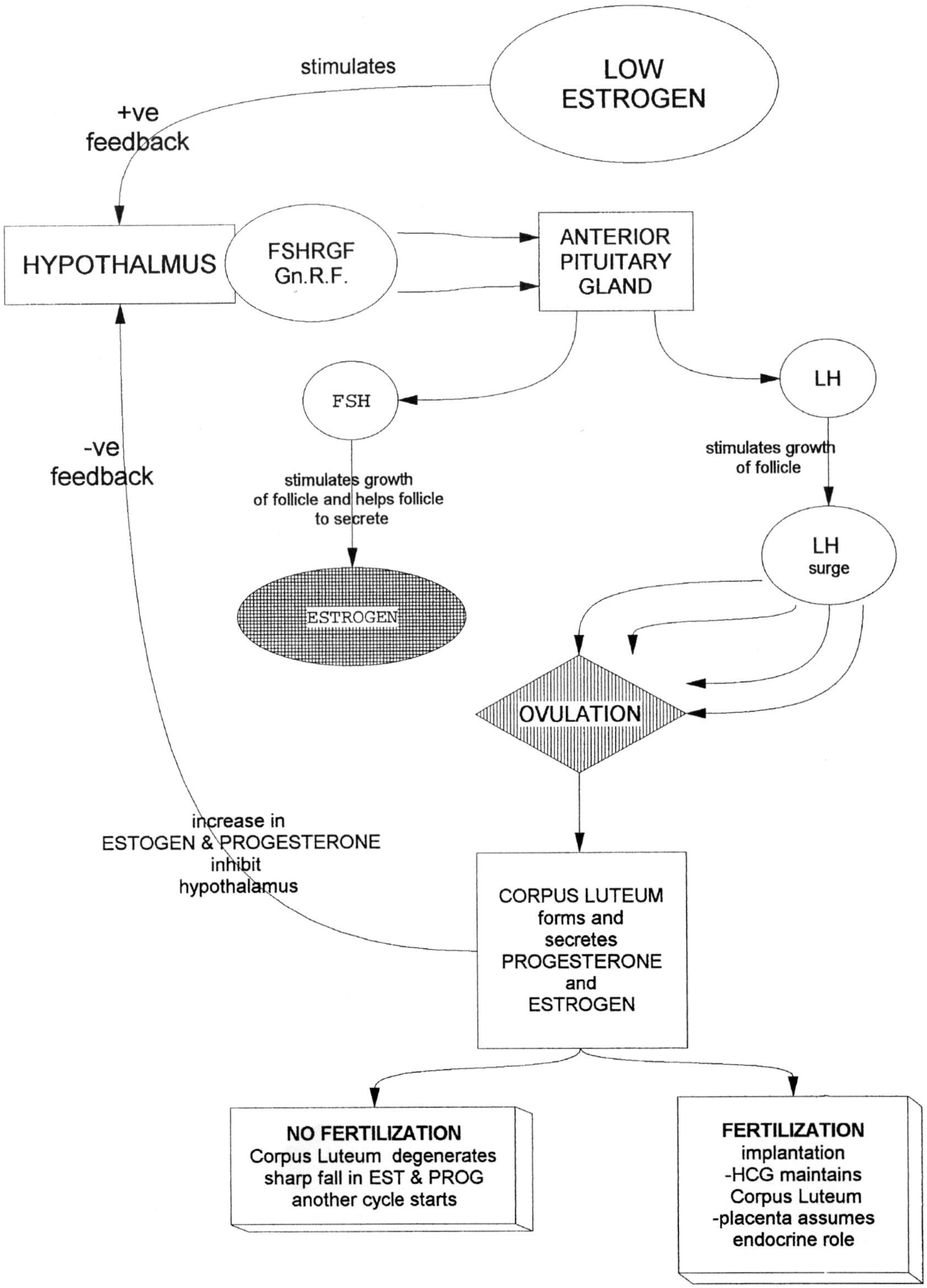

HORMONES AND PHARMACEUTICALS	
WHAT IT IS	WHAT IT DOES
CLOMID - CLOMIPHENE CITRATE -stimulates the pituitary to secrete increased amounts of FSH	-used in infertility for hormone induced ovulation -hCG may be used at point of ovulation to help release ovum
ESTROGEN -from granulosa cells lining the follicle within the ovary -peaks: 1st - just before ovulation 2nd - near mid luteal phase -creates -ve feedback on FSH -creates +ve feedback on LH	-stimulates growth, development and maintenance of female reproductive structures and secondary sex characteristics such as breast development, feminine body contours -cyclic changes in vagina, uterus -growth of arteries, glands in endometrium -myometrial growth -contraction of fallopian tubes -maintains calcium in bones
FOLLICLE STIMULATING HORMONE (FSH) -Gonadotropin produced by pituitary gland	-influences follicular growth and estrogen production and secretion by ovaries, provided that a small amount of luteinizing hormone is present
HUMAN CHORIONIC GONADOTROPIN -a pregnancy hormone produced by placental trophoblastic tissue -as the volume of trophoblastic tissue grown, the amount of serum b-hCG produced increases -levels rise exponentially, doubling every 48 hours until reaches peak at 6 weeks (8 weeks LNMP) leveling off until delivery -measured and referred either in either : 1. First International Reference Preparation 2. Second International Standard which are unequal units, therefore it is vital to know which standard is being use:	-maintain activity of the corpus luteum (output of estrogen and progesterone) -the continuous progesterone secretion is necessary for implantation of the gestational sac -secretion of HCG in urine serves as basis for most home pregnancy tests and can be detected 10 days after conception in a normal intrauterine pregnancy (day 25 LNMP) Abnormal Pregnancies -beta-hCG levels less than 2-3 standard deviations below mean, given menstral age, sac development or CRL suggest pregnancy failure -beta-hCG levels greatly above normal can suggest gestational trophoblastic disease, multiple pregnancy
LUTEINIZING HORMONE (LH) -Gonadotropin produced by pituitary	-stimulates further development of ovarian follicles, ovulation and the secretion of estrogen and progesterone secretion by the ovaries
ORAL CONTRACEPTIVES -hormonal method of birth control which has found widespread use	-several pills available: common one contains high concentration of progesterone and low concentration of estrogen which decrease FSH & LH by inhibiting GnRF -these low levels are not adequate to initiate follicle maturation and ovulation
PERGONAL (HMG)Human Menopausal Gonadotropin -natural hormone extracted from urine of post-menopausal women	-source of FSH & LH given to women who have not responded to clomid (pituitary not producing appropriate FSH levels) in hormone induced ovulation for infertility
PROGESTERONE -mainly produced by corpus luteum -creates negative feedback on LH -in pregnancy secreted also by placenta peak: 7 days after ovulation	-induces secretory activity in endometrium that was previously primed by estrogen in 2nd half of cycle -induces decidual hypertrophy in endometrium which will provide a thick moist environment for implantation -maintenance of pregnancy -development of mammary glands -increases basal body temperature 1°C

LEVEL OF PROGESTERONE, ESTROGEN AND b-hCG DURING PREGNANCY

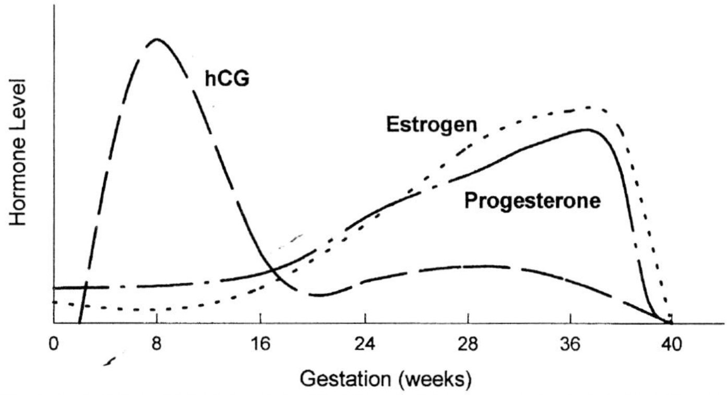

CHAPTER 7
EMBRYONIC AND EARLY FETAL DEVELOPMENT: FIRST TRIMESTER

A) NORMAL DEVELOPMENT

GAMETOGENESIS: maturation of male and female germ cells which undergo:
1. MEIOSIS- to reduce the number of chromosomes to half (46–23)
2. CHANGES- to alter their shape in preparation for fertilization

MALE (SPERMATOGENESIS) -development of spermatozoa which takes place in seminiferous tubules of testis	**FEMALE (OOGENESIS)** -development of the ovum within the ovary
primordial cells dormant in seminiferous tubules (teste) until puberty, then differentiate	primordial germ cells in ovary under go mitosis
⇓	⇓
SPERMATOGONIA (PRIMITIVE SPERM)	OOGONIA (PRIMITIVE OVA)
⇓	⇓
PRIMARY SPERMATOCYTE (2n-46 chromosomes) (XY)	PRIMARY OOCYTE (2n-46 chromosomes) (XX)
⇓	⇓
first meiotic division ⇓	at puberty finish meiotic division ⇓
2 EQUAL GROUPS 2 - SECONDARY SPERMATIDS (X) (Y)	2 equal groups
⇓ second meiotic division ⇓	1) SECONDARY OOCYTE (X) ⇓ receives all cytoplasm ⇓ ovulation ⇓ mitosis ⇓ 2) FIRST POLAR BODY(X) ⇓ degenerates nonfunctional
4 -SPERMATIDS (n-23 chromosomes) (X) (X) (Y) (Y) ⇓	**OVUM** (n 23X) large cell ready for fertilization 2nd polar body discarded
maturing process (formation of acrosome, neck, tail, condensation of nucleus and shedding most of cytoplasm) ⇓	
SPERMATOZOA (SPERM) (n 23X or 23Y)	

DEVELOPMENT OF THE OVUM	
PRIMORDIAL FOLLICLE	-oocyte plus surrounding epithelial cells -inner cell is granulosa cell layer and outer cell is theca cell layer -an oocyte starts with one layer of follicular cells which increase in number -grows under influence of follicle-stimulating hormone from the anterior pituitary gland
SECONDARY FOLLICLE	-small collection of fluid (antrum) fills and expands in the centre
MATURE GRAAFIAN / DOMINANT FOLLICLE	-atrium expands until only a layer of mature cells on the outermost part of the follicle -follicles are tense and liquid within is under pressure -cells secrete estrogen during proliferative phase -growth rate 2–4 mm/day until ovulation
CUMULUS OOPHORUS	-oocyte plus the surrounding granulosa cells
OOCYTE / OVUM	-day 14, ovum surrounded by zona pellucida, corona radiata bursts from the follicle into fimbriae of fallopian tube
CORPUS HEMORRHAGICUM	-walls collapse of empty follicle -some bleeding and clotting occurs and fills it
CORPUS LUTEUM	-follicle cells become luteinized by the retention of fluid which forms corpus luteum -secretes estrogen and progesterone during secretory phase in preparation of implantation of fertilized ovum corpus luteum of pregnancy: -with fertilization it continues to develop, maintained by hCG -produces sufficient estrogen and progesterone to inhibit further ovulation -will support pregnancy for up to 3 months when the placenta acquires the capability of progesterone and estrogen excretion
CORPUS ALBICANS	-no fertilization, corpus luteum involutes and degenerates into scar tissue

FERTILIZATION	
SPERM -Acrosome: enzymes secreted by acromsome to help dissolve zona pellucida -Sperm nucleus (in head): in ovum develops into male pronucleus -Plasma membrane -Tail: shed when enters ovum	OOCYTE -Corona radiata: several innermost layers of follicle cells -Zona pellucidum: gelatinous covering of ovum -disappears allowing blastocyst to attach to endometrium -Plasma membrane -Nucleus: develops into female pronucleus
<u>Acrosomal Reaction:</u> -as sperm approach ovum, perforations in acrosome release enzymes that separate and slough off corona radiata cells which facilitate passage of sperm through zona pellucida <u>Zona Reaction:</u> -as sperm contacts plasma membrane of ovum, changes in zona occur which prevent additional sperm from entering	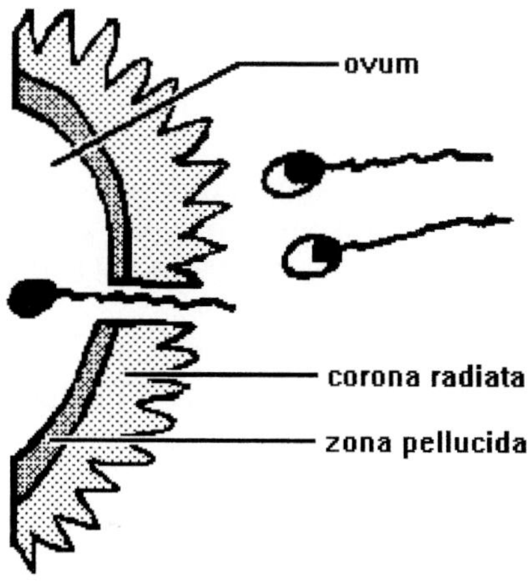

FIRST WEEK OF EMBRYONIC DEVELOPMENT		

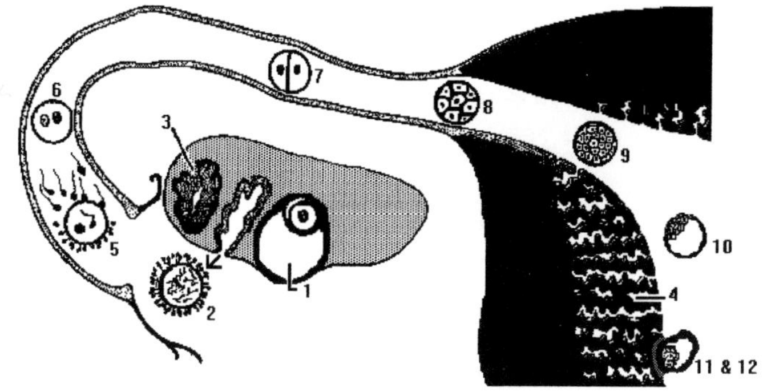

KEY AND DESCRIPTION TO ABOVE DIAGRAM OF FIRST WEEK OF EMBRYONIC LIFE		
1	GRAAFIAN FOLLICLE	-dominant follicle which enlarges until ovulation
2	OOCYTE / OVUM	-secondary oocyte released from ovary on about day 14
3	CORPUS LUTEUM	-collapsed follicle which secretes progesterone and some estrogen -maintained by hCG produced by syncytiotrophoblast
4	DECIDUAL REACTION	-hypertrophic changes of endometrial cells which provide nourishment to blastocyst
5	FERTILIZATION	-penetration of ovum by spermatozoon and subsequent union of sperm and ovum nuclei -occurs in distal fallopian tube, 12–24 hours after ovulation
6	ZYGOTE	-fertilized ovum, consisting of nucleus, cytoplasm and enveloping membrane
7	CLEAVAGE	-early rapid cell division of zygote -increases number of cell, not size of organism
8	BLASTOMERES	-2, 4, 8, cell stage of early zygote, approximately 30 hours old
9	MORULA	-12–16 cell embryonic mass which further differentiates into fluid-filled sphere -enters uterine cavity on day 18
10	BLASTOCYST	-forms by day 20 -inner cell mass + fluid filled cavity (blastocele) lined by trophoblastic cells -zona pellucida has disappeared
11	IMPLANTATION	-0.1 mm blastocyst implants into decidua, usually in fundus -occurs between days 21 and 23 (3 weeks LNMP), serum bHCG positive -inside blastocyst, primary yolk sac and amniotic sac form
12	CONCEPTUS	-products of conception; fetus, placenta and membranes -day 23-25: inside blastocyst inner cell mass gives rise to amnion, embryonic yolk sac, embryo (bilaminar disc) and umbilical cord

EARLY EMBRYONIC DEVELOPMENT

WEEK 4 -the bilaminar disc forms with fluid filled cavities on either side of it -smaller amniotic sac lies near the trophoblastic (placental) layer -yolk sac projected into chorionic cavity or sac and for a time is larger than the amniotic sac	4 weeks: Simple double bleb stage -bilaminar disc forms with fluid-filled cavities on either side -smaller amniotic sac lies near the trophoblastic (placental) layer -yolk sac projected into chorionic cavity and, briefly, is larger than the amniotic sac 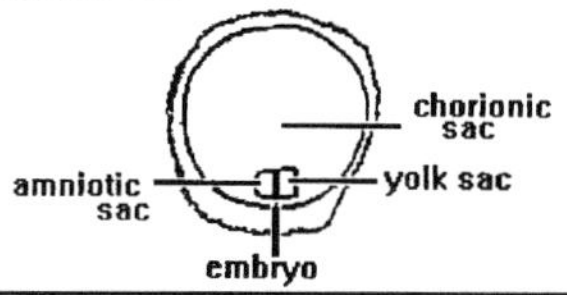
WEEK 5 -yolk sac becomes much smaller -amnion forms sac that encloses embryo -it contains amniotic fluid -this begins to expand to fill the chorionic cavity -gastrulation - trilaminar disc forms -neurulation - formation neural plate and closure to form neural tube -primitive heart begins to beat	4-5 weeks: Yolk sac and enlarging amniotic cavity within the chorionic sac 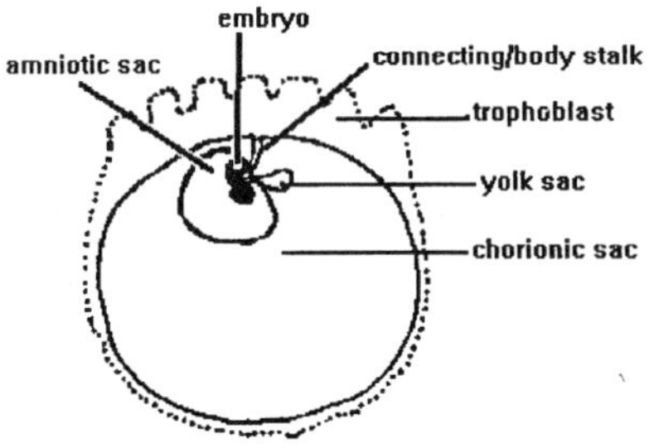
WEEK 6 -is beginning of embryonic period when all internal and external structures form -yolk sac is incorporated into embryo to form primitive gut -limb buds first appear	5-6 weeks: Sagittal midline section of embryo demonstrating the flexion of its body and the early formation of the heart, nervous system and gut 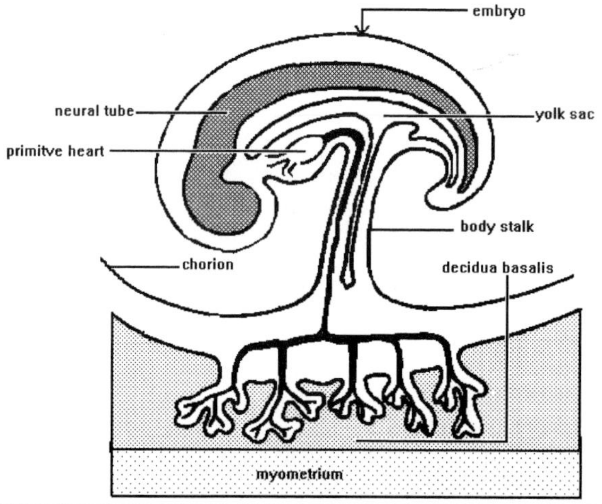

SONOGRAPHIC APPEARANCE OF NORMAL EARLY INTRAUTERINE GESTATION	
WEEKS-LMP SONOGRAPHIC FINDINGS	US APPEARANCES
3–4 weeks <u>DECIDUAL REACTION</u> -focal echogenic thickening of endometrium has been reported, but not a sonographic sign of pregnancy yet <u>INTRADECIDUAL SIGN</u> -small (< 5mm) sac becomes visible within one layer of endometrium <u>IMPLANTATION BLEEDING</u> -may follow implantation, due to erosion of uterine lining and could appear as a hypoechoic cleft in decidua near sac	transvaginal sagittal scans of early gestation sacs embedded in the endometrium of uterus 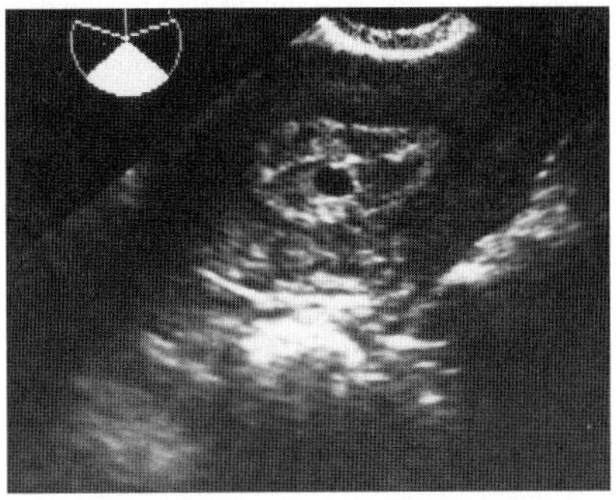 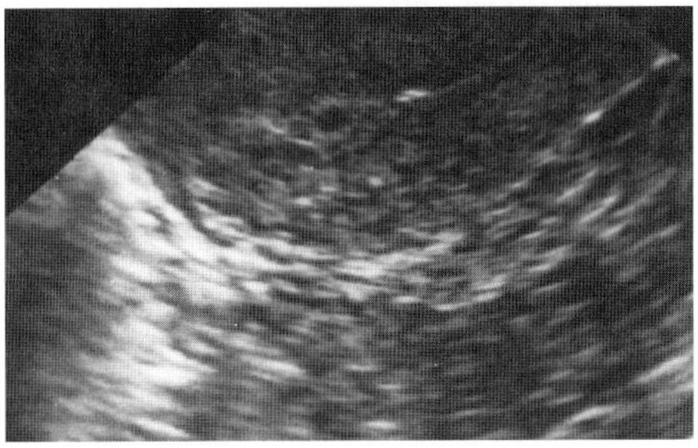
5 weeks **GESTATIONAL SAC DETECTED** -first reliable indicator of IUG is detection of gestational sac -no yolk sac or embryo yet -arises from blastocyst which implants into secretory endometrium <u>DECIDUA CHORIONIC RING SIGN or</u> <u>DOUBLE - DECIDUAL SIGN</u> -distinguishes true IUG from pseudogestational sac -two concentric hyperechoic rings adjacent to gestational sac: <u>1. inner ring</u>: decidua capsularis + chorion laeve <u>2. outer ring</u>: decidua vera -thicker at implantation site due to decidua basalis and chorion frondosum <u>3. sonolucent centre</u>: fluid-filled chorionic cavity	transvaginal axial scan of uterus containing small gestation sac with decidua chorionic ring sign 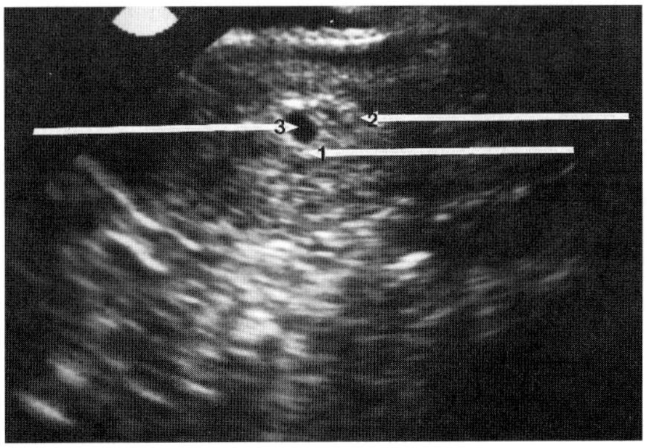

ULTRASOUND FINDING	US APPEARANCE
5.5 weeks **SECONDARY YOLK SAC DETECTED** -first structure seen; 2–5 mm in size -rounded sonolucent structure (outside amniotic cavity) within chorionic cavity between amnion and chorion -largest between 5 and 9 weeks <u>DOUBLE BLEB SIGN</u> -uncommon transient phenomenon -first demonstration of amnion -2 tiny sacs: represent the amnion and secondary yolk sac separated by embryonic disc	transvaginal scan of 5 1/2 week gestation with secondary fetal yolk sac inside (arrow) 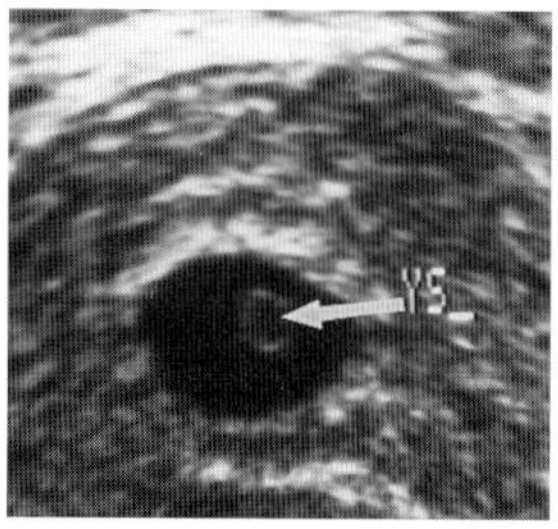
6-7 weeks **EMBRYONIC (FETAL) POLE DETECTED** CRL: 2–4 mm seen adjacent to yolk sac -a tiny fetal pole (1–2 mm) may be seen 3–7 days after visualization of yolk sac with transvaginal sonography **CARDIAC ACTIVITY DETECTED** -although heart first contracts on about day 37, cardiac activity first seen sonographically a few days later -the rate and rhythm can be measured on M-mode -first seen adjacent to yolk sac -cardiac activity can often be observed prior to embryo identification as embryo next to gestational sac wall can sometimes make it difficult to define	transvaginal scan of uterus with calipers demarcating a tiny 1–2 mm embryo adjacent to the yolk sac 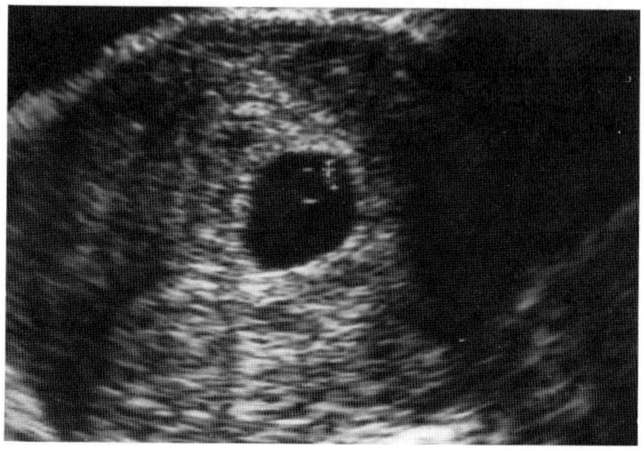

<table>
<tr><th>ULTRASOUND FINDING</th><th>US APPEARANCE</th></tr>
<tr><td>

7-9 weeks

EMBRYO
-CRL: 12–14 mm
-embryo seen with amnion snugly around it
-early umbilical cord is connecting stalk attaching embryo to well seen developing placenta (chorion frondosum)
-limb buds first appear

Central Nervous System:
-brain is seen as a single ventricle (telencephalon) partitioned by falx at 7 weeks
-falx seen at 8–9 weeks and lateral ventricles fill with echogenic choroid
-spine can be seen from week 9

Midgut:
-normal migration of bowel into umbilical cord occurs from 7th to 11th week

AMNIOTIC MEMBRANE
-curvilinear echogenic line within chorionic sac snugly around embryo
-fills chorionic cavity by 14-16 weeks
-fuses with chorionic membrane by 16 weeks
-chorionic fluid is more echogenic than amniotic fluid

</td><td>

transvaginal scan of fetus with yolk sac (Y) outside the amnion (arrow) in the chorionic cavity

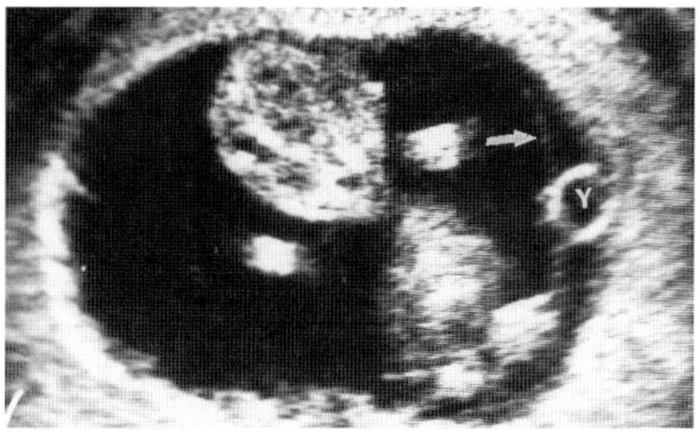

transvaginal scan showing amnion (arrow) separating the echogenic chorionic sac (C) from the amniotic sac (A)

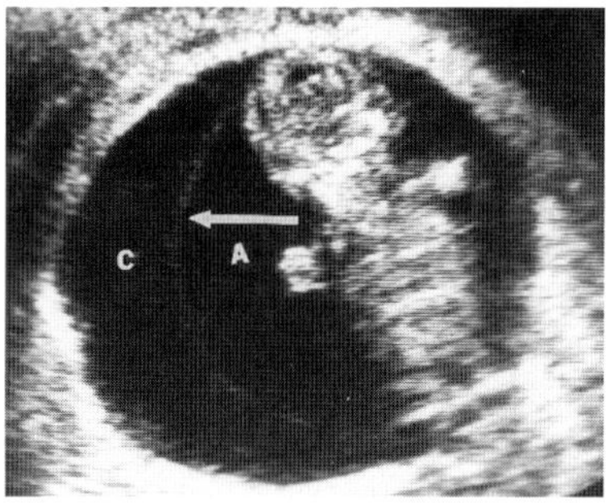

transabdominal scan of 9-week fetus demonstrating the head, body and limbs and yolk sac

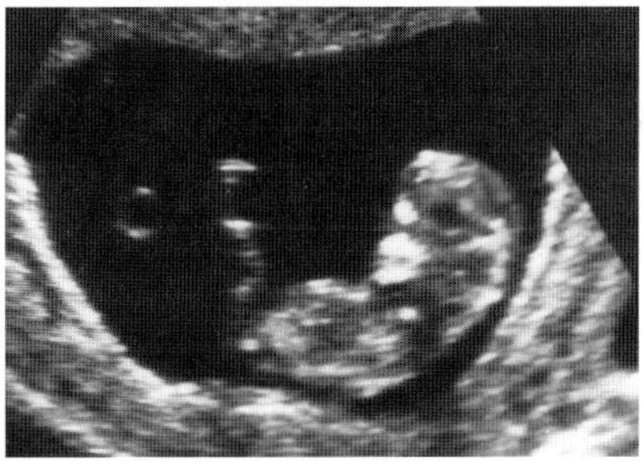

</td></tr>
</table>

ULTRASOUND FINDING	US APPEARANCE
10-12 weeks **EMBRYO** -beginning of fetal stage Extremities: -head and limbs well identified -can be evaluated and appearance -long bones can be evaluated after 11 weeks Central Nervous System: -small cystic structure in posterior cranium represents the hindbrain (rhombencephalon) -at 10 to 11 weeks the thalami and cerebellum can be seen Midgut: -after 11 weeks, bowel returns to abdominal cavity completing a 270° counterclockwise rotation -smaller, compressed yolk sac GU system: Week 11 - Kidneys reach adult position in abdomen **AMNIOTIC MEMBRANE** -amnion reaches chorionic membrane	11 weeks fetus 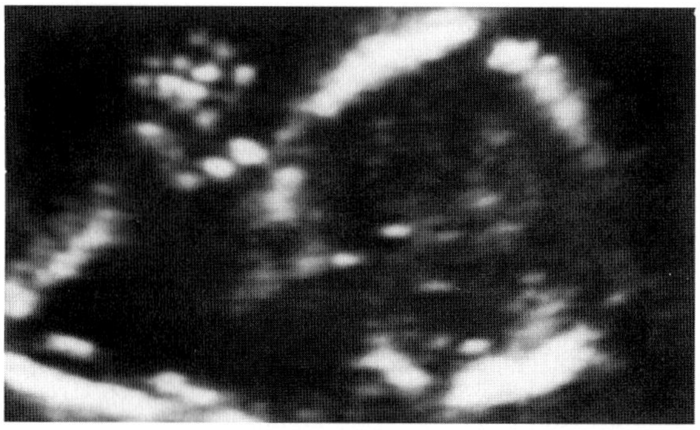 transvaginal scan of 12-week fetal spine; with the bony centers now ossifying, systems such as the spine can now begin to be evaluated 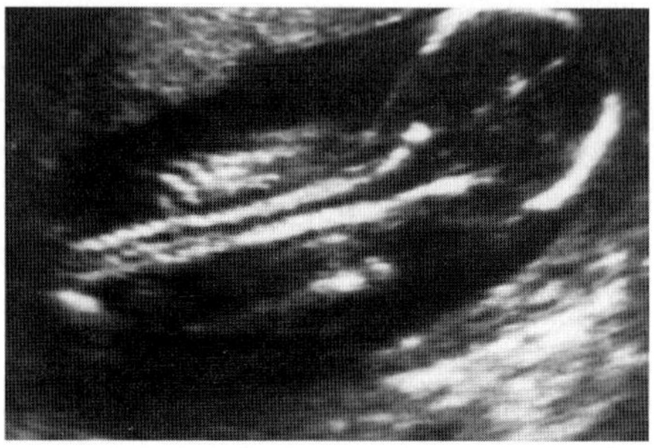

SONOGRAPHIC DISCRIMINATORY LEVELS
-levels above which a normal intrauterine pregnancy should be observed sonographically
-caution is suggested in strict implementation of these values to avoid a false negative ultrasound examination
-beta-hCG is in IRP -First International Reference Preparation

SONOGRAPHIC FINDING	OBSERVED WHEN THE:	TRANSABDOMINAL	TRANSVAGINAL
GESTATIONAL SAC	menstrual age is	35 days	30–32 days
	beta-hCG level is > than	3600 mIU/ml	2,000 mIU/ml
	mean sac diameter is	5 mm	2–3 mm
YOLK SAC	mean sac diameter is	20 mm	6–10 mm
	menstrual age is	42 days	35 days
	beta-hCG level is > than	not correlated with b-hCG	>7200 mIU/ml
EMBRYONIC POLE	mean sac diameter is	25 mm	16 mm
HEART ACTIVITY	crown rump length is	9 mm	5 mm
	beta-hCG level is > than	not correlated with b-hCG	10,800 mIU/ml
	menstrual age is	45–48 days	36–40 days
	mean sac diameter is	25 mm	> 10 mm

FETAL MEMBRANES -membranes arising from development of zygote which lie outside embryo and protect and nourish embryo	
YOLK SAC	-endoderm-lined membrane that surrounds yolk of gestation -responsible for early blood formation (hematopoiesis), transfer of nutrients, formation of primitive gut, development of sex glands -shrinks as pregnancy progresses as eventually embryo receives nourishment from endometrium -becomes pinched off as it is compressed between amnion and chorion at the end of the first trimester -becomes incorporated into gut of embryo -if persists, becomes an outpouching of the ileum in adults, known as Meckel's diverticulum
ALLANTOIS	-small vascularized membrane which is a diverticula of yolk sac -its vessels serve as connections in the placenta between mother and fetus -becomes umbilical cord
AMNION	-thin protective membrane that initially lies over embryonic disc -formed 1 week after fertilization -grows and becomes filled with amniotic fluid -eventually surrounds fetus and fuses to inner layer of chorion
CHORION	-derived from trophoblast cells of blastocyst and its associated mesoderm -surrounds embryo -eventually becomes main part of placenta

B) ABNORMALITIES

SONOGRAPHIC PREDICTORS OF EARLY EMBRYONIC DEMISE		
FINDING	**NORMAL CRITERIA**	**ABNORMAL CRITERIA**
AMNION	-seen when embryo = 13 mm	-visualization of amnion without embryonic visualization
CHORIO-DECIDUA REACTION	-no doppler signal in trophoblastic tissue -double decidual sac sign	-degenerating trophoblastic tissue generates a low resistive flow pattern -incompletely or poorly formed decidual reaction
EMBRYO	-should appears in chorionic sac next to yolk sac before the MSD reaches 16 -18 mm (TV) -normal growth rate = 0.8 mm per day	-embryo with no fetal heart beat by 6.5 weeks
HEART RATE	-cardiac activity seen when embryo seen but this often depends on equipment and operator, therefore can be normal to see no FH with 2-4 mm CRL -seen always after CRL = 4 mm Normal rate: 5-6 weeks = 100 BPM 8-9 weeks = 140 BPM	Bradycardia -embryos at 5-8 weeks with a heart rate < 85 BPM may be associated with spontaneous miscarriage -normal fetal cardiac activity after 8 weeks associated with >95% pregnancy continuation rate
GESTATIONAL SAC SIZE Mean Sac Diameter (MSD)	Double Decidual Sac Sign -should be seen when MSD = 10 mm (TA) yolk sac + amnion Yolk sac -should be seen within gestation sac when MSD =20 mm (TA) or 13 mm (TV)	Abnormally Small Sac Size Criteria (Oligohydramnios) -small mean sac diameter compared to the CRL is associated with spontaneous abortions -uncertain etiology -MSD < 5 mm at 5.5 -9 weeks
	Embryo -should be seen within gestational sac when MSD = 25 mm (TA) or 16-18 mm (TV)	Abnormally Large Sac Size Criteria MSD > 8 mm without a yolk sac (TV) > 16-18 mm without embryo (TV)
SAC GROWTH	Normal Growth Rate = 1.1 mm per day	Abnormal Growth rate < 0.6 mm per day
SAC SHAPE	-elliptical shape -may be distorted by contractions and external pressures	-distorted, bizarre, irregular sac shape
SAC POSITION	-sac embedded in the decidual endometrium, usually in fundus	-"sac" in central uterine cavity -low position in uterus or positioned in cervix
SUBCHORIONIC HEMORRHAGE	-extrachorionic hematoma is detected in 18% of women with 1st trimester vaginal bleeding -caused by abruption at the placental margin resulting in venous bleeding that strips placental membranes away from myometrium -MAY BE associated with poor outcome especially if it has a volume > 60 cc. US Appearance: -extrachorionic crescent fluid collection between the gestational sac and the uterine wall -collection begins at edge of placenta and does no usually extend behind, within or in front of it	
YOLK SAC	1. Size: < 6 mm 2. Shape: rounded with thick echogenic wall 3. Duplication: one yolk sac per embryo 4. Appearance: thin echogenic rim around a sonolucent center which remains constant in appearance until 10 weeks, when it starts to regress in size	-abnormalities of the yolk sac may be associated with poor outcome, although not universally accepted i.e.:- yolk sac < 2 mm. between 8-12 weeks - yolk sac > 5.6 mm between 5-10 weeks - solid echodense yolk sac - non visualization of yolk sac in presence of embryo

Blighted Ovum: transvaginal scan of a large gestational sac with a large yolk sac, and no fetal pole

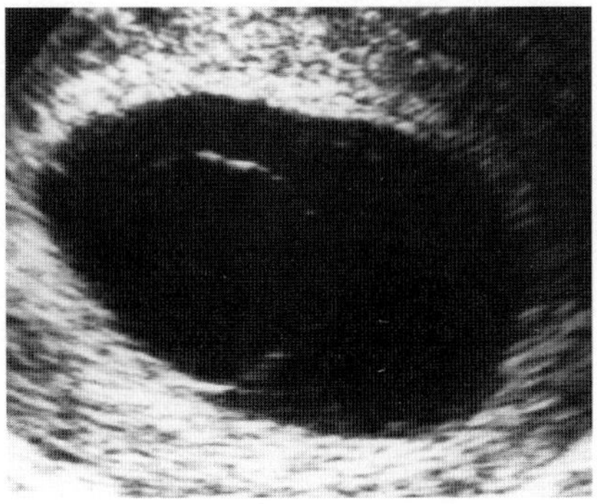

Abnormal Gestational Sac: transvaginal scan of uterus with an irregularly shaped gestational sac secondary to fetal demise

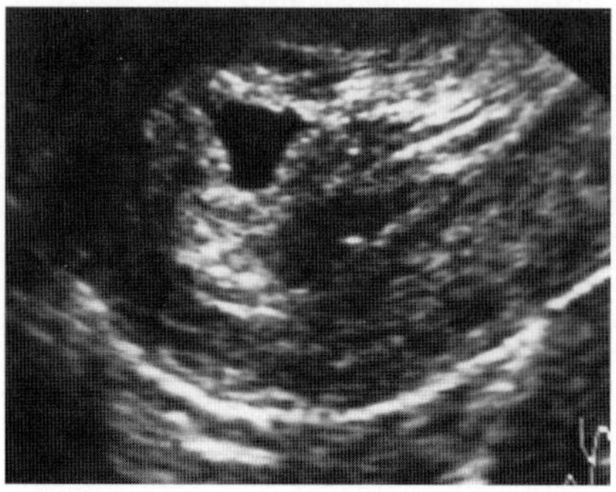

UNSUCCESSFUL FIRST TRIMESTER PREGNANCIES

ABORTION (MISCARRIAGE)....termination of pregnancy before viability

0–10 weeks: OVULAR DEFECTS- failed or defective development of embryo, abnormal implantation of early placenta

11 weeks until term: MATERNAL DEFECTS- infection (TORCH), nutrition, endocrine anomalies, maternal uterine anomalies, emotional stress, physical trauma

COMPLETE	-entire products of conception expelled
HABITUAL	-more than 3 consecutive miscarriages - can be due to maternal environment, incompetent cervix, chromosome anomalies
INCOMPLETE	-partial expulsion of products of conceptus from uterus with some retained conceptus, usually placenta
INDUCED	-artificial: some types are known as therapeutic, elective, criminal -suction curettage is a method for terminating an early pregnancy -hypertonic saline, hysterectomy, oxytocin are methods for termination after 12 weeks
INEVITABLE - IMPENDING - IMMINENT	-cervix dilated, severe pain, uterine contractions, membranes protruding, low gestation sac position -cannot be halted
MISSED	-embryonic or fetal death with retention of products of conceptus within uterus for any amount of time -definitions vary: used to originally mean death occurring before 28 weeks with retention of fetus for > 2 months
SPONTANEOUS	-occurring without apparent cause -can occur with advanced maternal age (chromosome anomalies) fibroids, uterine anomalies, women whose mothers were exposed to diethylstilbestrol during pregnancy
THREATENED	-clinical term defined as a pregnancy with vaginal spotting, mild cramping, closed cervix <20 weeks -most common indication for 1st trimester ultrasound -includes a broad spectrum of conditions: ectopic pregnancy, missed abortion, blighted ovum, normal intrauterine pregnancy, an abnormal living intrauterine pregnancy

SONOGRAPHIC APPEARANCES OF MISCARRIAGE:

-depends on when it is scanned and at what point in pregnancy it occurs

-embryo and gestational sac become smaller and more disorganized

-sometimes, sonograms alone cannot make certain diagnosis

-see gestational sac criteria for abnormal pregnancy

threatened abortion: transvaginal scan of an irregularly shaped, collapsing gestation sac with poor trophoblastic decidual reaction low in the uterus

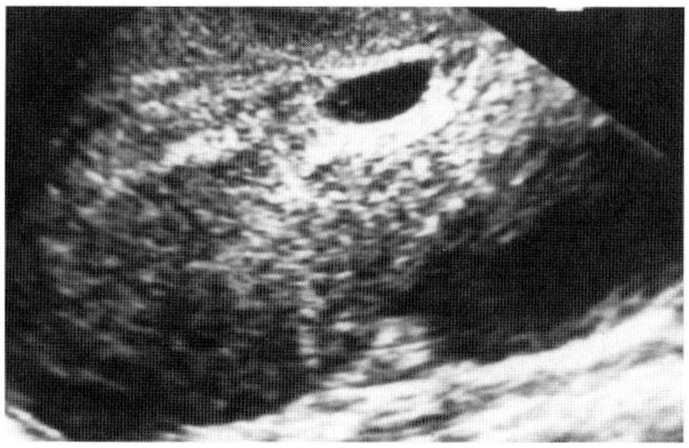

impending: transabdominal sagittal scan of an irregularly shaped gestation sac containing an embryo with no heart activity

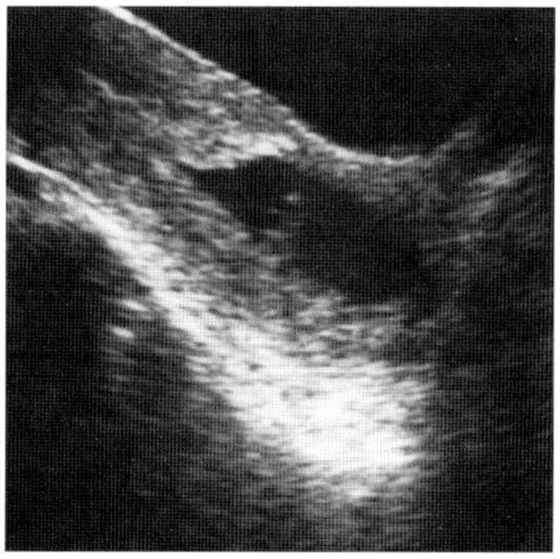

inevitable: transvaginal scan of a gestation sac partially protruding through the endocervical canal. The sac contains an irregularly shaped fetal pole with no fetal heartbeat

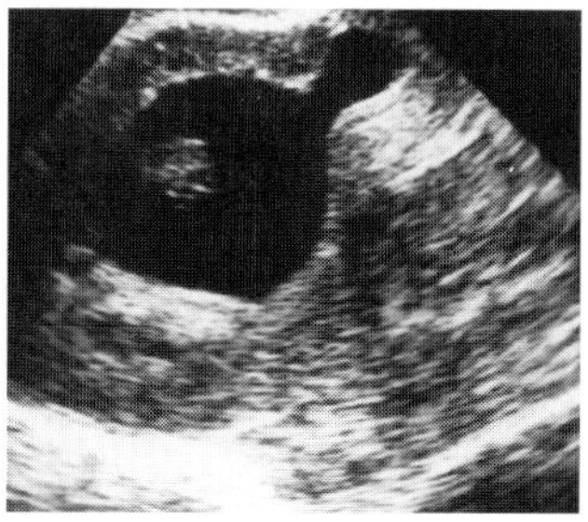

FIRST TRIMESTER BLEEDING DIFFERENTIAL	
WITH INTRAUTERINE CONCEPTUS IDENTIFIED	-blighted ovum -vanishing twin syndrome -implantation bleed -threatened abortion -gestational trophoblastic disease -normal pregnancy -pseudogestational sac with an ectopic pregnancy
WITH EMPTY UTERUS + beta-hCG > 1800 mIU/ml	-recent spontaneous abortion -ectopic pregnancy
WITH EMPTY UTERUS + beta-hCG < 1800 mIU/ML	-early intrauterine pregnancy -ectopic pregnancy

UNSUCCESSFUL FIRST TRIMESTER PREGNANCIES	US APPEARANCE
BLIGHTED OVUM (ANEMBRYONIC PREGNANCY / EMBRYONIC RESORPTION) -fertilized ovum development arrested because of failure of inner cell mass to develop -trophoblast continues to function, therefore, sac grows, although at a diminished rate -often demonstrate chromosomal anomalies SS -spotting decrease in pregnancy type symptoms -12–14 week size uterus with no fetus -lower than normal b-hCG levels US -large gestation sac without an embryo: Transvaginal: MSD >16 mm with no embryo Transabdominal: MSD > 25 mm with no embryo -poor gestational sac growth -poor trophoblastic reaction	transabdominal scans of a large (3 x 6 x 3 mm) irregularly shaped empty gestational sac 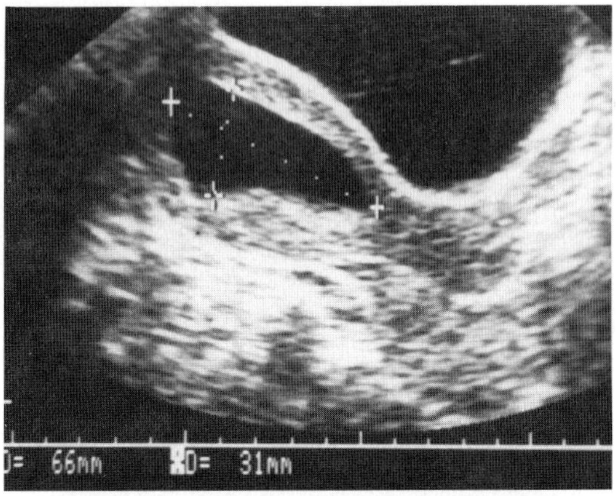 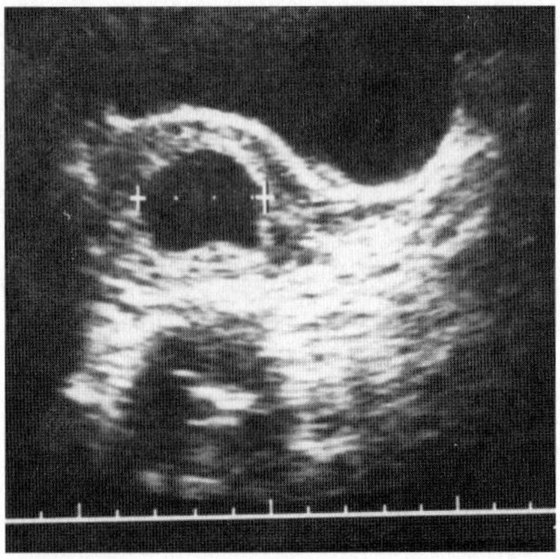

UNSUCCESSFUL FIRST TRIMESTER PREGNANCIES

ECTOPIC PREGNANCY

-any pregnancy located outside endometrial cavity
-causes approximately 25% of maternal deaths (interstitial tubal ectopics have most serious consequences due to forcible expulsion, rupture and hemorrhage)
-contributing factors include pelvic inflammatory disease, tube malfunction due to scarring, adhesions or disease, IUCD, artificial insemination, endometriosis
-25% chance of recurrence
-qualitative beta HCG useful in diagnosis
<u>Heterotopic Pregnancy</u>: rare occurrence of simultaneous intrauterine and ectopic pregnancy

SS
-classic triad: bleeding, pelvic pain, adnexal mass
-positive pregnancy test
-lower levels and lower rise of beta-HCG compared with normal IUG
-possible shoulder pain from intraperitoneal bleeding with diaphragmatic irritation

US
-free fluid (hemoperitoneum) in the pelvis and possibly abdomen
-hematosalpinx (blood within fallopian tube)
-visible extra uterine gestational sac with or without fetal activity
-ellipsoid tubal ring-like adnexal mass (concentric echogenic rim with hypoechoic center)
-enlarged empty uterus with possible thickened endometrium
-absent or irregular choriodecidual reaction with possible pseudogestational sac
<u>PSEUDOGESTATIONAL SAC</u>
-irregular sac-like structure identified in endometrial canal which has been created by the decidual reaction and bleeding which creates an anechoic fluid center

<u>Doppler</u>
-a uterine gestation sac has high-velocity low-impedance flow around its periphery, which also could be present in an extrauterine gestation sac
-increased vascularity around periphery of gestation sac has a waveform similar to normal luteal flow in an ovary, therefore, low impedance flow must be seen separate from ovarian vessel flow to positively identify flow within an ectopic gestational sac
-placental flow is never associated with pseudogestational sac

US APPEARANCE

transvaginal scan of ectopic gestation with a live fetus (calipers) at approximately 7 weeks in the right adnexa; uterus (U)

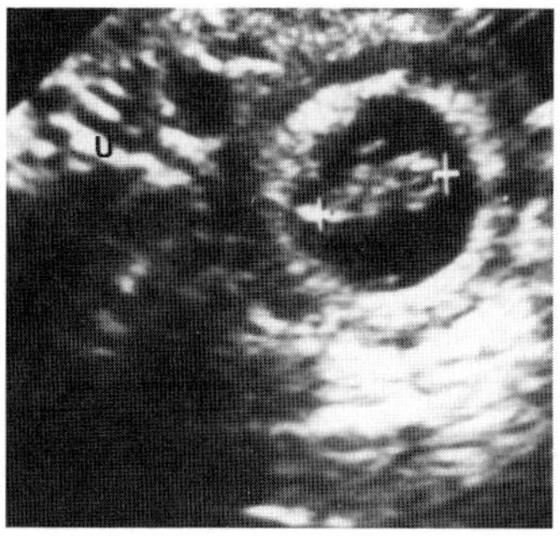

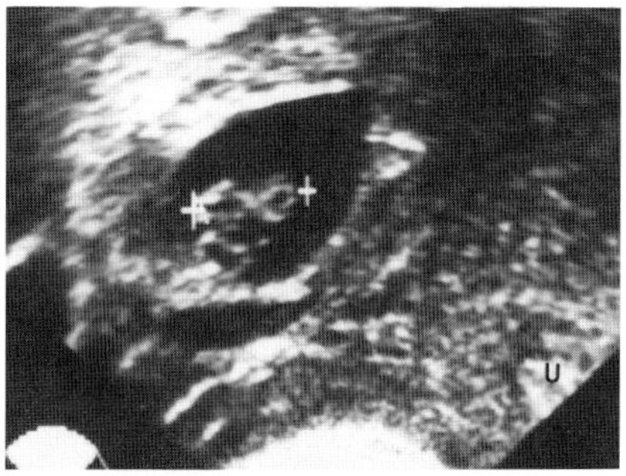

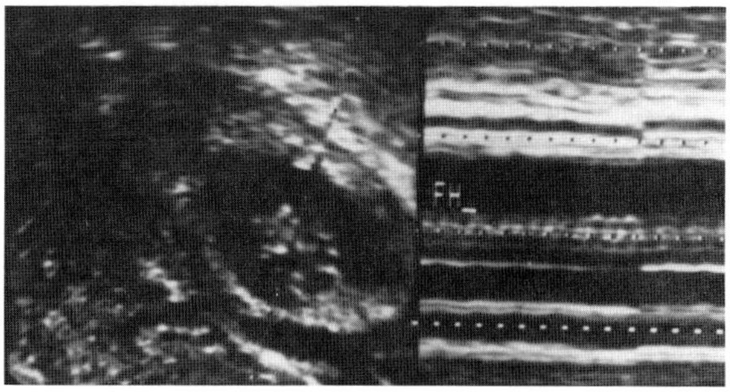

<u>LOCATION:</u>
1. Tubal - 95%
 a) ampulla (most common site)
 b) isthmus
 c) interstitial

Other - 5%
2. Abdomen (interligamentary)
3. Ovary
4. Cervix

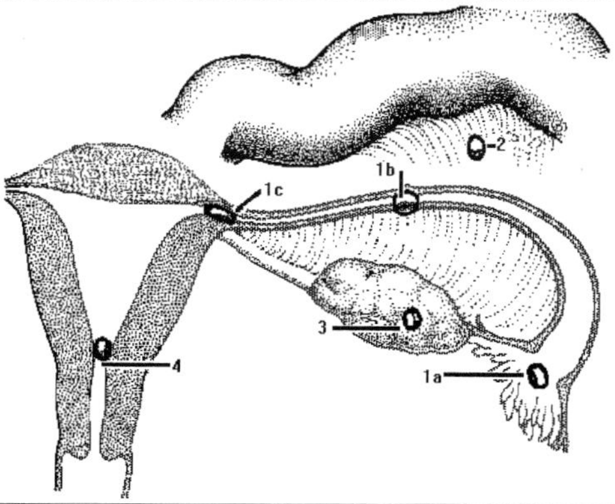

CHAPTER 8 - FETAL DEVELOPMENT: SECOND TRIMESTER

SECTION 1. DIGESTIVE SYSTEM, SPLEEN AND ADRENAL GLANDS

A) NORMAL ANATOMY AND DEVELOPMENT

DEVELOPMENT OF DIGESTIVE SYSTEM, SPLEEN AND ADRENAL GLANDS	
6 weeks	-primitive gut forms
8 weeks	-intestines herniate into umbilical cord
10 weeks	-adrenal cortex encapsulates medulla
12 weeks	-intestines return rapidly to abdomen
14 weeks	-bile formed and secreted

DEVELOPMENT OF DIGESTIVE SYSTEM

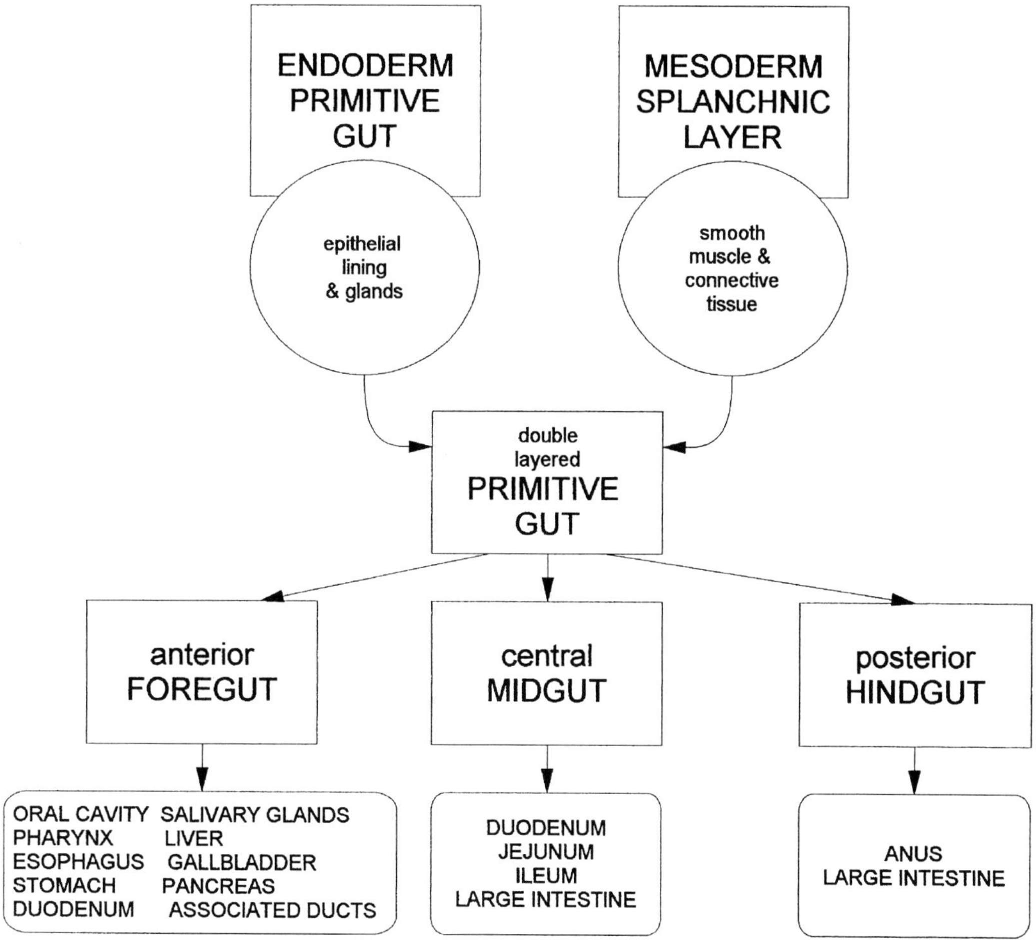

ANATOMY	US DESCRIPTIONS	US APPEARANCE
ADRENAL GLANDS -relatively large in fetus -at birth 20 times their relative adult size	-seen in 3rd trimester -curvilinear structures along posterior abdominal wall -consist of hypoechoic outer area (cortex) with a thinner echogenic zone (medulla)	transverse scan of 3rd trimester fetal abdomen showing normal adrenal gland (arrows) 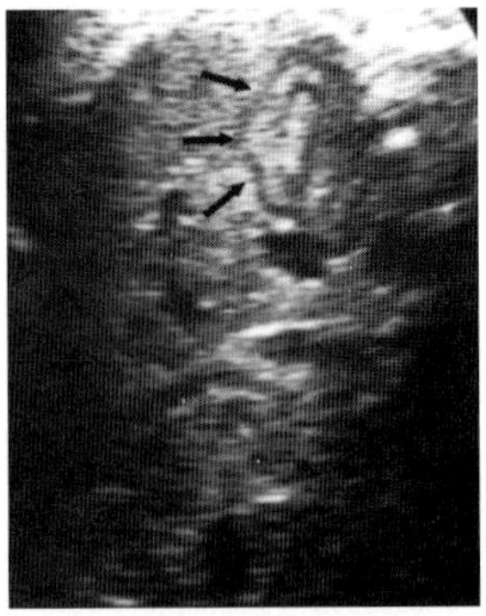
BOWEL After 20 Weeks -should be able to distinguish between large and small bowel Large Bowel -reservoir for meconium (epithelial cells, mucous, bile) from small bowel, therefore, diameter increases during pregnancy -normal bowel can be mistaken for dilated bowel, renal cysts and other pelvic masses -echogenic meconium can be a normal variant appearing often as a "pseudomass" or can associated with fetal pathologies such as Meconium ileus or peritonitis Small Bowel -small bowel loops are seen occasionally by third trimester -they should not exceed 6 mm in diameter 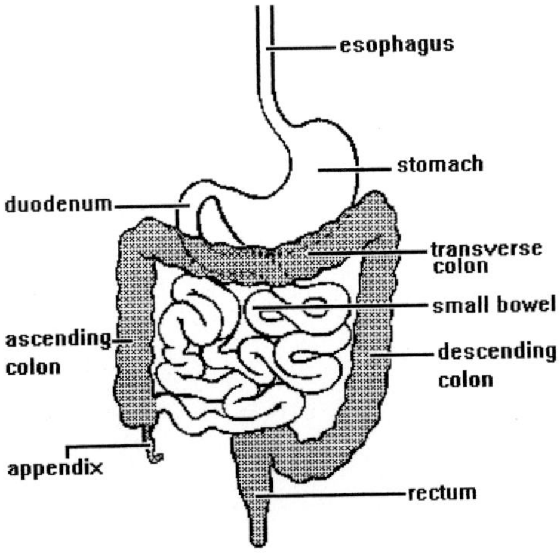 	First & Second Trimester -ill-defined area of increased echogenicity in mid to lower abdomen Large Bowel -long tubular hypoechoic structure located usually in periphery of abdomen -does not usually show peristalsis -enlarges progressively throughout pregnancy Small Bowel -more echogenic than large bowel until late 3rd trimester as with more swallowed amniotic fluid it can appear more sonolucent -appears more centrally in abdomen -can peristalsis	in this cross section of a 32-week abdomen, normal fetal bowel appears as a hypoechoic tubular structure around periphery of fetal abdomen 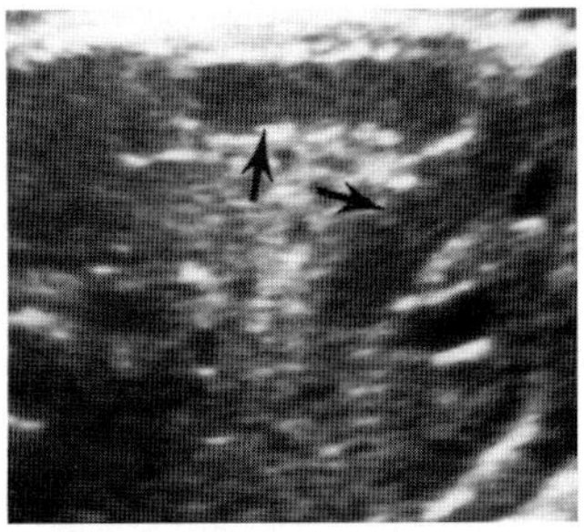 sagittal image of fetal abdomen with echogenic small bowel 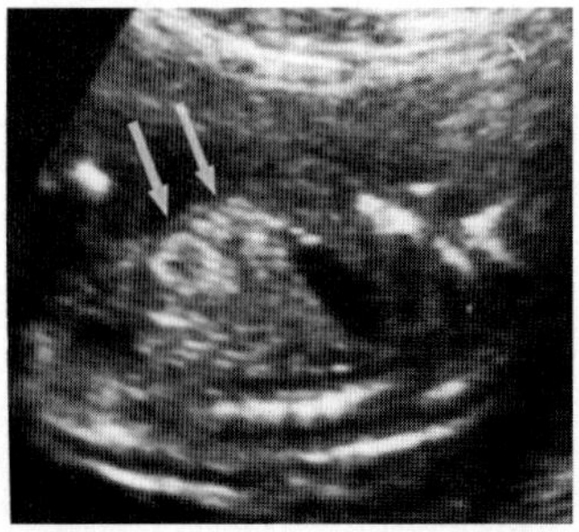

ANATOMY	US DESCRIPTIONS	US APPEARANCE
GALLBLADDER -forms at about 7 weeks -passive role in fetus	-visualized at about 20 weeks -small oval anechoic structure within liver -should be seen to the right of the portal/umbilical vein	transverse scan of fetal abdomen with gallbladder (arrow) 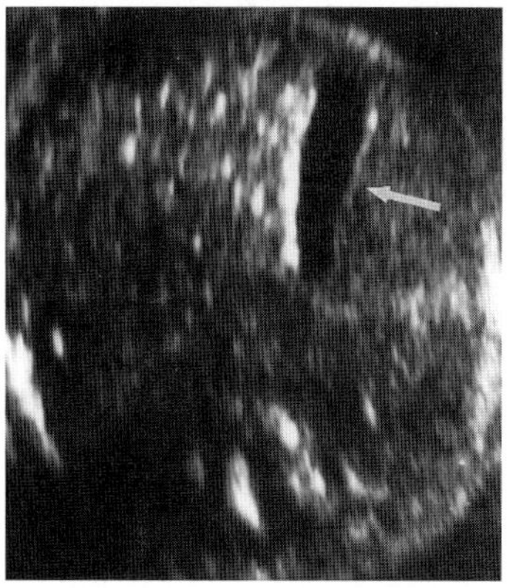
LIVER -proportionately larger in fetus than in child or adult -site of hematopoiesis by 8th week -bile formation begins at end of 1st trimester -hepatic vessels can be distinguished within -contributes to size of abdominal circumference (small in conjunction with IUGR, large with macrosomia)	2nd trimester: -large homogenous structure beneath diaphragm on right side of abdomen -margins are rarely distinct	transverse oblique scan through fetal abdomen showing hepatic veins within the echogenic liver (L) draining into IVC 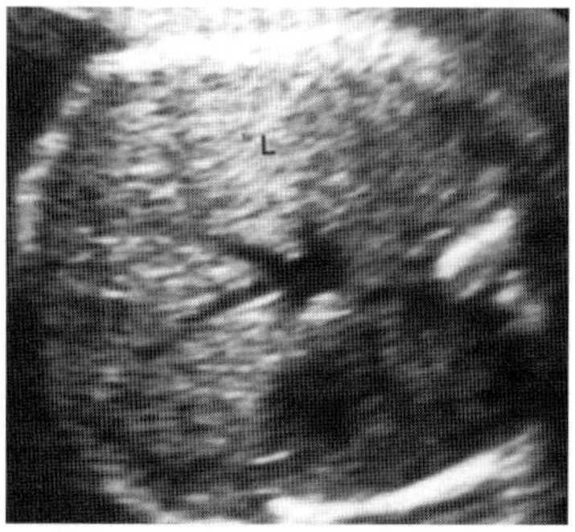
SPLEEN -increases in size during gestation -posterolateral to stomach -not usually part of routine obstetrical sonographic evaluation	-visualized between 18 and 40 weeks -homogenous structure beneath diaphragm on left side of abdomen -isoechoic to liver	transverse scan of fetal abdomen showing an ill-defined spleen in the left upper quadrant (arrow) 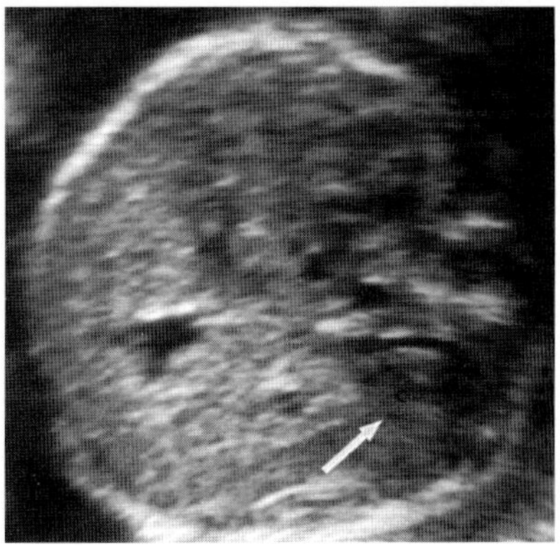

ANATOMY	US DESCRIPTIONS	US APPEARANCE
STOMACH -fetus begins to swallow amniotic fluid at about 16 weeks, therefore, should be seen routinely in all normal fetuses after 18 weeks -can be seen as early as 13 weeks -size varies depending on fluid recently swallowed	-fluid-filled stomach "bubble" is seen as an anechoic crescent-shaped structure in the left hemiabdomen	1st trimester fetal stomach (arrow) in left upper quadrant of abdomen 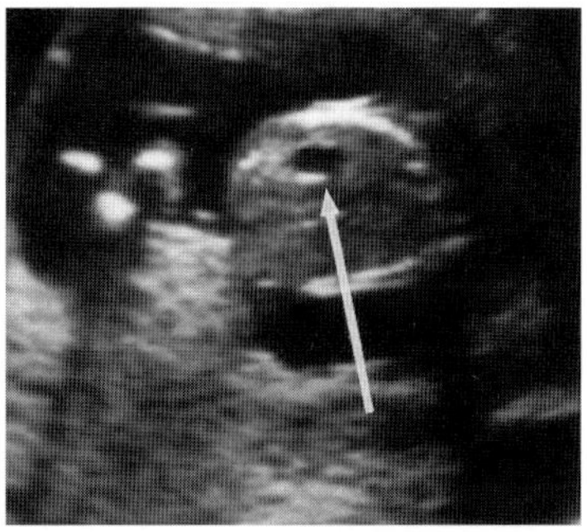 transverse 3rd trimester fetal abdomen showing stomach (S) in its normal position on the left 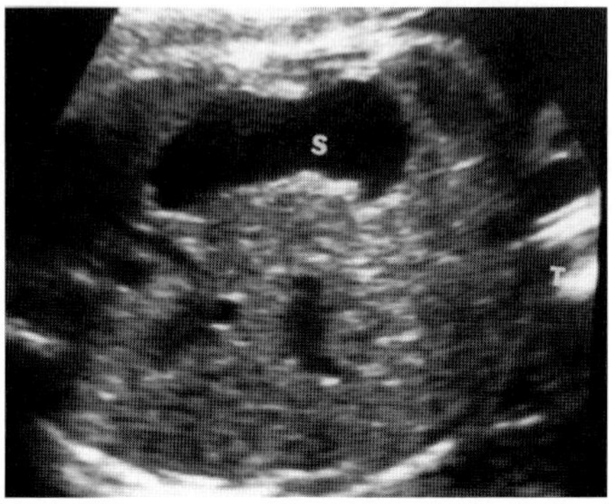

B) ABNORMAL DEVELOPMENT

ANOMALY	US FINDINGS	US APPEARANCE
ABDOMINAL CYSTS -differential includes ovarian cysts, enteric or duplication cysts, choledochal cysts, meconium pseudocysts and dilated bowel	-cystic mass located in abdomen of fetus	a scan of the lower abdomen of a female fetus shows a cystic mass, most likely an ovarian cyst (arrow) 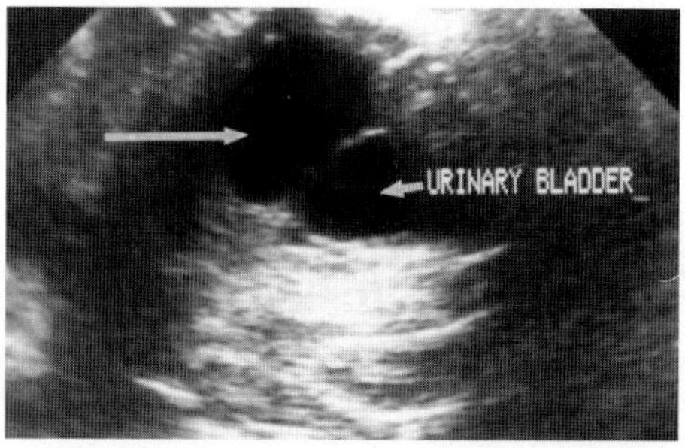

ANOMALY	US FINDINGS	US APPEARANCE
ASCITES & HYDROPS -true ascites is always abnormal -associated with hydrops fetalis, pleural effusions, pericardial effusions, bowel perforations, urinary tract rupture, glycogen storage disease Pitfall: Pseudo Ascites-abdominal musculature can appear as a thin hypoechoic rim along the anterior surface of the fetal abdomen, which must not be interpreted as fluid	-can outline ligaments -fluid seen in plural, pericardial, and peritoneal spaces	-peritonium and pleura are filled with fluid -fluid surrounds the abdominal organs, diaphragm, heart, lungs, and ligaments 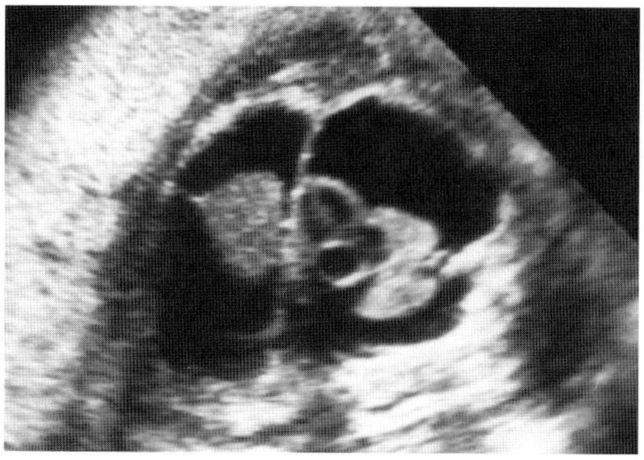 -huge amount of ascites filling fetal abdomen and surrounding liver 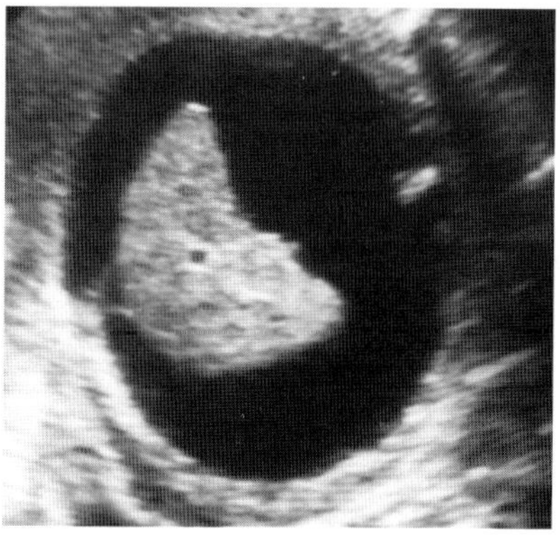
ATRESIA <u>Esophageal Atresia</u> -usually accompanied by a tracheo-esophageal (TE) fistula -associated with VACTERL and trisomies 18,21,13 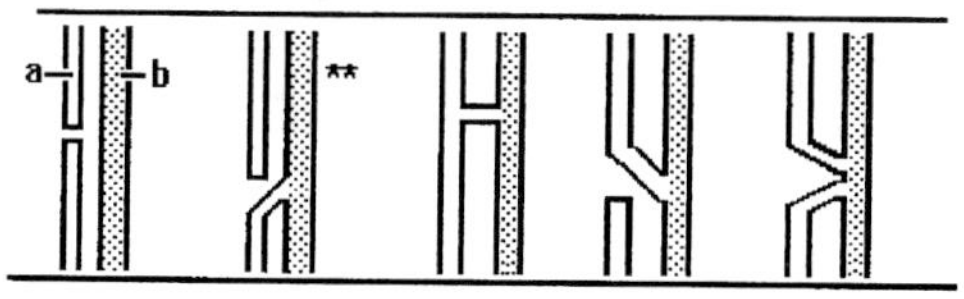 **Esophageal Atresia and Tracheoesophageal Fistula** **..type of a=esophagus b=trachea** **** = most common** <u>Duodenal Atresia</u> -results from failure of recanalization of duodenum -highly associated with other anomalies: trisomy 21, morphologic abnormalities, congenital heart disease <u>Jejunal-Ileal Atresia</u> -etiology thought to be sporadic, therefore not concurrent with other anomalies	<u>Duodenal Atresia</u> -"double bubble sign": distended stomach and proximal duodenum -polyhydramnios -I.U.G.R. -seen usually after 24 weeks <u>Esophageal Atresia</u>: -absence of fluid-filled stomach as fetus cannot swallow amniotic fluid -polyhydramnios -small abdomen circumference with fistula -stomach bubble can be seen <u>Jejunal-Ileal Atresia</u> -a triple or quadruple "bubble" sign may be visualized which is a cross-section cut through several dilated loops of bowel	transverse scan demonstrates characteristic "double bubble" with fluid-filled stomach (S) and dilated duodenum (D) (**) 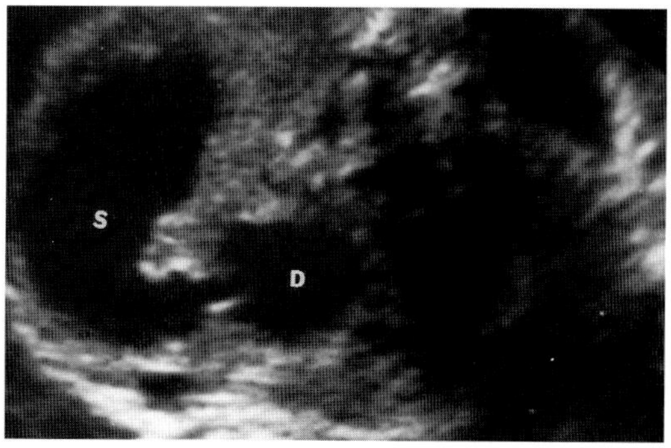

ANOMALY	US DESCRIPTION	US APPEARANCE
BOWEL OBSTRUCTION -may be caused by stenosis, volvulus, enteric duplication, meconium ileus, Hirschsprung disease MECONIUM ILEUS -form of small bowel obstruction that results from meconium impacted in distal ileum -associated with cystic fibrosis	-small bowel dilatation proximal to site of obstruction -multiple distended bowel loops -polyhydramnios (not seen in distal intestinal obstruction) Meconium Ileus: -hyperechoic intraluminal meconium -dilated ileum, microcolon	meconium peritonitis: an image of the abdomen at 29 weeks shows a single loop of abnormal dilated bowel (arrows) with volvulus 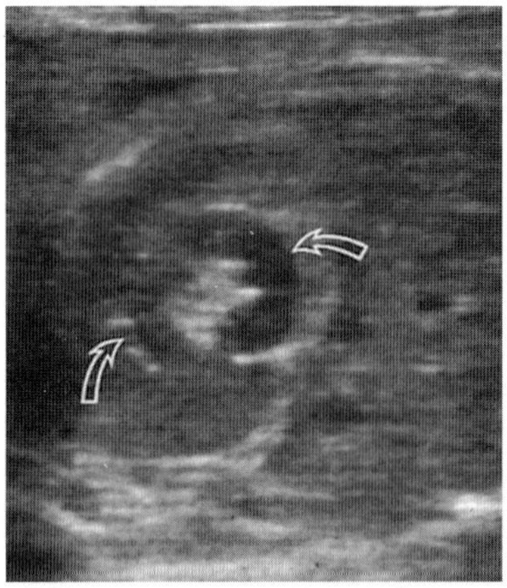 an image of the abdomen at 30 weeks shows the same loop of abnormally dilated bowel (arrow) and some mild ascites (A), liver (Li) 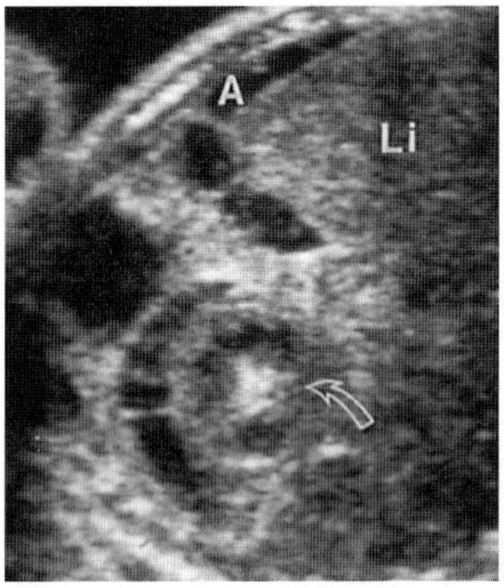
GALLSTONES -most likely an incidental finding as no clinical significance has been correlated to fetal "gallstones" -unknown etiology	-tiny echogenic foci/focus within gallbladder	multiple tiny echogenic foci fill the gallbladder on this transverse scan of a fetal abdomen (**) 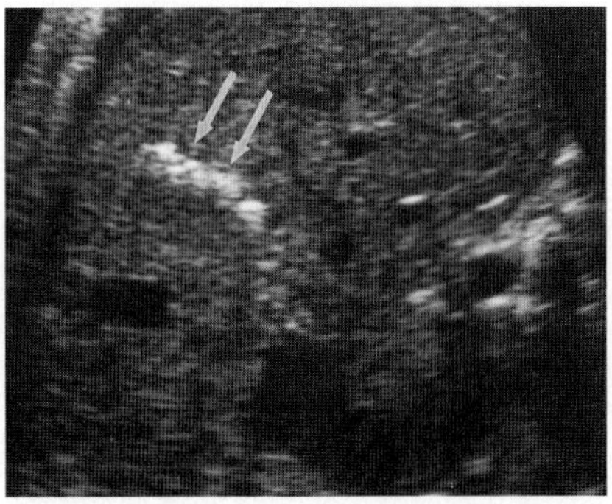

<table>
<tr><th>ANOMALY</th><th>US DESCRIPTION</th><th>US APPEARANCE</th></tr>
<tr>
<td>

GASTROSCHISIS

-anterior abdominal wall defect where fetal viscera protrude through a paraumbilical defect to the right of a normal closed umbilical ring
-not diagnosed until after 14 weeks when bowel loops can be expected to have re-entered abdominal cavity from their normal physiological herniation
-elevated maternal serum alphafetoprotein
-not usually associated with anomalies, therefore, survival rate is good, approaching 100% in tertiary care hospitals

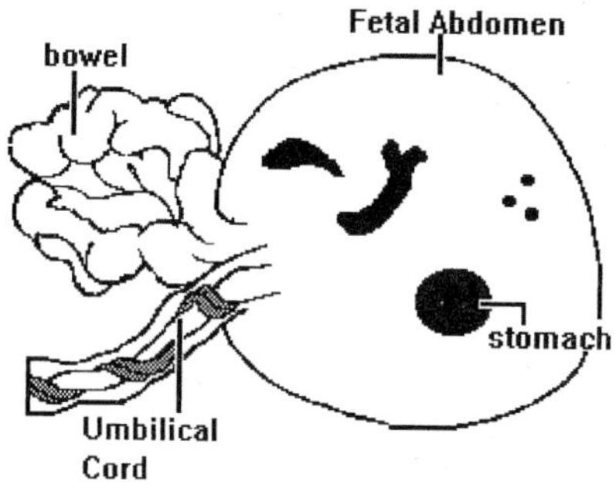

</td>
<td>

-multiple loops of small and large bowel floating freely in amniotic fluid with no covering membrane
-"ragged" edge to mass
-occasionally other organs such as stomach and rarely liver may also herniate
-normal insertion of umbilical cord to the left of mass
-stomach and bladder close together due to absence of abdominal contents
-polyhydramnios

</td>
<td>

sagittal scan through anterior abdomen shows mass of bowel (B) projecting into amniotic fluid

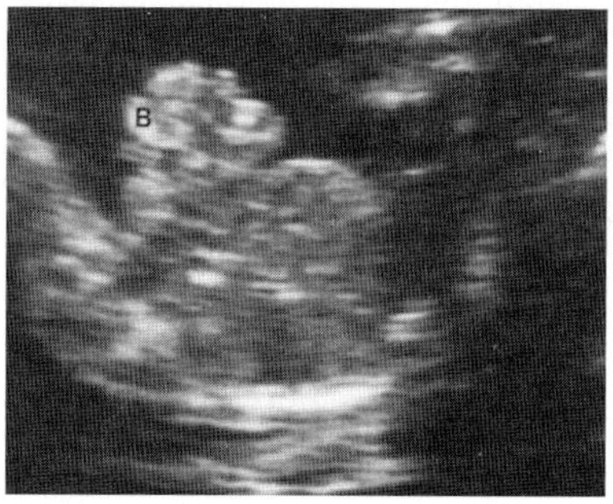

transverse scan through fetal abdomen shows bowel (short arrows) eviscerated through a defect to the right of the umbilical cord (long arrows)

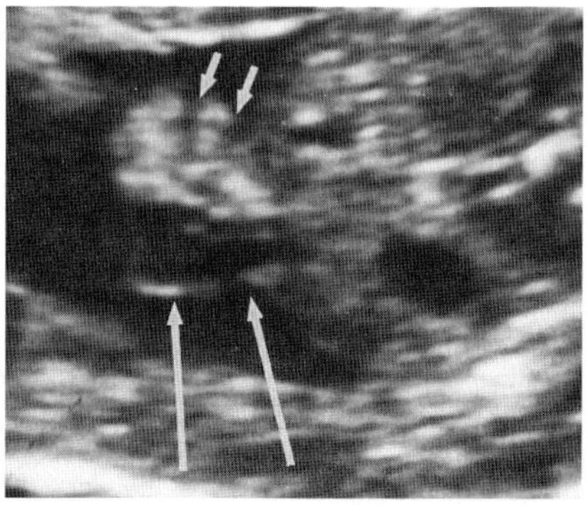

bowel loops floating freely in the amniotic fluid at about 34 weeks

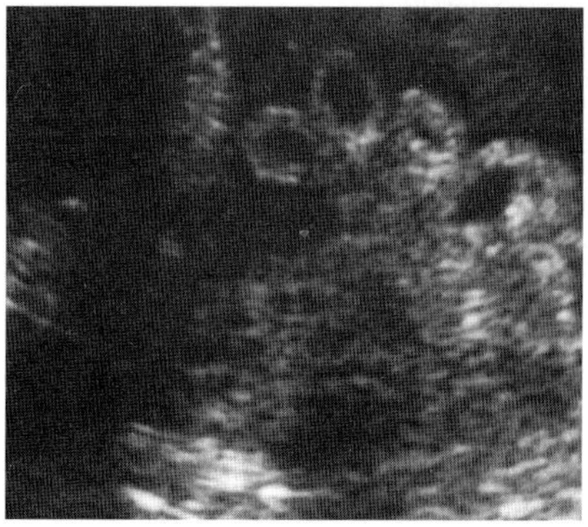

</td>
</tr>
</table>

ANOMALY	US DESCRIPTION	US APPEARANCE
OMPHALOCELE -anterior abdominal wall defect where abdominal contents herniate into base of umbilical cord -also described as malformation of umbilical cord where intestinal contents extrude through the umbilical ring -elevated maternal serum AFP -not diagnosed until after 14 weeks when bowel loops can be expected to have re-entered abdominal cavity from their normal physiological herniation -highly associated with anomalies trisomies 13, 18, 21, Turners, Kleinfelter Syndrome, Pentalogy of Cantrell, Cloacal Exstrophy, Beckwith Widermann Syndrome -outcome related to associated anomalies 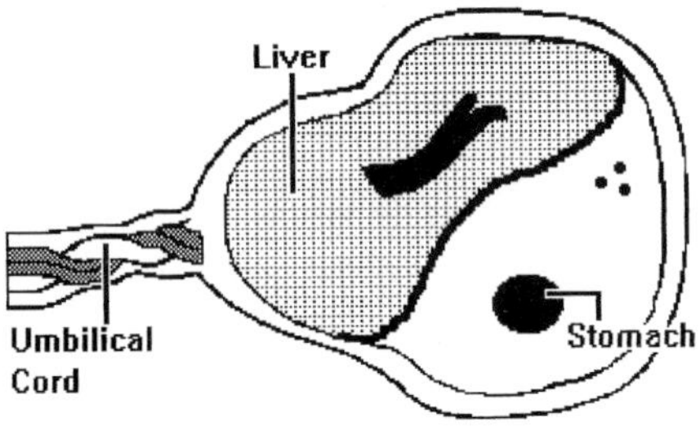 	-anterior midline mass with covering membrane -herniation of abdominal viscera at base of cord (can contain liver, bowel and/or stomach) -chromosomal abnormalities are more likely when only bowel seen in omphalocele sac -umbilical cord enters mass/defect -umbilical vein within mass -fetal ascites	scans in longitudinal plane show large omphalocele which contains liver with covering membrane (arrow) 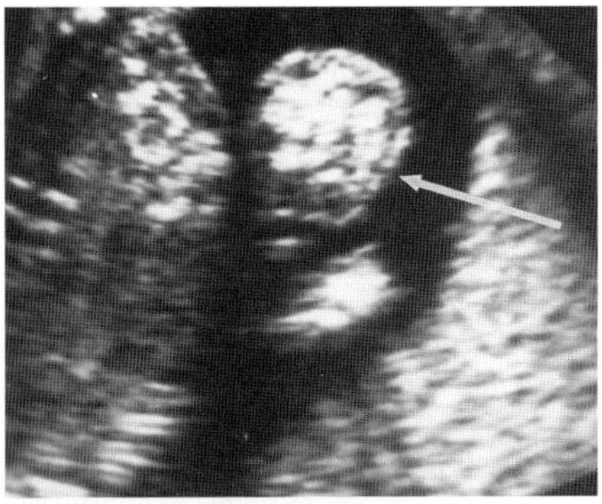 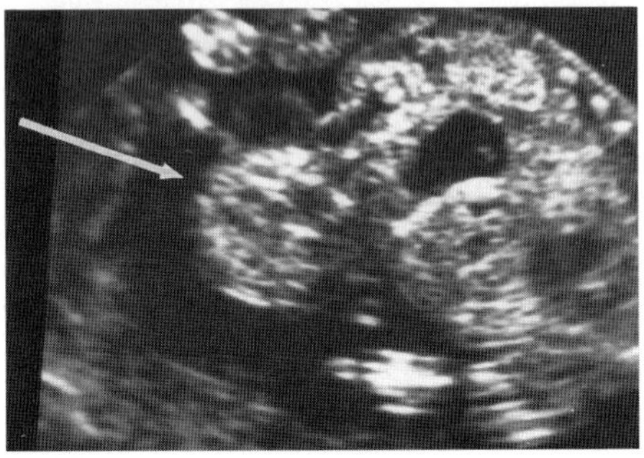

COMPARISON OF GASTROSCHISIS AND OMPHALOCELE CHARACTERISTICS	
GASTROSCHISIS	OMPHALOCELE
-**no** membrane covering mass -cord inserts on abdominal wall -bowel herniates, but stomach can also herniate -no association with other defects	-membrane covering mass -cord inserts onto membrane -liver usually herniates, but bowel and stomach can as well -high association with other congenital anomalies

SONOGRAPHIC EVALUATION OF FETAL DIGESTIVE SYSTEM

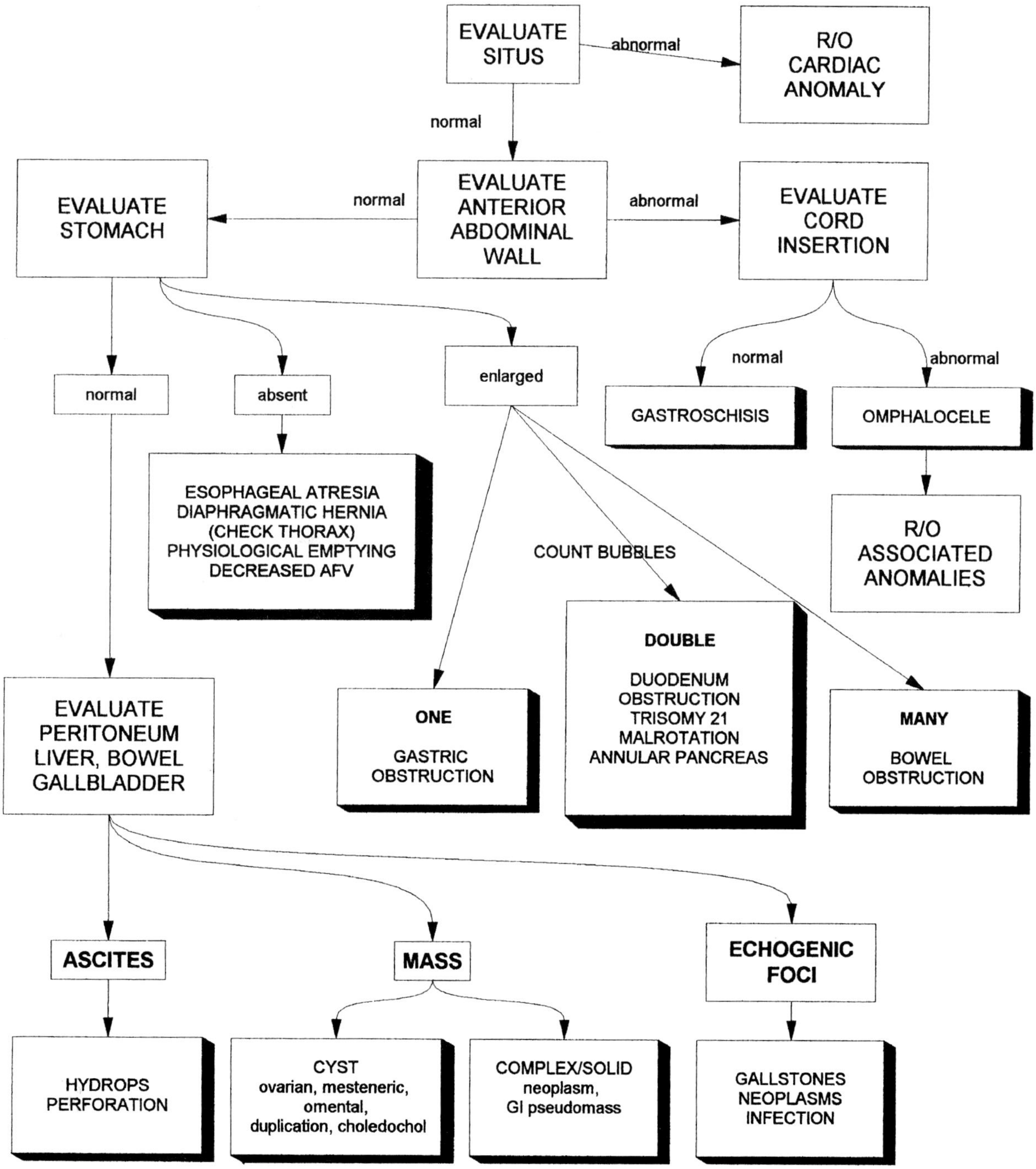

A) NORMAL ANATOMY AND DEVELOPMENT

DEVELOPMENT OF G.U. TRACT	
7 weeks	-kidneys begin to develop
8 weeks	-bladder forms from cloaca and ureters open into bladder
10 weeks	-kidneys ascended to permanent position
11 weeks	-kidneys begin to form urine, but not major source until 14-16 weeks -external genitalia begins to differentiate
12 weeks	-urinary bladder is completely developed
14 weeks	-external genitalia are fully formed
28-30 weeks	-testes begin to descend
32-34 weeks	-testes enter scrotal sac

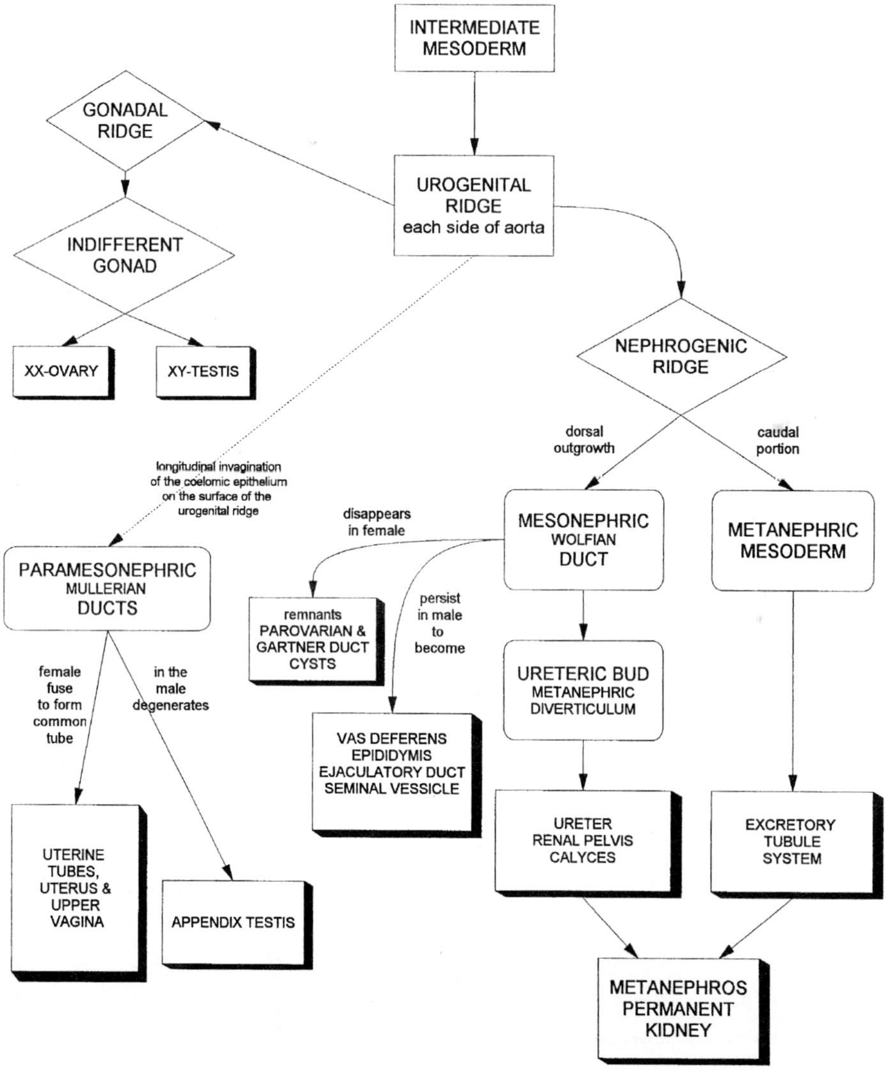

DEVELOPMENT OF THE GENITOURINARY SYSTEM

ANATOMY	US FINDING	US APPEARANCE
KIDNEYS -develop in pelvis and gradually migrate upward into the retroperitoneal space of abdomen -produce amniotic fluid which permits normal lung development -size is function of gestational age -ratio kidney circumference : abdominal circumference = 0.27– 0.30 URETERS -not routinely identified and visualization should suggest pathologic process -dilated ureters are identified but must be differentiated between other abdominal structures such as the psoas muscle or vessels NORMAL URINARY TRACT Male: 1. KIDNEY 2. RENAL PELVIS 3. URETER 4. BLADDER A. TRIGONE OF BLADDER 5. PROSTATE 6. URETHRA 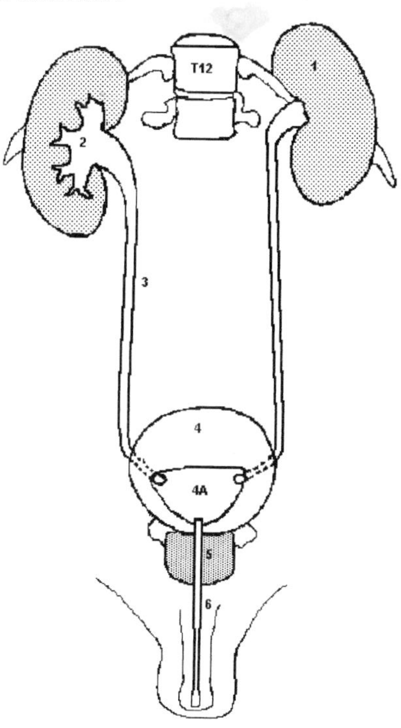	-longitudinal: elliptical shape -transverse: circular shape -hypoechoic medullary pyramids -echogenic renal cortex -kidneys can be seen at 14 weeks (TA) 12 weeks (TV) and should be seen routinely by 20 weeks in their paraspinous position	transverse scan of the posterior 3rd trimester fetal abdomen shows the right and left kidneys on either side of the fetal spine (S) 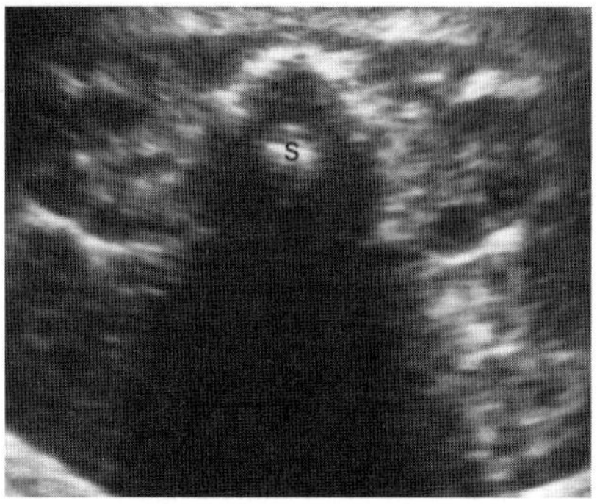 longitudinal scan shows the reniform normal shape of a fetal kidney 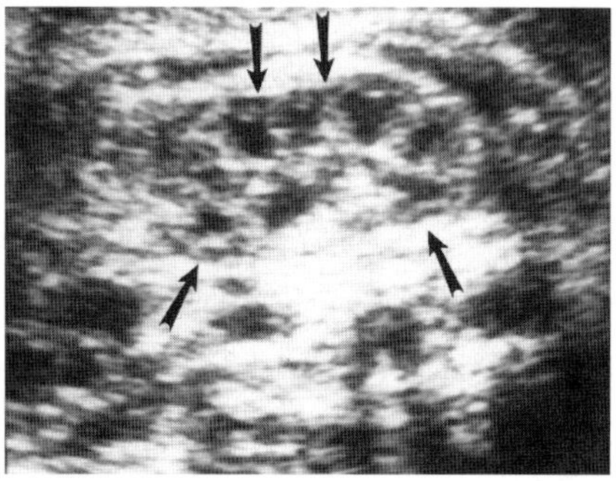 longitudinal view of fetal abdomen shows the left kidney (arrows) lying below fetal stomach (S) 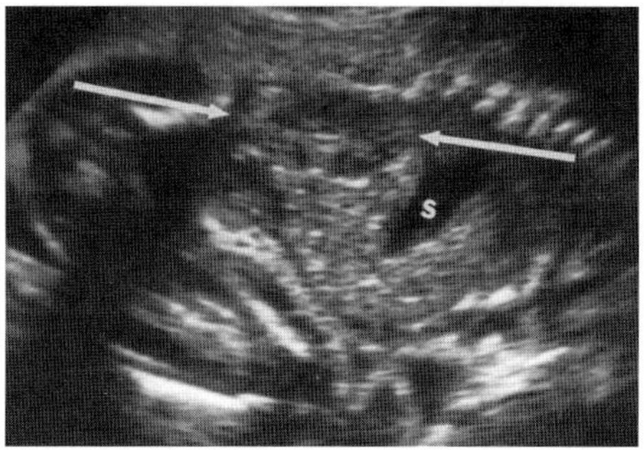

ANATOMY	US DESCRIPTION	US APPEARANCE
REPRODUCTIVE TRACT -fetal gender can be determined as early as 16 weeks -identification accuracy varies according to gestational age, fetal position -can be seen in early second trimester -usually not of clinical significance -exceptions: monozygotic twinning, urinary tract obstruction, x-linked disorders (eg. Turners syndrome)	<u>Male</u> -sex is confirmed by depiction of penis, scrotum and testicles -testes can be visualized after they have descended into scrotum in early 3rd trimester -prostate not seen	a transverse scan shows the scrotum and penis between the legs of a male fetus 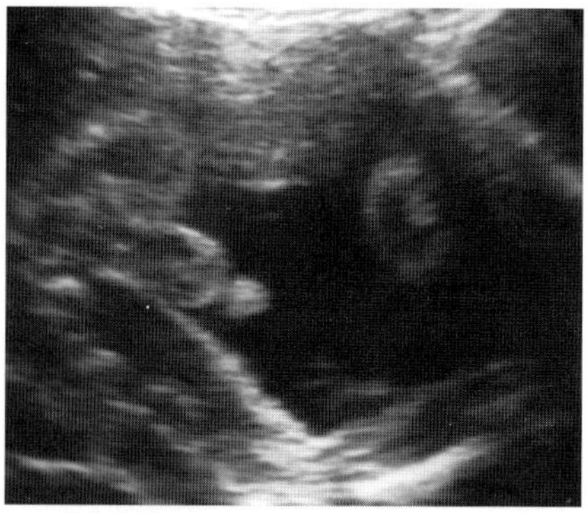 cross-section of scrotum shows teste (T) with a normal amount of fluid surrounding it 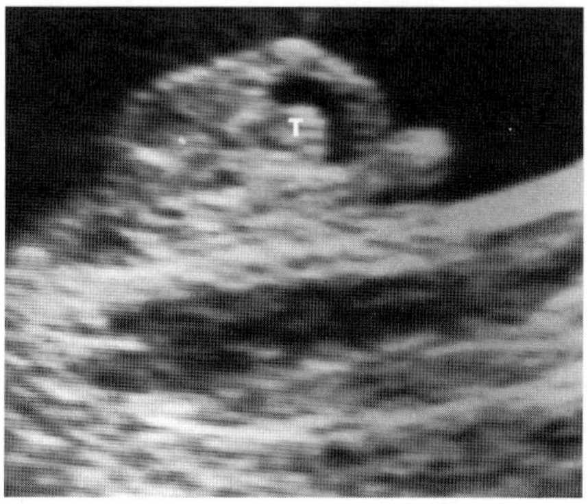
	<u>Female</u> -gender is confirmed by depiction of labia -uterus, vagina and ovaries not routinely visualized	at 30 weeks, a transverse scan of female genitalia shows the labia major (arrows) 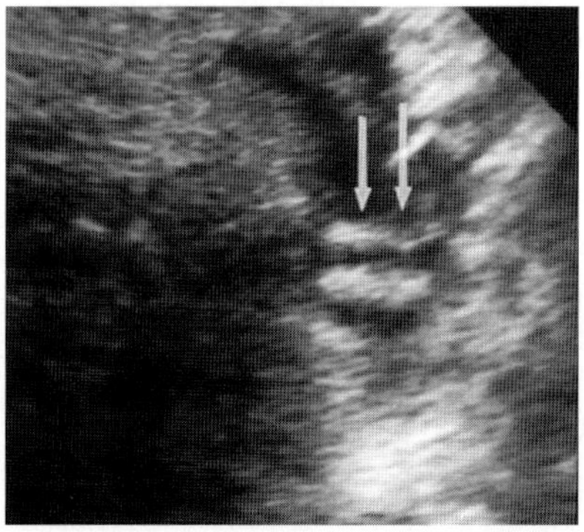

ANATOMY	US DESCRIPTION	US APPEARANCE
URINARY BLADDER -fills and empties every 30–45 minutes, therefore, during sonographic evaluation its volume will vary -seen routinely after 14 weeks (should be observed by 16 weeks in a 60-minute observation period)	-thin-walled anechoic structure in pelvis that varies in size -spherical or elliptical when distended -internal iliac arteries course around lateral margins of bladder	transvaginal scan of 11-week fetal bladder (BL) 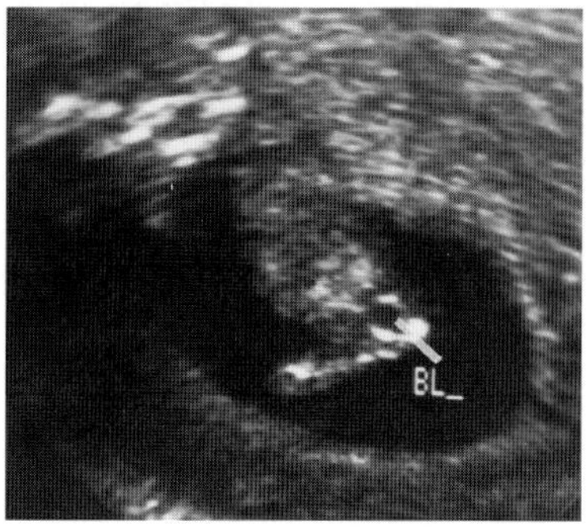 transverse scan of pelvis shows fluid-filled-urinary bladder (B); note iliac arteries (A) adjacent to side walls of bladder 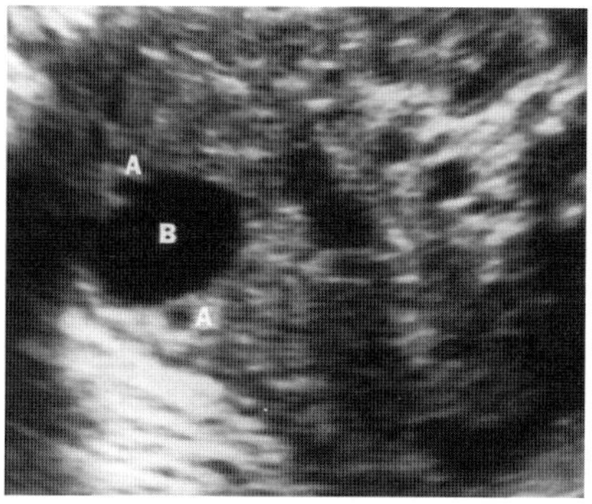

B) ABNORMAL DEVELOPMENT

<table>
<tr><th>ANOMALY</th><th>US FINDINGS</th><th>US APPEARANCE</th></tr>
<tr>
<td>
ABNORMAL POSITION or SHAPE

Crossed Fused Ectopic
-may mimic unilateral agenesis

Duplication of Collecting System
-occurs in up to 4% of population and is the most common major GU anomaly
-ureteroceles are associated with duplication of ureters

Horseshoe Kidney
-fusion of upper or lower poles
-kidneys may be malrotated

Pelvic Kidney
-may mimic unilateral ageneis but kidney found adjacent to bladder
-can be associated with other anomalies

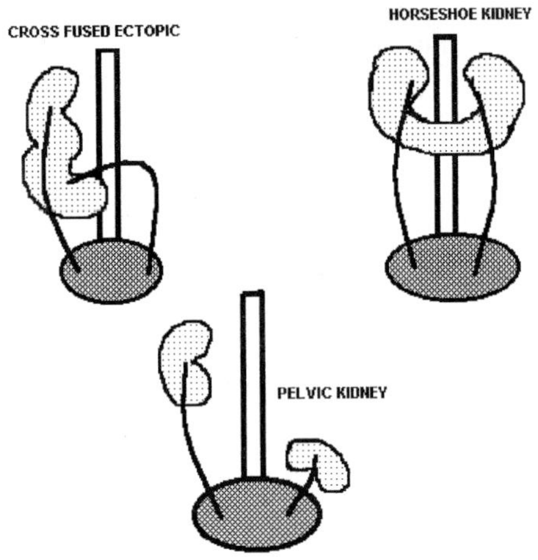

</td>
<td>
-a kidney that is not present in its usual position in the renal fossa
-kidney may have abnormal shape and size
</td>
<td>
horseshoe kidney: a transverse scan at the level of the kidneys shows a band of renal tissue (arrows) across the abdomen representing a horseshoe kidney (the kidney on the fetal side down is partially obscured by the spine)

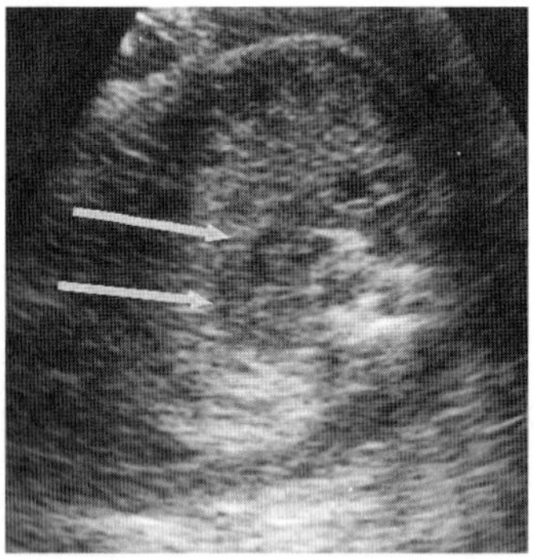

double collecting system: longitudinal kidney (between calipers) of 28-week fetus measured 50 mm. in length and demonstrates 2 prominent renal pelves

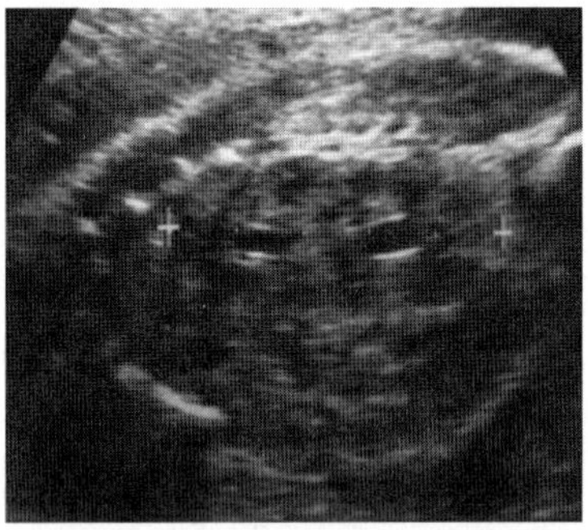

longitudinal scan of a kidney with a duplicated collecting system and dilated ureter (U) associated with an ureterocele (**)

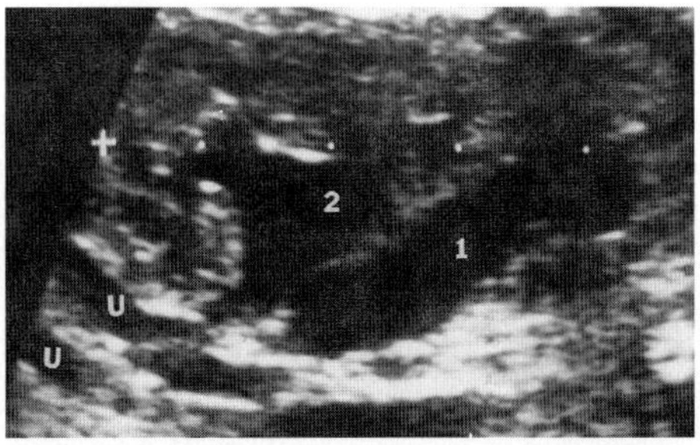

</td>
</tr>
</table>

ANOMALY	US DESCRIPTION	US APPEARANCE
CYSTIC KIDNEYS Adult Polycystic Kidney Disease-APKD(Potter type III) -autosomal dominant of 100% penetrance but variable expression—usually in adult life -rare event in utero	APKD -large echogenic kidneys -with or without resolvable cysts	IPKD: sagittal scan of a neonatal, shows IPKD (kidney beneath liver) 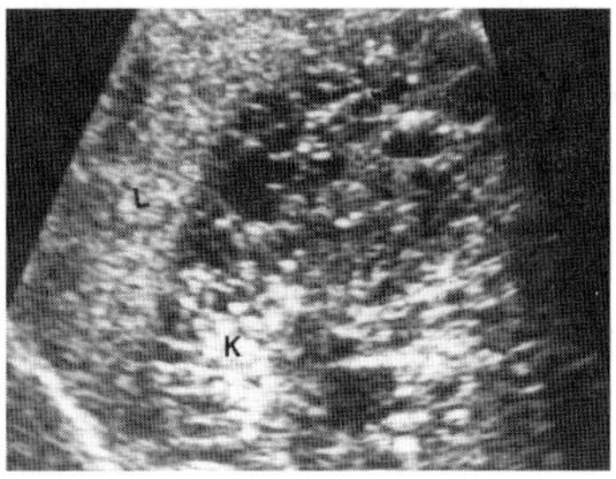
Infantile Polycystic Kidney Disease-IPKD (Potter type I) -autosomal recessive -bilateral -collecting tubes filled with multiple tiny 1–2 mm cysts -variable degree of genetic expression -massive nephromegaly and oligohydramnios -is lethal from pulmonary hypoplasia	IPKD -bilateral, enlarged, reniform shaped hyperechogenic kidneys -cysts tend not to be resolved with ultrasound -oligohydramnios	MCDK: transverse scan of kidneys with multiple cysts of varying size 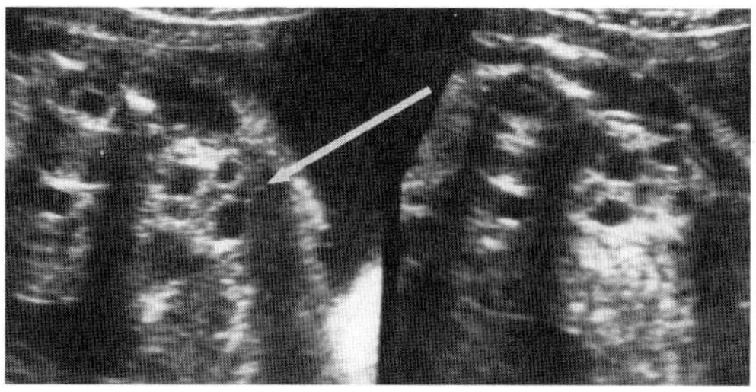
Multicystic Dysplastic Kidney Disease -MCDK (Potter type II) -uni (75%) or bilateral -may be some renal function but usually not -bilateral it is a lethal anomaly -males affected more often than females -associated with contra lateral UPJ obstruction	MCDK -large kidney -multiple noncommunicating cystic structures of varying size -no recognizable renal parenchyma -reniform shape is lost -severe oligohydramnios if bilateral	MCDK: in some incidences can give similar appearance to hydronephrosis 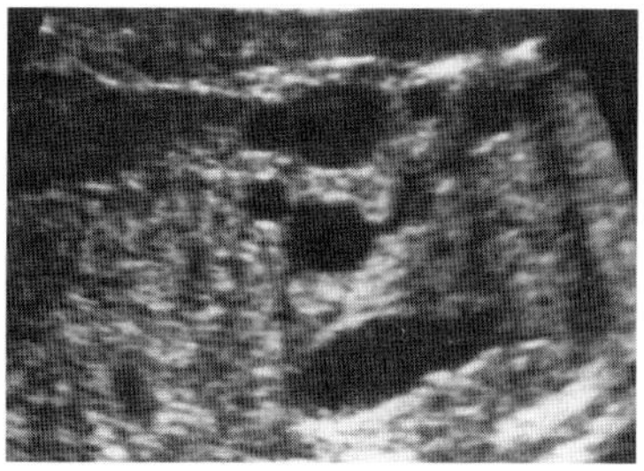
Obstructive Uropathy Causing Renal Cystic Dysplasia (Potter type IV) -associated with urethral level obstruction ASSOCIATED DISORDERS WITH CYSTIC DISEASE: Meckel–Gruber Syndrome, Trisomy 13, Trisomy 18	Potter type IV -hyperechogenic kidneys with or without visible cysts	renal cystic dysplasia: transverse fetal abdomen of an echogenic fetal kidney (between arrows) with a couple of larger cysts (Potter IV) 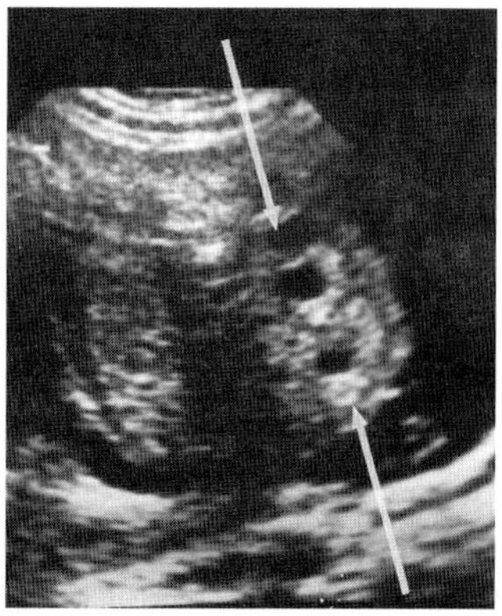

<table>
<tr><th>ANOMALY</th><th>US DESCRIPTION</th><th>US APPEARANCE</th></tr>
<tr><td>HYDROCELE
-excessive accumulation of fluid in the tunica vaginalis due to overproduction or mechanical obstruction
-can be a normal variant or a sign of physiological abnormalities
-no pathologic significance of isolated hydrocele in fetus</td><td>-excessive fluid in scrotal sac surrounds entire testicle</td><td>scan of male genitalia shows fluid within the scrotal sac surrounding each testicle (T)
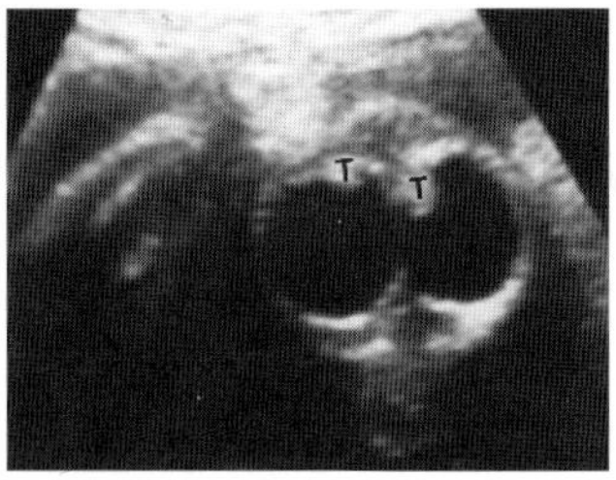</td></tr>
<tr><td>HYDRONEPHROSIS
-mild fetal pyelectasis is not uncommon
-hydronephrosis is the most common fetal renal anomaly

neonatal follow-up when:
renal pelvis AP diameter is:
1. > 1 cm
2. > 50% of corresponding AP diameter of kidney
3. calyces become visible

appearances depend on level of obstruction:
1. UPJ - obstruction at renal pelvis–ureter junction
2. UVJ - obstruction at level of ureter insertion into bladder</td><td><u>UPJ obstruction</u>
-usually mild and unilateral renal pelvis dilation
-normal ureter and bladder

<u>UVJ obstruction</u>
-can be associated with a duplex renal collecting system
-with a duplex system there can be an ectopic urterocele where the duplex ureter inserts into bladder
-this can result in secondary hydronephrosis and secondary dilation of upper collecting system</td><td>transverse scan through a kidney shows a normal mild pyelectasis (arrow)
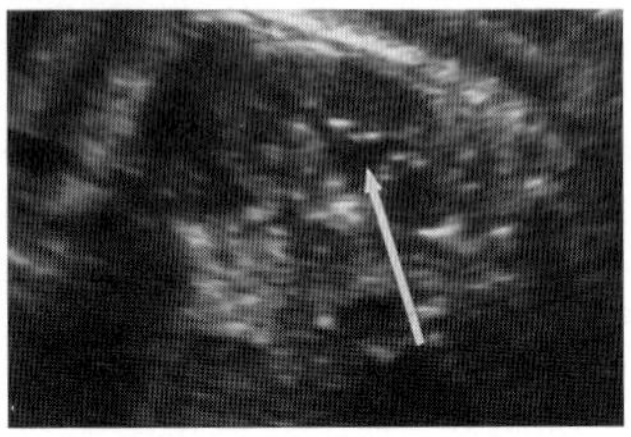
bilateral mild hydronephrosis in 24-week fetus (arrows)
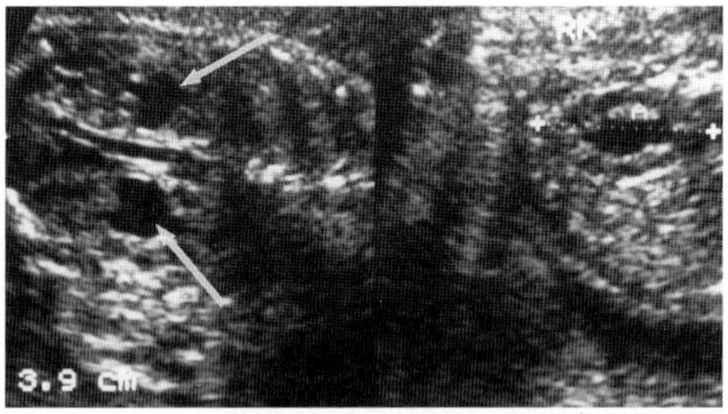
longitudinal scan through a fetal kidney shows a moderate amount of hydronephrosis present (arrow)
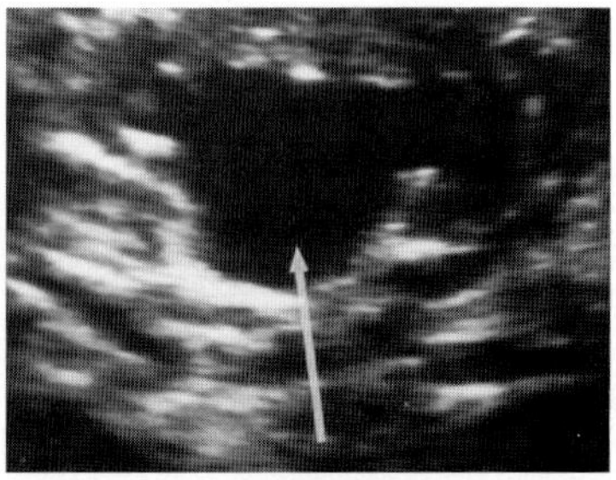</td></tr>
</table>

ANOMALY	US DESCRIPTION	US APPEARANCE
HYDRONEPHROSIS contd.		longitudinal scan of kidney with massive hydronephrosis that is obscuring normal renal parenchyma; dilated convoluted proximal ureter (U) 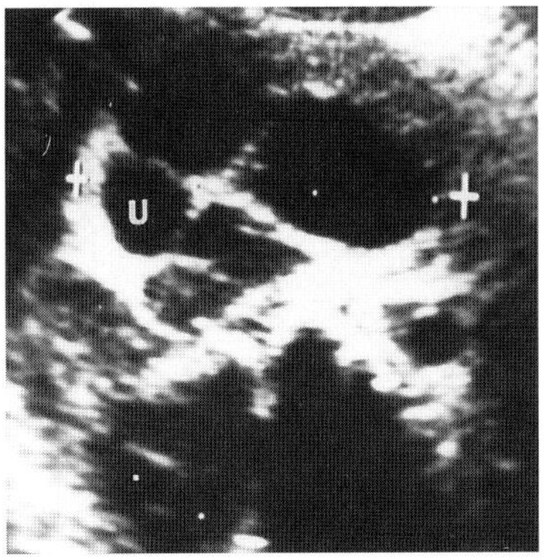
RENAL AGENESIS <u>Bilateral</u> -congenital absence of both kidneys -lethal anomaly resulting from pulmonary hypoplasia <u>Potters Syndrome</u> -renal agenesis, plus facial deformity, limb contractures, pulmonary hypoplasia <u>Unilateral Renal Agenesis</u> -more common than bilateral -contralateral kidney can be enlarged due to compensatory hypertrophy	<u>Bilateral</u> -severe oligohydramnios (hinders visualization) -failure to see kidneys (adrenal glands must not be mistaken for kidneys) -persistent non-visualization of fetal bladder <u>Unilateral</u> -normal amount of amniotic fluid, and bladder seen	coronal scan of the fetal abdomen shows no kidneys in the renal fossi and severe oligohydramnios 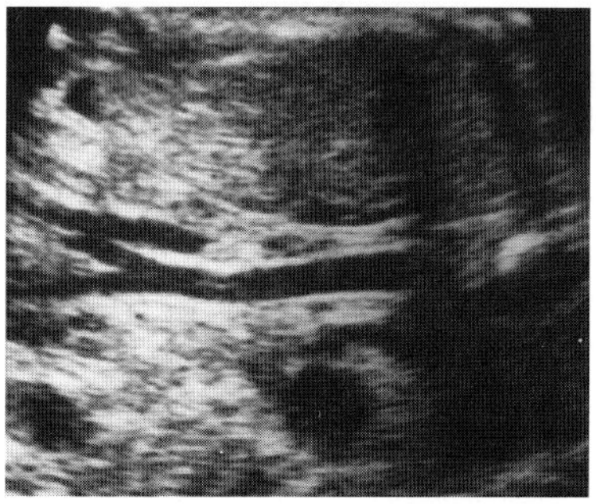
URETHRAL LEVEL (BLADDER OUTLET) OBSTRUCTION <u>Posterior Urethral Valves</u> -bladder outlet obstruction in males -formation of rudimentary valves (membranous flaps) in region of posterior urethra <u>Other Causes</u> -urethral atresia or stricture -cloacal persistence -caudal regression anomaly -megacystis-intestinal hypoperistalsis syndrome	-bilateral hydronephrosis -bilateral hydroureter -thick walled dilated bladder that fills pelvis and does not empty (may decompress with rupture) -distended proximal urethra -"key hole" defect -oligohydramnios <u>Prune Belly Syndrome</u> triad of anomalies: 1. bladder outlet obstruction 2. abdominal wall laxity 3. cryptorchidism in males	fetal kidney shows a dilated ureter (U) and gross hydronephrosis (**) 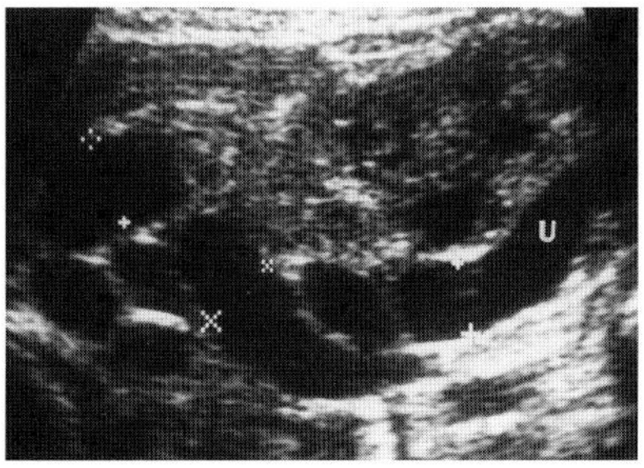 coronal scan of a male fetus shows a dilated urinary bladder (B) with a thickened wall and a dilated posterior urethra (UR) giving a "key hole" appearance; both dilated ureters (U) are seen in cross section adjacent to the bladder (**) 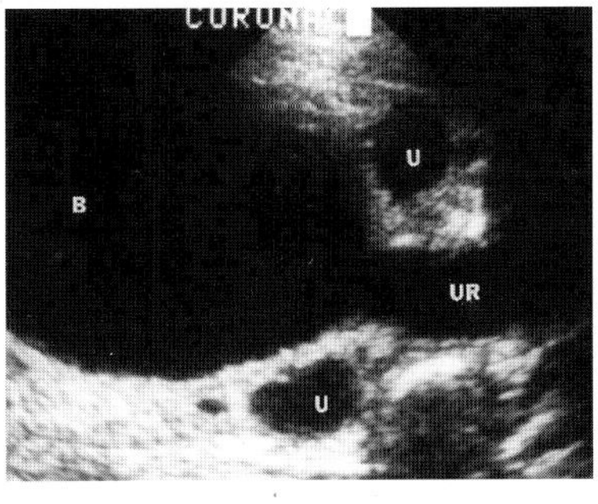

ANOMALY	US DESCRIPTION	US APPEARANCE
URETEROCELE -a cystic-like dilatation of the distal ureter into the bladder -associated with duplication of the renal collecting system -can be ectopic (ureter inserts into bladder in abnormal location)	-thin walled cyst is present at the site of entry of a duplicated ureter into the bladder	sagittal scan of the urinary bladder shows an associated thin walled cystic (arrow) which represents the site of entry of a dilated duplicated ureter 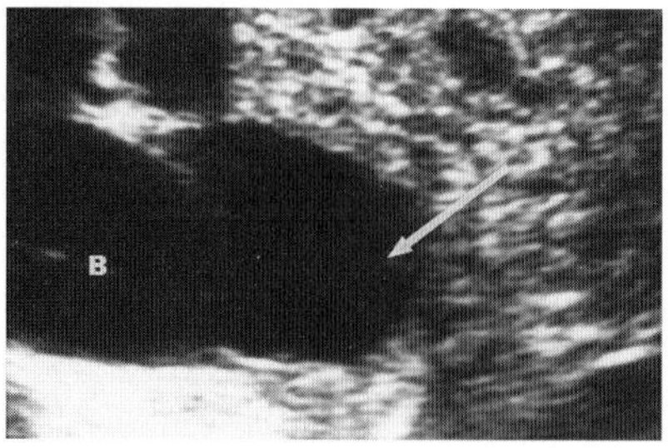

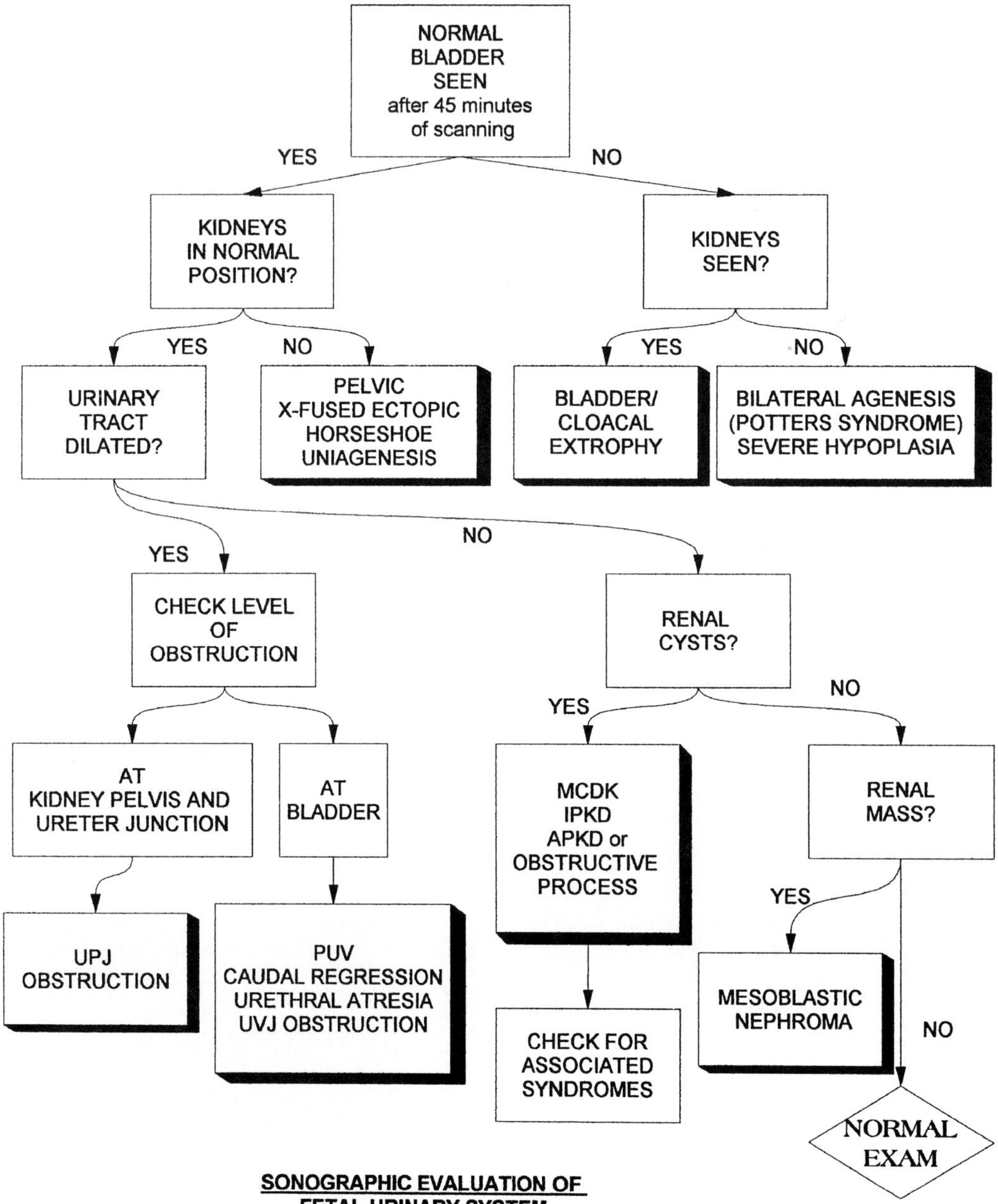

SONOGRAPHIC EVALUATION OF FETAL URINARY SYSTEM

SECTION 3. HEAD (CRANIUM AND FACE) AND NECK

A) NORMAL ANATOMY AND DEVELOPMENT

DEVELOPMENT OF FETAL BRAIN	
5 weeks	-neurulation begins: formation of neural plate and its closure to form neural tube
6 weeks	-neural tube closed and main divisions of CNS are formed: prosencephalon, mesencephalon, rhombencephalon
7 weeks	-prosencephalon divides into telencephalon and diencephalon and rhombencephalon divides into metencephalon and myelencephalon -CNS seen as a single ventricle
8 weeks	-falx grows into single ventricle -choroid plexus begins to form in entire ventricular system except aqueduct and frontal and occipital horns
10 weeks	-interhemispheric fissure separates cerebral hemispheres
11 weeks	-choroid plexus fills most of lateral ventricles
12 weeks	-extraventricular development of cerebellum begins -following structures are present: cerebral hemispheres, thalami, midbrain, cerebellum, ventricles, medulla oblongata and pons
13 weeks	-corpus callosum is developed

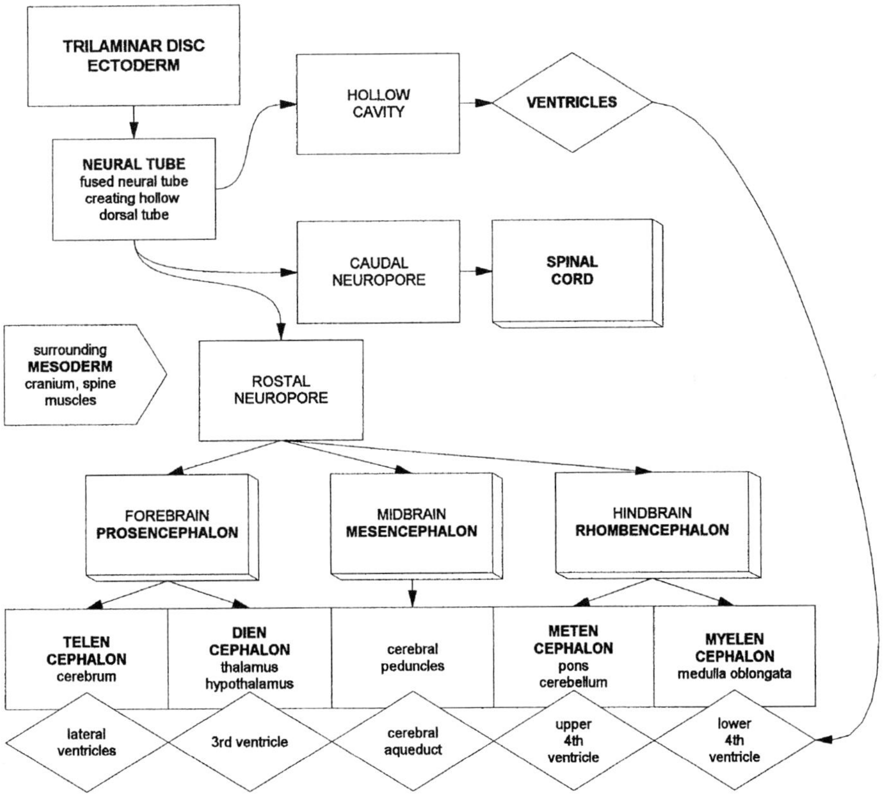

DEVELOPMENT OF FETAL NEURAL SYSTEM

DEVELOPMENT OF FETAL FACE	
6 weeks	mandible form and eyes, inner ears and nose begin to develop
7 weeks	lips fuse and achieve final shape
8 weeks	external ear begins to develop
10-11weeks	features of fetal face start to be seen on sonographically - orbits
13 weeks	fetal profile seen
14 weeks	fusion of palate is complete

coronal scan of 10–week fetal face

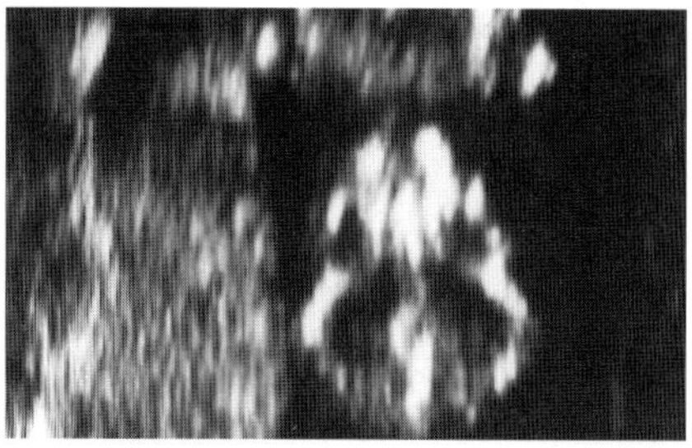

profile of 3rd trimester fetal face

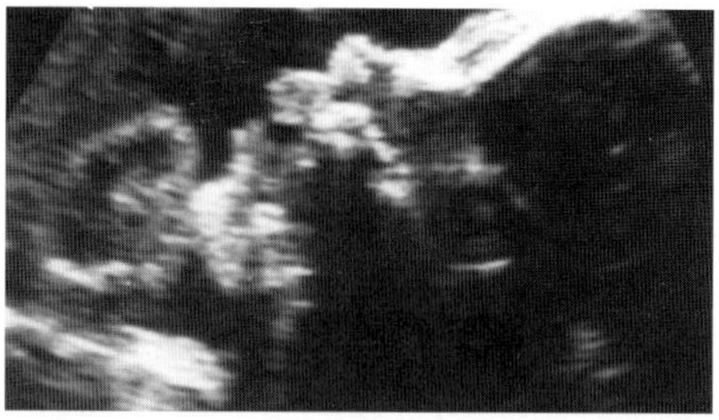

coronal scan of fetal face

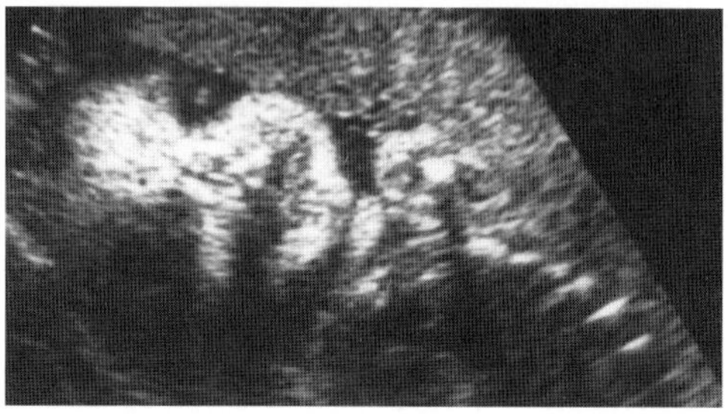

coronal scan of 3rd trimester fetal nose, cheeks, chin and lips

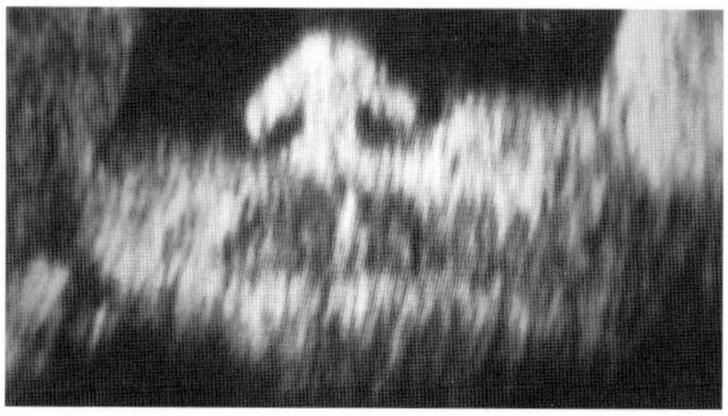

tongue (arrow) seen on fetal profile

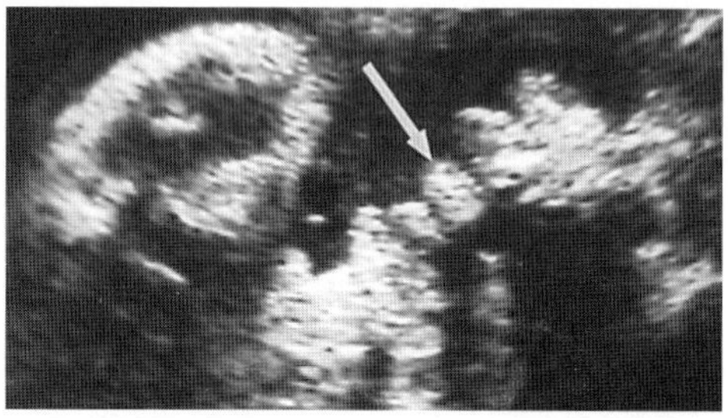

lens of eye (arrow)

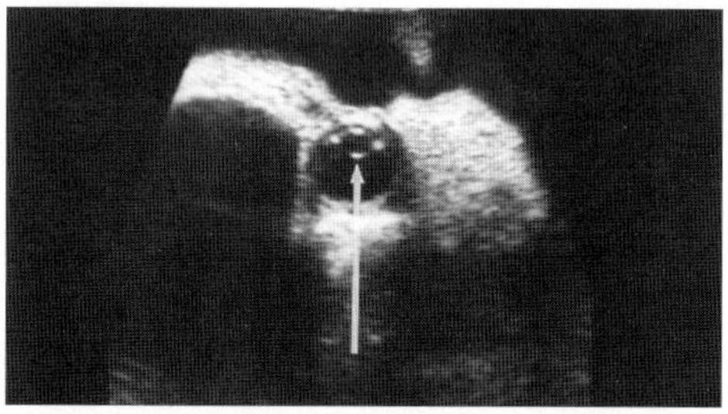

ear

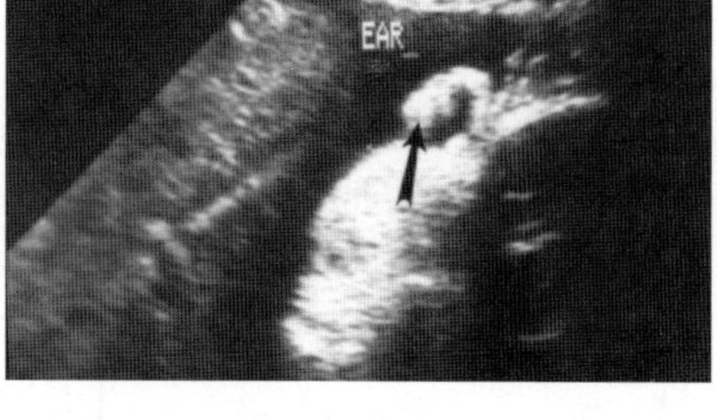

hair (arrows-outer layer), skin (middle), skull (inner echogenic layer)

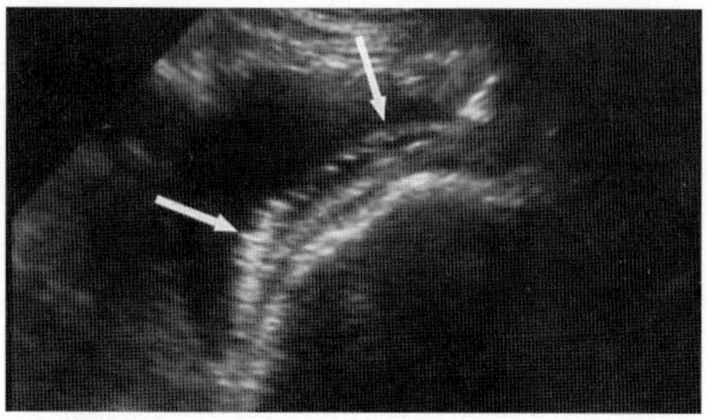

VENTRICULAR SYSTEM OF BRAIN	
VENTRICLES	-spaces lying within brain formed from the canal of the embryonic brain tube -assist in protecting the central nervous system -contain cerebrospinal fluid -membrane lining the ventricles is the ependyma
1. lateral ventricles-consist of a. body b. anterior horn (in frontal lobe) c. posterior horn (in occipital lobe) d. inferior lobe (in temporal lobe)	-two in number -largest of ventricles -extend into cerebral hemispheres -communicates with 3rd ventricle and rest of system via interventricular′foramen of monro
2. Atrium (Trigone)	-site where anterior, occipital and temporal horns of lateral ventricles join
3. Foramen of Munro	-cavity that connects lateral ventricles to 3rd ventricle (interventricular foramen)
4. Third Ventricle	-small slit-like midline cavity which lies between the thalami -communicates laterally with lateral ventricles and posteriorly with Aqueduct of Sylvius
5. Cerebral Aqueduct of Sylvius	-midline narrow cavity which passes through midbrain connecting 3rd and 4th ventricles -communicates superiorly with 3rd ventricle and inferiorly with 4th ventricle
6. Fourth Ventricle	-midline diamond-shaped space -lies anterior to cerebellum and posterior to pons and upper half of medulla oblongata -communicates with subarachnoid space in spinal column via three openings b) Foramina of Luschka - two lateral openings c) Foramen of Magendie - one medial opening -superiorly through Aqueduct of Sylvius communicates with 3rd ventricle

SAGITTAL PLANE

sagittal plane

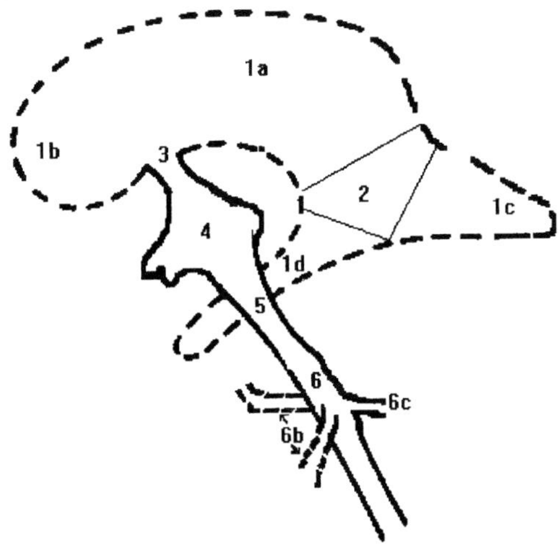

CORONAL PLANE

coronal plane

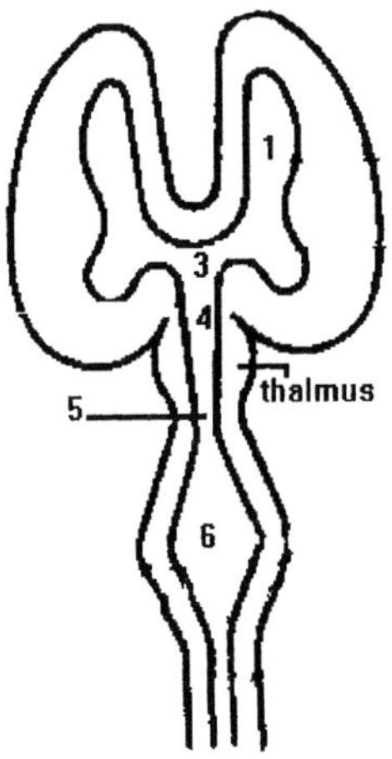

coronal scan on neonatal head with dilated ventricles to demonstrate ventricular anatomy

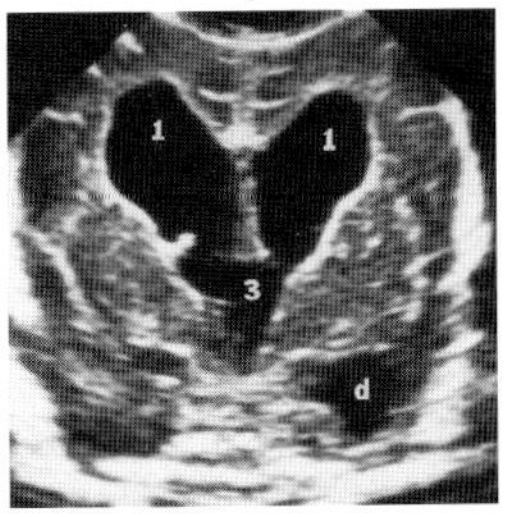

sagittal scan of neonatal head with dilated ventricles to demonstrate ventricular anatomy

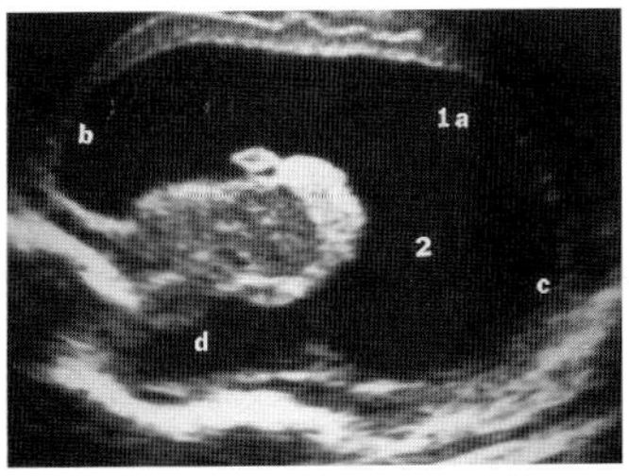

sagittal scan of fetal head with normal ventricles

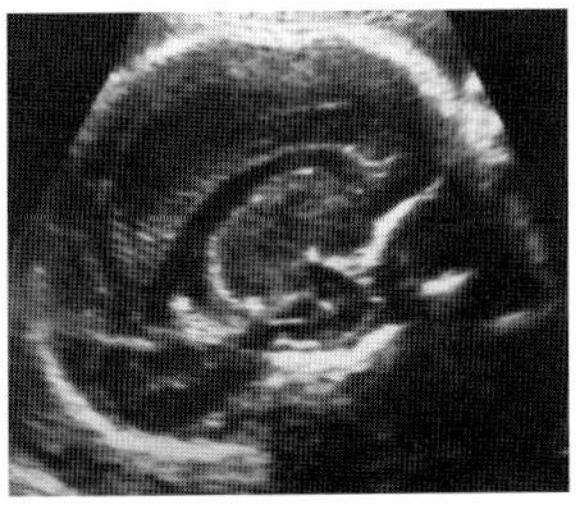

ANATOMY	US APPEARANCE
FIRST TRIMESTER -choroid plexus (C) - echogenic material that fills lateral ventricles except front horns	transvaginal scan of 11-week fetus; normal choroid (C) filled lateral ventricles 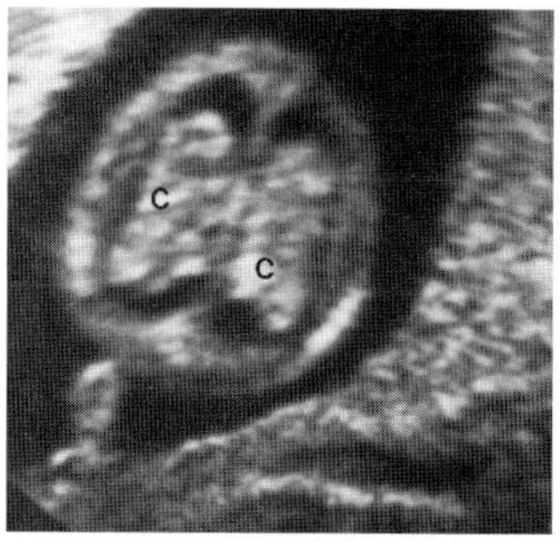
BIPARIETAL DIAMETER LEVEL 1. THALAMI (T) -paired bilateral midline triangular-shaped structures of moderate echogenicity encircling superior portion of third ventricle -joined across midline by massa intermedia 2. CAVUM SEPTI PELLUCIDI (C) -short parallel echogenic lines between anterior horn of lateral ventricles -formed by corpus callosum, it stretches between corpus callosum and fornices 3. CAVUM VERGAE -posterior to foramina of Munro 4. 3RD VENTRICLE -midline specular reflector 5. FALX CEREBRI (INTERHEMISPHERIC FISSURE) -midline specular reflector which is a vertical fold of dura lying in longitudinal fissure between cerebral hemispheres 6. CHOROID PLEXUS -prominent echogenic structures filling most of lateral ventricles (not in anterior or occipital horns-OH)	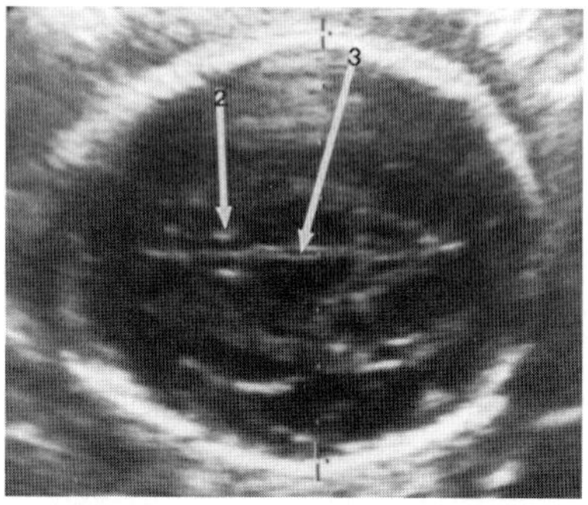 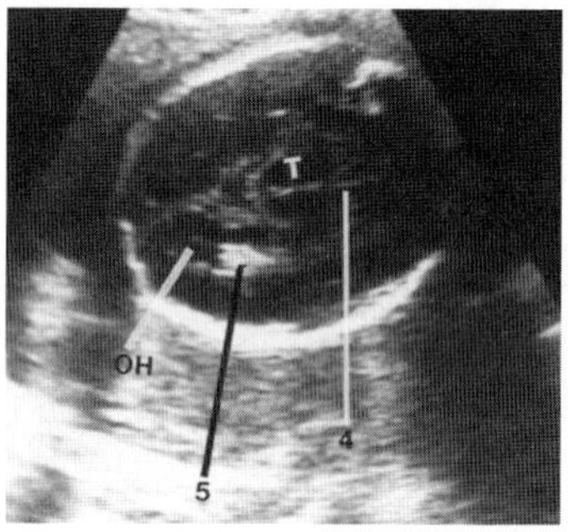
POSTERIOR FOSSA VERMIS OF CEREBELLUM -echogenic linear structure inferior to tentorium in mid cerebellum CEREBELLAR HEMISPHERES (2) -paired round structures of moderate echogenicity, either side of vermis -lies posterior to pons and medulla oblongata below tentorium CISTERNA MAGNA (3) -fluid filled space between cerebellum and posterior cranium -best identified from 15 to 28 weeks gestation FALX CEREBELLI -small fold of dura on the vermis between the cerebellar hemispheres below the tentorium STRAIGHT SINUS (5) -midline echo in cisterna magna	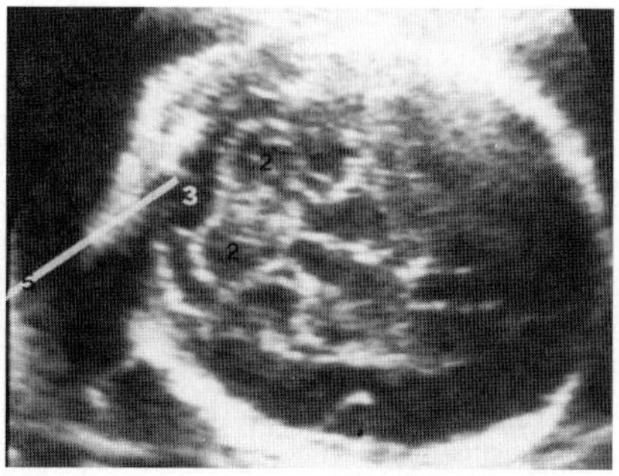

B) ABNORMAL DEVELOPMENT

ANOMALY	US DESCRIPTION	US APPEARANCE
AGENESIS OF CORPUS CALLOSUM -ranges from complete to partial, but only complete agenesis is diagnosed sonographically in utero -fibers that were supposed to cross in corpus callosum, run longitudinally along medial walls of lateral ventricles -poorly developed cerebrum around atria and occipital horns of lateral ventricle -commonly associated with other anomalies; holoprosencephaly, Dandy–Walker malformations	-lateral ventricles widely separated and medial walls appear indented -elongation and high placement of 3rd ventricle -enlarged atria and occipital horns of lateral ventricle -absence of cavum septi pellucidi -falx present -normal thalami -normal cerebral cortex	transaxial scan with high placement of 3rd ventricle between the thalamus (**) 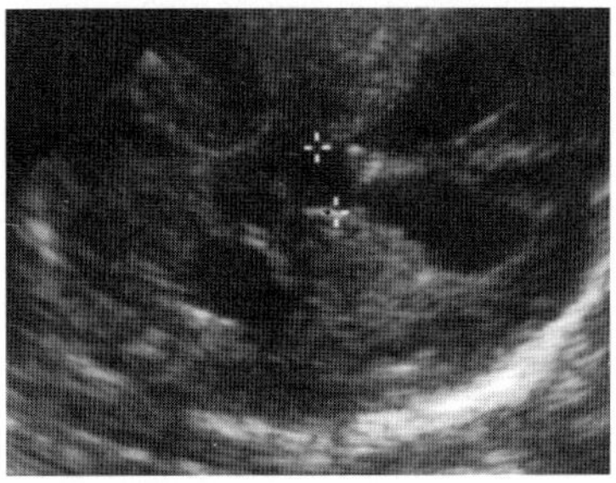 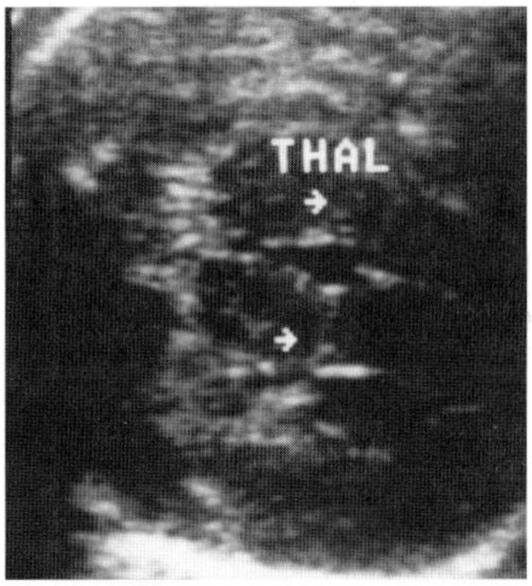 abnormally shaped lateral ventricle 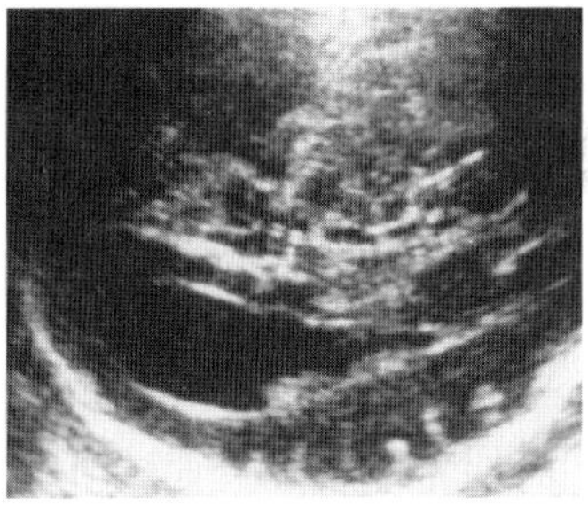
ANENCEPHALY -absence of cranial vault (acrania) and brain tissue due to failure of rostral portion of neural tube to close at 6 weeks -most common and severe form of failure of neural tube closure -rudimentary brainstem and portion of basal ganglia usually present -lethal anomaly -associated with spina bifida, spinal dysraphism, meningocele, myelomeningocele, cleft palate, umbilical hernia, polyhydramnios -elevated alpha-fetoprotein	-polyhydramnios -absence of cranium and cerebral ventricles -occiput, facial bones and orbits often present -increased fetal activity	coronal view of fetal head showing absence of cranium 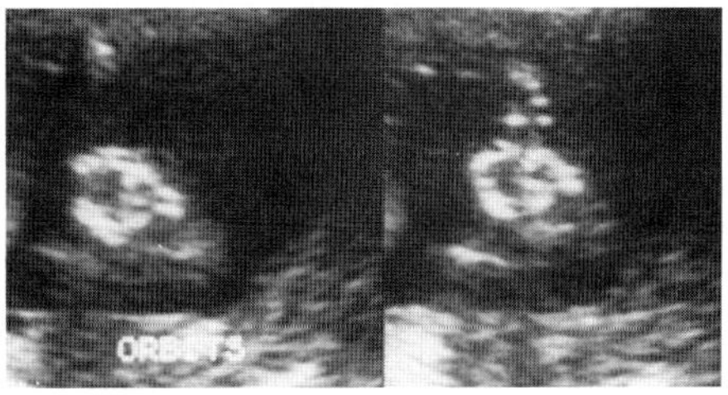

ANOMALY	**US DESCRIPTION**	**US APPEARANCE**
CEPHALOCELES/ MYELOCELES -herniation of some part of neural tube through bony defect in skull or spinal column -variety depends on location and on what part of neural tube is involved <u>Encephalocele</u> -herniation of meninges and brain tissue <u>Encephalocystomeningocele</u> -herniation of meninges, brain and ventricles <u>Meningocele</u> (meningo= membranes covering spinal cord or brain) -herniation of meningeal sac and meninges <u>Meningoencephalocele</u> -herniation of brain and meninges <u>Meningomyelocele/Myelomeningocele</u> -herniation of meninges and spinal cord <u>Myelocele</u> -herniation of spinal cord <u>Myelocystocele</u> -spina bifida containing spinal cord substance <u>Myelocystomeningocele</u> -herniation of spinal cord and meninges <u>Myeloschisis</u> -splayed spinal cord open to amniotic fluid	-separation and splaying outward of posterior ossification sites of spine or a bony cranial defect -loss of normal skin contour with a mass/sac protruding from spine of calvarium which can contain meninges and/or spinal cord -can be seen with Chiari II malformations -can be seen with hydrocephalus and polyhydramnios	transverse scans through fetal head shows an encephalocele at the posterior aspect of the fetal skull 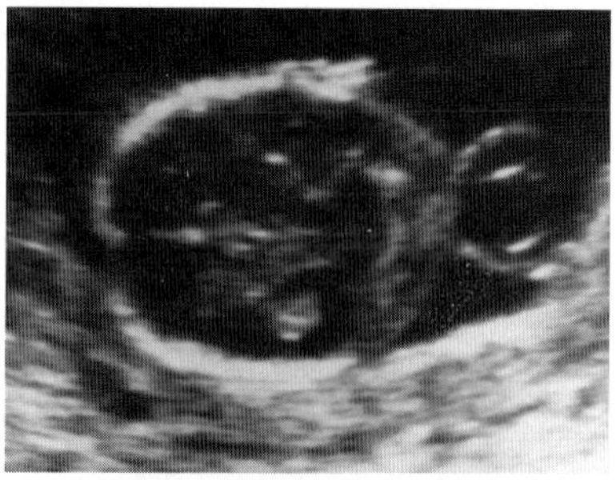 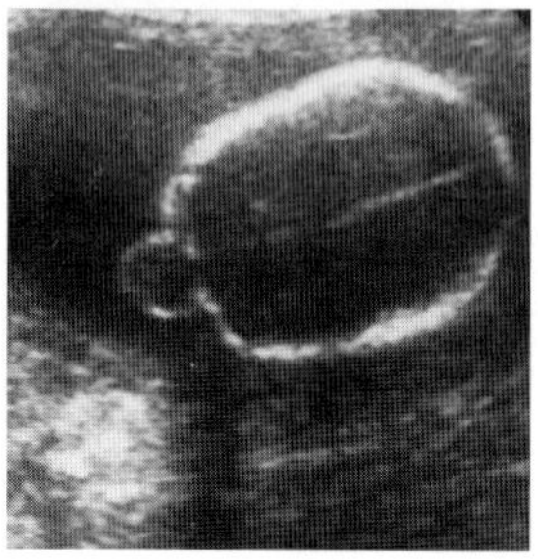 sagittal scans of fetal head with a posterior encephalocystomeningocele (**) 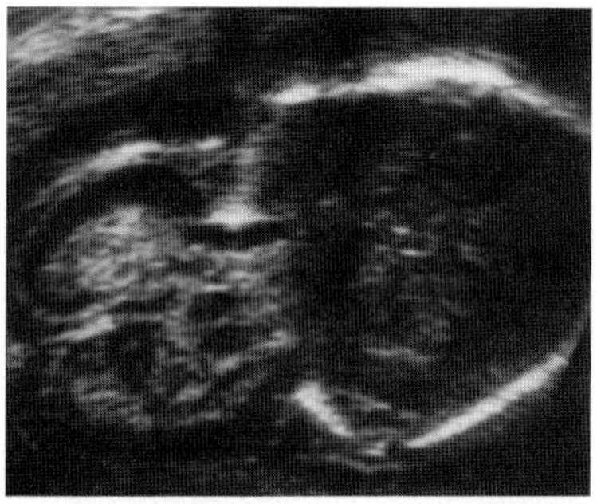 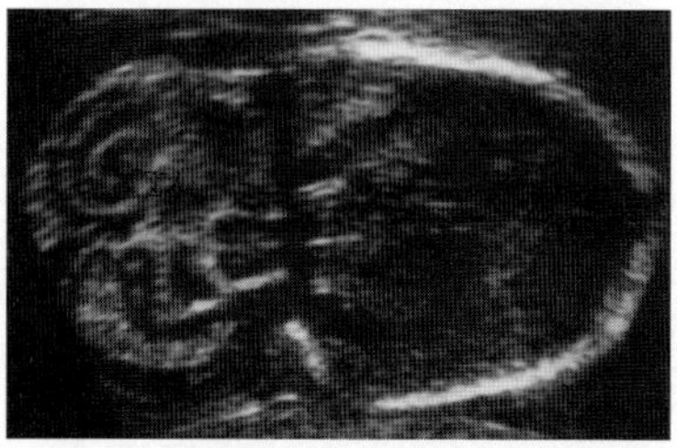

ANOMALY	US DESCRIPTION	US APPEARANCE
CHIARI MALFORMATION <u>Chiari I Malformation</u> -adults and older children -medulla displaced caudally with cerebellar tonsillar herniation -not associated with myelomeningocele <u>Chiari II Malformation</u> -most commonly referred to type -found in association with spinal dysraphia, myelomeningocele and anterior and posterior neural tube closure defects -caudal displacement of the brainstem and cerebellum through the foramen magnum into the cervical spine canal	<u>Chiari II</u> -"lemon" shaped head -obliterated cisterna magna -compressed posterior fossa creating "banana" shaped cerebellum -cerebellar tonsillar herniation into spinal canal -elongation and caudal displacement of 4th ventricle -hydrocephalus (3rd and lateral ventricles) -"Batwing" appearance/ pointing of frontal horns -meningomyelocele	abnormally shaped cranium; "lemon shaped" head (black arrows) with posterior meningomyelocele (arrow) 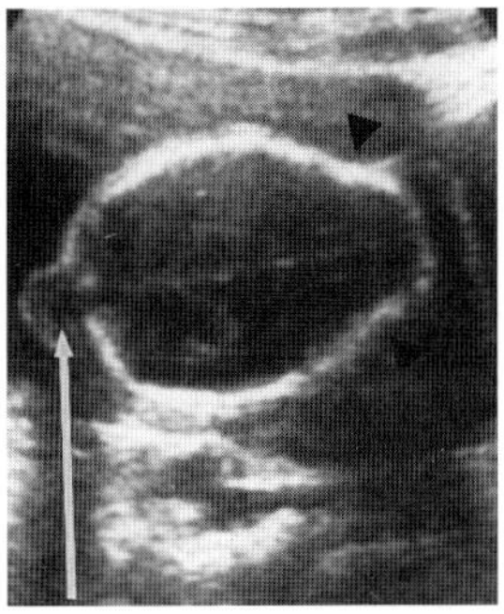 coronal scan of fetal head and upper spine; cerebellum (between arrows) has herniated into spinal canal (**) 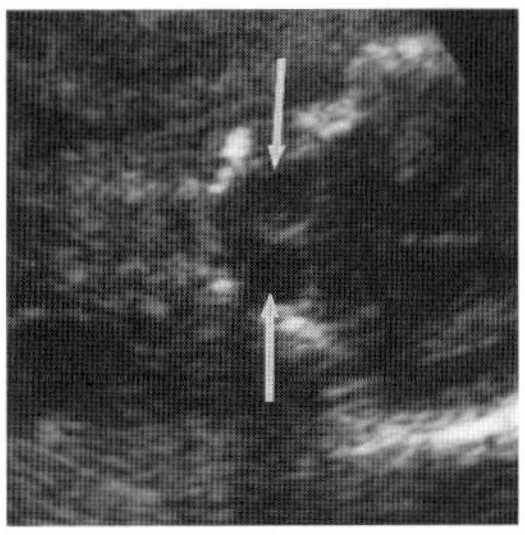 transaxial view of posterior fossa; "banana" shaped (between arrows) cerebellum and obliterated cisterna magna 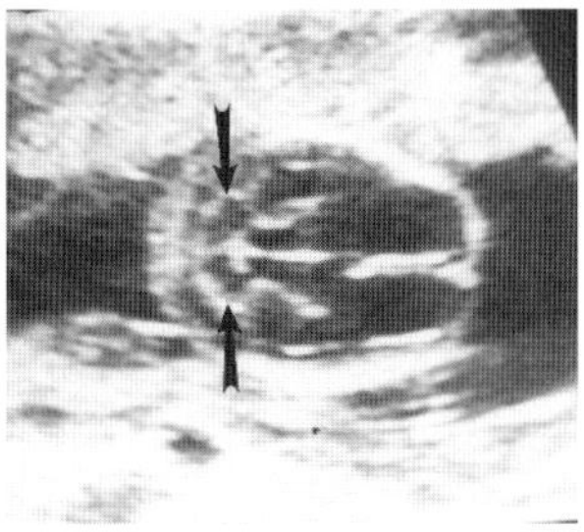

ANOMALY	US DESCRIPTION	US APPEARANCE
CYSTIC HYGROMA (CAVERNOUS LYMPHANGIOMA) -lymphatic channels filled with lymph creating a large fluid filled cystic mass -80% occur in cervical region -can also appear in axilla, groin, mediastinum -secondary to an obstruction between the lymphatic and venous pathway in the cervical area -associated with generalized edema, fetal hydrops, pleural effusions, ascites -associated with chromosomal anomalies: Turners Syndrome, trisomy 18, 21	-thin walled, multi-septated, fluid filled mass posterior/lateral aspect of head and neck -vary widely in size -mimic cervical meningocele or low occipital cephalocele -associated findings: hydrops fetalis	sagittal scan through 2nd trimester fetus shows huge multiseptated cystic mass (arrows) projecting at the back of the head (H) 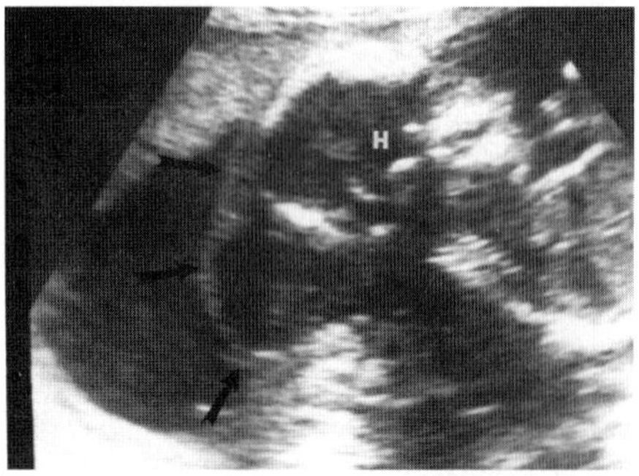 transverse of fetal cervical spine (S) with huge cystic mass (arrows) surrounding it 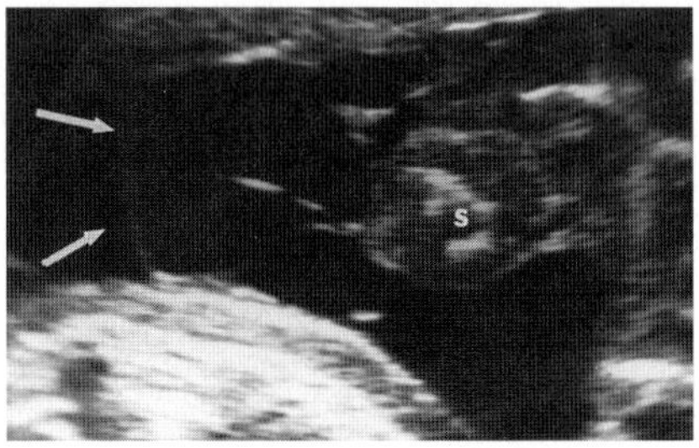
DANDY–WALKER CYST -abnormal development of cerebellum and 4th ventricle -enlargement of 4th ventricle probably due to atresia of Luschka & Magendie foramina -agenesis or hypoplasia of cerebellar vermis and hemispheres	-enlarged posterior fossa (large posterior fossa cyst) continuous with dilated 4th ventricle -hydrocephalus (3rd & lateral ventricle) -splaying of cerebellar hemispheres -complete or partial absence of cerebellar vermis	transaxial scan of fetal head shows an enlarged posterior fossa (arrow) with splaying of the cerebellar hemispheres (C) (**) 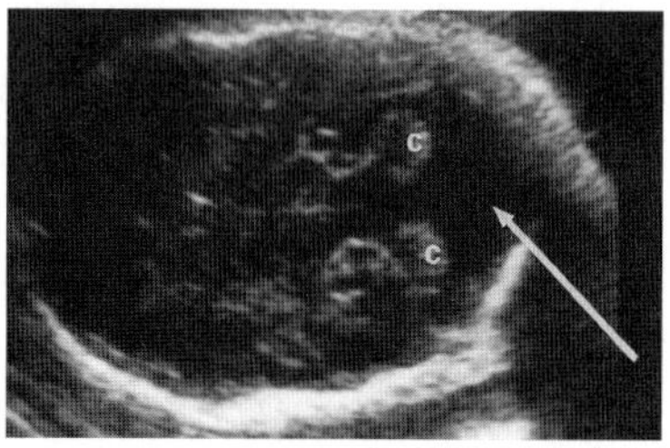

ANOMALY	US DESCRIPTION	US APPEARANCE
HOLOPROSENCEPHALY -spectrum of midline malformations resulting from failure of cleavage of prosencephalon into separate hemispheres to varying degrees -normal mid and hindbrain -associated with chromosomal anomalies <u>Alobar</u> -most severe -undivided holosphere and monoventricle communicating with dorsal sac	<u>Alobar</u> -single large ventricle -absent interhemispheric fissure, falx, 3rd ventricle, corpus callosum -fused thalami -severe midfacial abnormalities, hypotelerism	profile of fetal head showing large ventricle (H) occupying most of cranium (**) 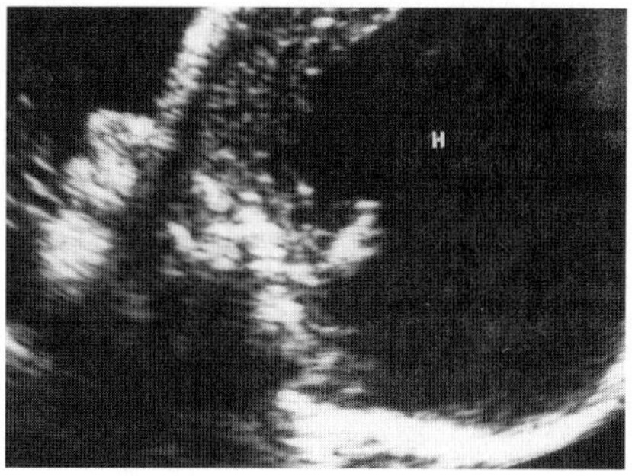
<u>Semilobar</u> -intermediate form -small brain, incomplete interhemispheric fissure, absent or incomplete corpus callosum -cleft palate and lip	<u>Semilobar</u> -partial separation of single ventricle into occipital and temporal horns -more cerebral tissue present -fused thalami	sagittal midline scan of bladder (B) and uterus with fetus in cephalic presentation; large cystic space in cranium (H) 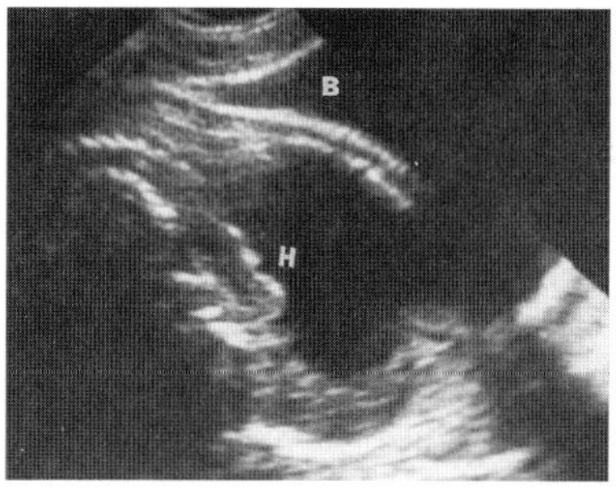
<u>Lobar</u> -mildest form -two separate hemispheres -mild facial deformities	<u>Lobar</u> -separation of ventricle except at frontal horns which are fused -slightly dilated lateral ventricles	coronal scan of fetal head; fusion of ventricles (**) 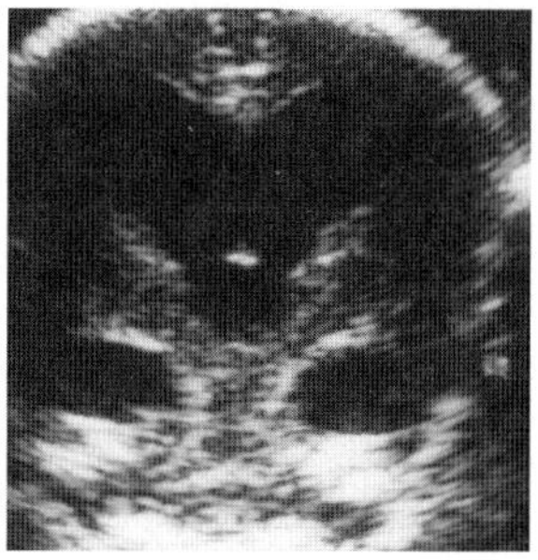
		coronal image of head shows an abnormal monoventricular lateral ventricular system (arrows) that surrounds the fused thalami (T); cerebral cortex is present (C) (**) 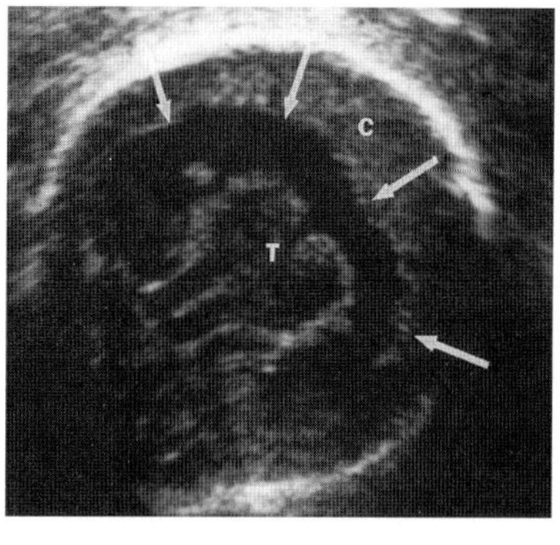

ANOMALY	US DESCRIPTION	US APPEARANCE
HYDRAENCEPHALY -replacement of cerebral hemispheres by large membranous sac filled with cerebral spinal fluid -normally developed skull -acquired destruction usually by a vascular accident or infection -preservation of some intracranial structures supplied by basilar vessels and some collateral flow -not associated with other anomalies	-absent ventricles and cerebral hemispheres -fluid filled large cranial vault -intact cerebellum and midbrain -falx usually present -absent internal carotid circulation -polyhydramnios	coronal and transaxial views of fetal head with absent ventricles and cerebral hemispheres; falx present (**) 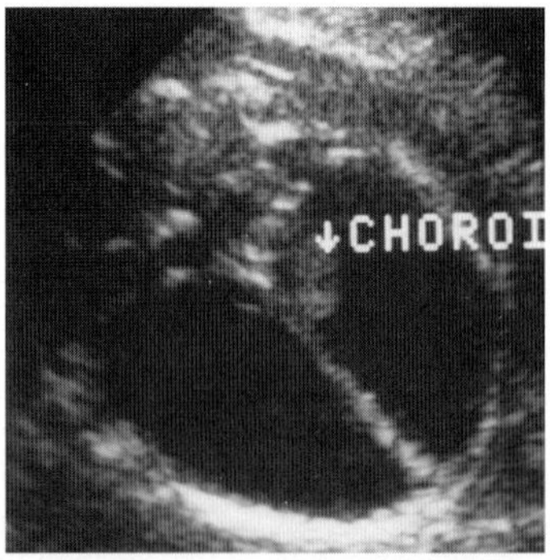 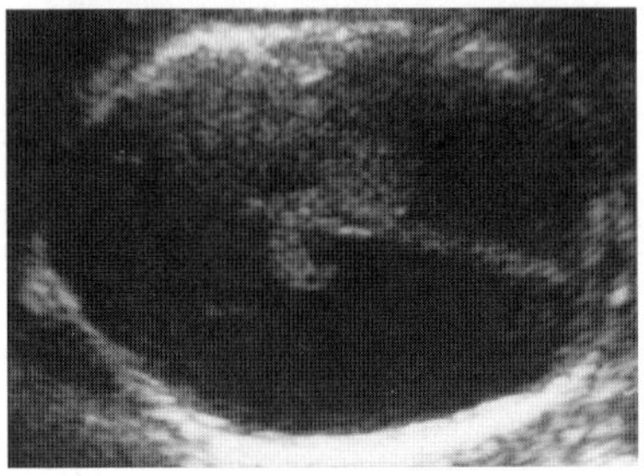
INFECTION (congenital) TORCH (**to***xoplasmosis,* **r***ubella,* **c***ytomegalic inclusion disease,* **h***erpes simplex virus*) -cross placenta to infect fetus -fetal encephalitis with varying degrees of cerebral destruction can result	-microcephaly -ventriculomegaly -hepatosplenomegaly (CMV) -diffuse or focal pattern of calcification	parasagittal scan through neonatal head shows multiple echogenic foci from a CMV infection 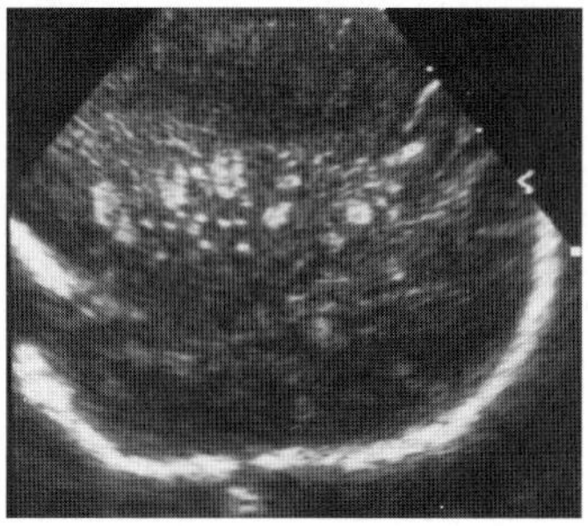
PORENCEPHALY PORENCEPHALIC CYSTS -destruction of previously formed brain tissue that forms a cavitation or CSF filled cyst in brain which communicates with a ventricle -caused by vascular occlusion, birth trauma, ventricular puncture, inflammatory disease, vascular insults SCHIZENCEPHALY -bilateral clefts in cerebrum -etiology uncertain, may be related to vascular occlusion or primary mal-development	Porencephaly -no mass effect -single or multiple cystic areas within cerebrum that can communicate with lateral ventricle Schizencephaly -bilateral symmetrical areas of cystic necrosis	large cyst (arrow) in posterior aspect of head adjacent to lateral ventricle (V) (**) 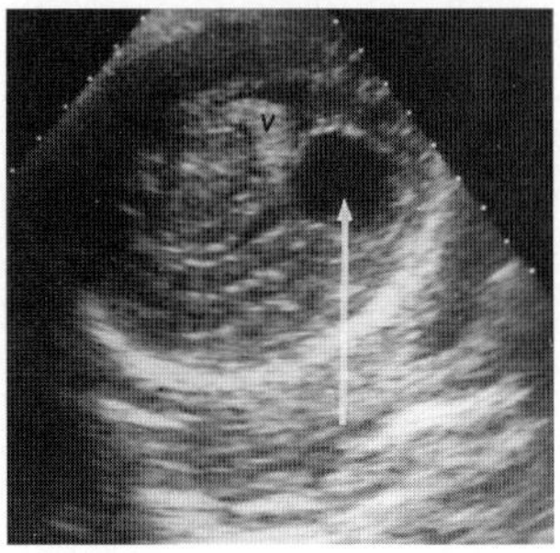

ANOMALY	US DESCRIPTION	US APPEARANCE
SPACE-OCCUPYING LESIONS <u>ARACHNOID CYST</u> -arachnoid lined cyst caused by congenital invagination or inflammatory entrapment of the pia layer -most common location is in the region of Sylvian fissure <u>CHOROID PLEXUS CYST</u> -common, benign cystic lesion located in choroid of lateral ventricle -can be normally seen at 16–21 weeks, and usually resolve spontaneously -some association with chromosomal anomalies <u>VEIN OF GALEN ANEURYSM</u> -result of an arteriovenous malformation -failure of embryonic A-V shunts to be replaced by capillaries	<u>Arachnoid Cyst</u> -creates mass effect and does not communicate with lateral ventricle <u>Choroid Plexus Cyst</u> -bi or unilateral -0.5–2 cm in size -located in lateral ventricle near glomus of choroid plexus <u>Vein of Galen Aneurysm</u> -tortuous cystic structure posterior to foramen of Monroe, near midline, superior to 3rd ventricle, contains doppler signal	arachnoid cyst: transaxial view of fetal head; large cystic structure (arrow) in right side of cranium (**) 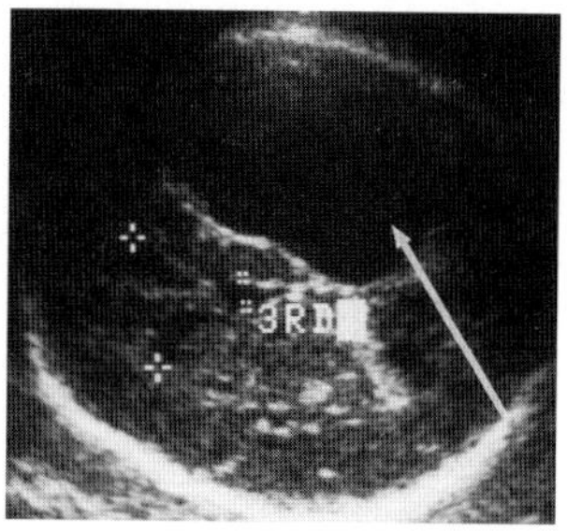 choroid plexus cyst(s) - coronal scan through 2nd trimester fetal head, shows bilateral choroid plexus cysts (arrows) 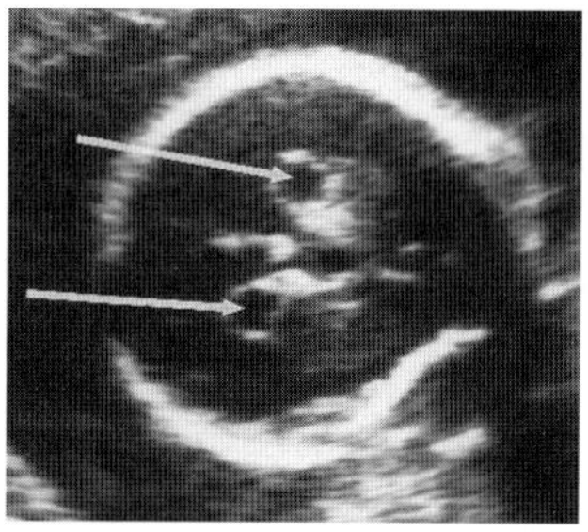
TERATOMAS -neoplasms composed of a wide variety of tissue foreign to the site where they grow -usually benign, but have malignant potential -can occur in the sacrococcygeal region, retroperitoneum, face <u>SACROCOCCYGEAL TERATOMA</u> -arises from coccyx -most common fetal tumor	-complex mixed, cystic and solid lesion -can have areas of calcification -can be quite large -polyhydramnios -lower tumors can displace urinary bladder anteriorly and may obstruct kidneys	sagittal scan through 2nd trimester fetal head shows a large echogenic teratoma (M-between arrows) that is creating a mass effect 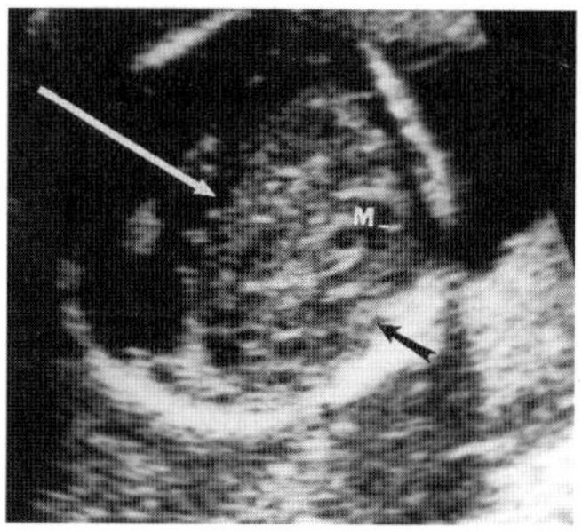

ANATOMY	US DESCRIPTION	US APPEARANCE
VENTRICULOMEGALLY -enlargement of ventricles -2 types: A) PASSIVE -due to cerebral atrophy or dysgenesis (HYDROCEPHALUS EX VACUO) -passive dilation of ventricles B) HYDROCEPHALUS -abnormal increase in volume of ventricles due to increased amount of CSF or from obstruction of CSF flow	-dilated ventricular system -early features include enlargement of occipital horn and trigone region of ventricles -choroid plexus that fails to fill transverse diameter of the body of the lateral ventricle -midline displacement of the medial wall of the lateral ventricle -often accompanies neural tube defect	transaxial view of fetal head; hugely dilated ventricle with suspended choroid (C), thin mantle of brain tissue (B) (**) 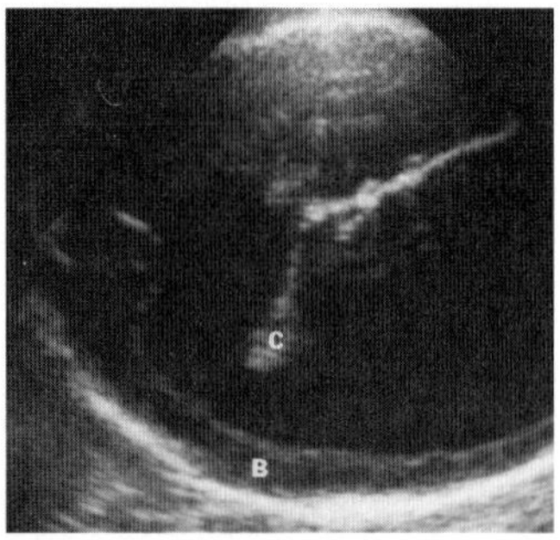 coronal scan through frontal horns showing ventricular enlargement (**) 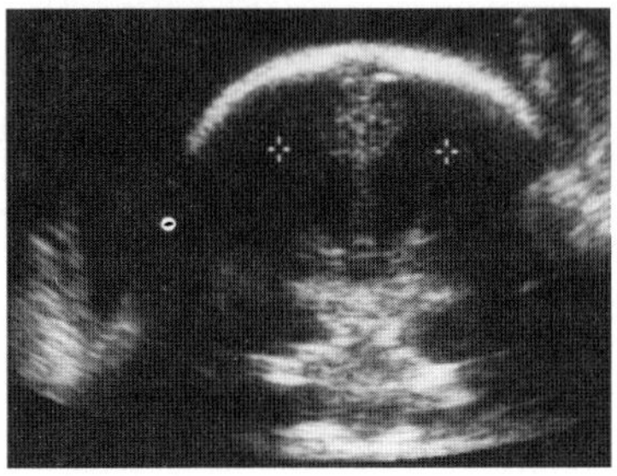

HEAD AND NECK ANOMALIES AND VARIANTS - TERMINOLOGY	
ACRANIA (EXENCEPHALY)	-partial or complete congenital absence of cranium -associated with anecephaly
ANENCEPHALY	-absent brain and cranial vault
BRACHYCEPHALY	-short wide head -caused by cranial dystosis or oligohydramnios or can be a variant of normal
CRANIOSYNOSTOSIS	-premature fusion of cranial sutures causing abnormal cephalic index and mis-shapen skull
DOLICHOCEPHALY	-narrow head -caused by cranial dystosis or oligohydramnios or can be a variant of normal
HOLOANENCEPHALY	-complete absence of brain and cranial vault
KLEEBLATTSCHADEL (CLOVERLEAF SKULL)	-premature fusion of coronal and lambdoidal sutures associated with fetal triploidy and some dwarfisms -on ultrasound seen as bulging of parietal bones, prominent forehead
MACROCEPHALY	-head circumference is abnormally large for true gestational age -associated with hydrocephaly or hydranencephaly
MEROANENCEPHALY	-a form of anencephaly where the brain may not be totally absent and cranial vault may be more formed
MICROCEPHALY	-head smaller than 5th %tile or less than 3 standard deviations below the mean for true gestational age -caused by TORCH, genetic anomalies, environment insults
SCAPHACEPHALY	-premature fusion of sagittal sutures creating a narrow head

FACIAL ANOMALY	US FINDINGS
EPINATHUS -rare pharyngeal teratoma arising from palate -varies in size and texture	-mass extending through mouth -creates an anterior complex/solid/cystic mass
FACIAL CLEFTS -several types: unilateral or bilateral and incomplete or complete cleft palate -lack of fusion of facial grooves creating a congenital fissure in the roof of the mouth -this forms a communicating passageway between mouth and nasal cavities -can be associated with chromosomal and congenital anomalies (trisomy 13, 18)	-best seen on modified coronal view of face -gap in upper lip and nose -mass effect of the budding upper lip -nose flattened and widened <u>Cleft Lip (Harelip)</u> -separation of upper lip, which may be associated most frequently with club foot
HYPOTELERISM -orbits close together -manifestation of severe brain malformation such as holoprosencephaly <u>HYPERTELERISM</u> -orbits too far apart caused by craniosynostoses or anterior cephalocele <u>ANOPHTHALMIA</u> -congenital absence of one or both eyes <u>MICROPHTHALMIA</u> -abnormally small eyes	-perform quantitative orbital measurements when subjective scanning suggests abnormality -coronal oblique is best scan plane to visualize these defects
MACROGLOSSIA -hypertrophied, congenital condition of the tongue -associated with Beckwith–Weidemann Syndrome	-seen in sagittal profile of face or coronal anterior section through lips and nose -large, protruding tongue from open mouth
MICROGNATHIA -abnormal mandible development that results in a small, receding chin resulting in considerable overbite -associated with several syndromes and trisomy 13,18	-best seen on sagittal view of profile of face -small chin -prominent nose and upper lip area
cleft palate & lip-sagittal of fetal face showing space in upper lip (**) 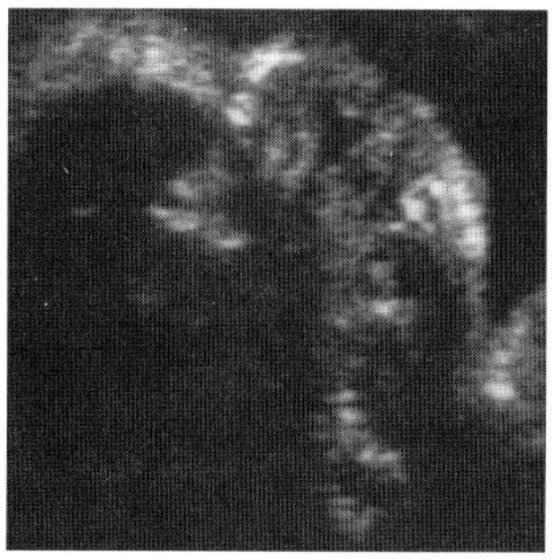	cleft palate: coronal view of fetal face shows abnormal maxilla (**) 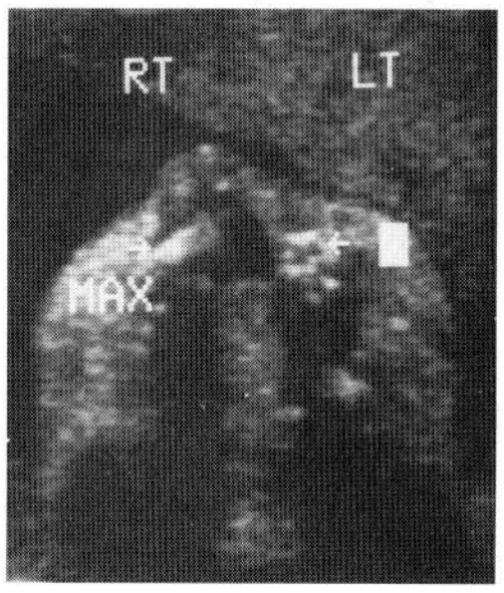

SONOGRAPHIC FINDINGS OF HEAD AND NECK ANOMALIES		
SONOGRAPHIC SIGN	**WHAT IT INDICATES**	**US APPEARANCE**
ABNORMAL CISTERNA MAGNA -anterioposterior diameter is abnormally increased (>1 cm) or decreased in size -normal range is from 4–10 mm	<u>Small/ Obliterated</u> 1. Arnold Chiari malformations <u>Enlarged</u> 1. normal variant 2. communicating hydrocephalus 3. cerebellar hypoplasia 4. retrocerebellar arachnoid cyst 5. Dandy–Walker cyst 6. trisomy 18	obliterated cisterna magna (arrow); no fluid seen between banana shaped cerebellum (C) and skull 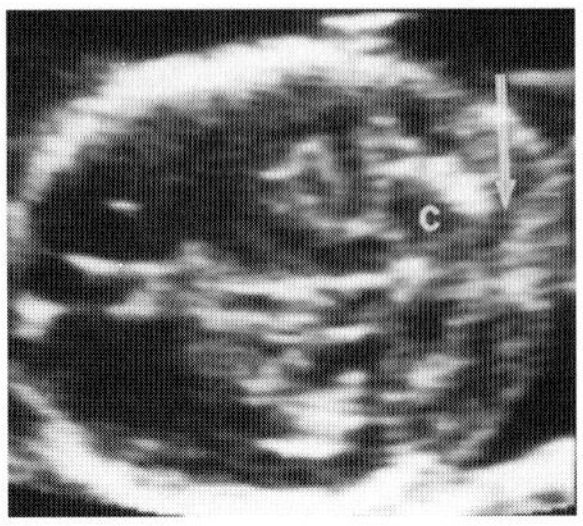 cisterna magna that is at the upper limits of normal, measuring 10 mm (cerebellum = C) 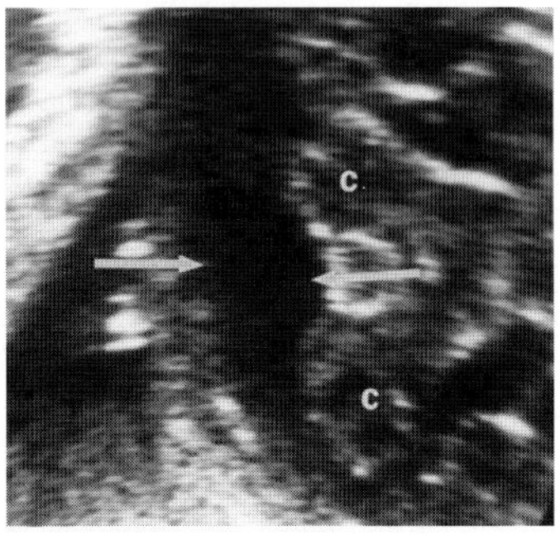
BANANA SIGN -abnormal cerebellum -posterior cerebellar margin is smoothly curved and convex rather than bilobar which indicates obliteration of cisterna magna	-Arnold Chiari malformation secondary to spinal meningomyelocele (spina bifida) -compression of posterior fossa	"banana" shaped cerebellum (between arrows) 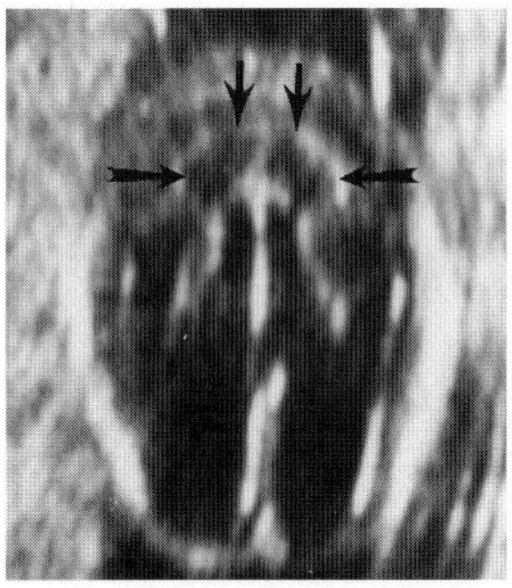

SONOGRAPHIC SIGN	WHAT IT INDICATES	US APPEARANCE
DANGLING CHOROID SIGN -choroid normally lies in body, atrium and temporal horn of ventricle -choroid is not firmly held in lateral ventricle therefore assumes a gravitational dependent position -choroid must "dangle" or "hang-down" until it meets resistance from brain parenchyma at lateral ventricular wall -when the ventricles are grossly dilated the choroid appears suspending within them	-enlarged ventricles Pitfall: Pseudo Dangling Choroid -technical factors can cause the brain parenchyma to appear isoechoic to the ventricles "creating" an enlarged ventricle -the choroid appears to be dangling within this created large ventricle which simulates dangling choroid -therefore if "dangling" choroid is seen, be aware of artifact simulation	true dangling choroid-enlarged lateral ventricle with choroid (C) seemingly suspended in the fluid 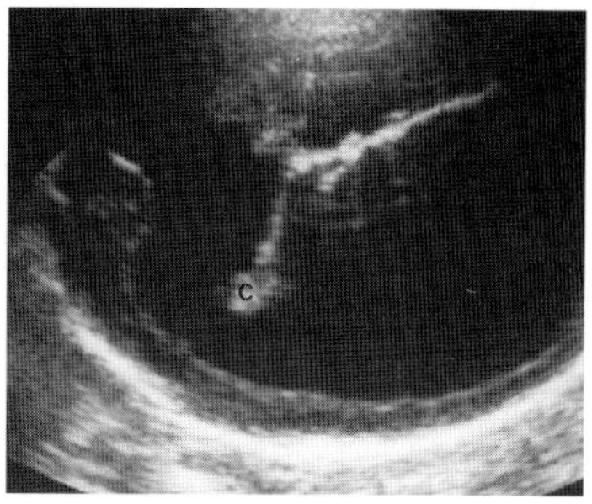 PSEUDO DANGLING CHOROID-normal head; lateral ventricular wall is not well seen and parenchyma appears anechoic (arrow) due to technical factors which makes the choroid (C) appear to be suspended, rather than rest on the ventricle wall 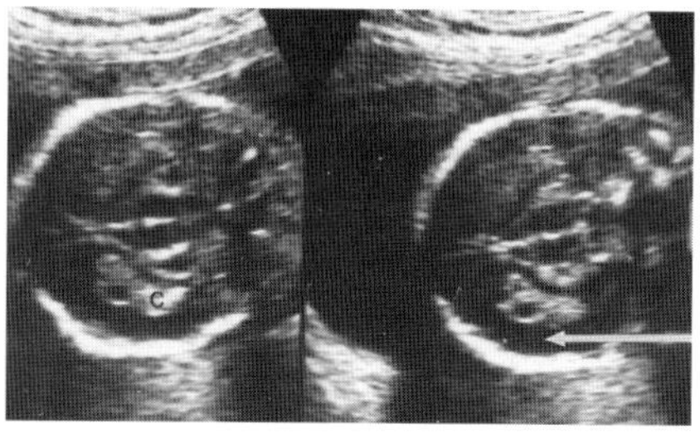
LEMON SIGN Lemon Shaped Head -abnormal skull shape -bifrontal indentations of skull which causes skull shape to be similar to that of lemon -concave deformity of cranium at the approximate level of the coronal sutures	-associated with spinal meningomyelocele (spina bifida) -Chiari II malformation Pitfall: Pseudo Lemon Sign -normal skull can appear to be abnormal if the transducer angle is such that it cuts through the frontal sutures creating a lemon shaped skull -if the scanner can make the skull appear both normal and an abnormal lemon shape, it is most likely a normal cranium	true lemon sign-transaxial scan of skull with concave deformity of frontal bones (arrows) creating a "lemon" shaped head 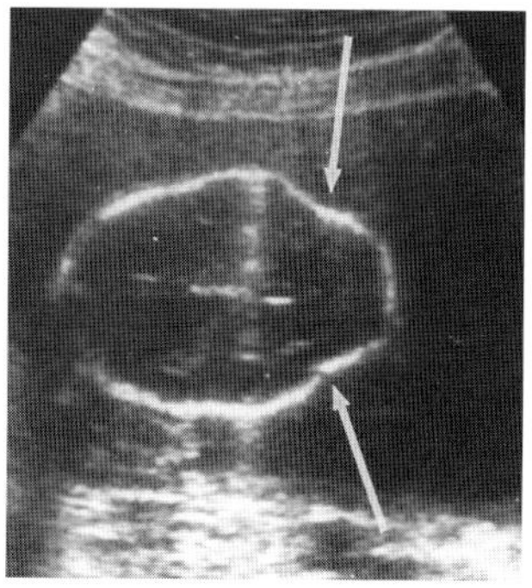 PSEUDO LEMON SIGN-transaxial scan of skull with normally shaped cranium; which appears slightly concave due to the angle of the transducer on this scan plane 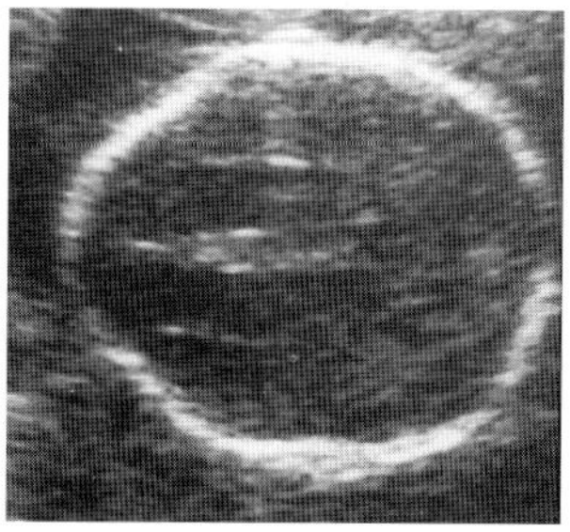

SONOGRAPHIC SIGN	WHAT IT INDICATES	US APPEARANCE
NUCAL SKIN FOLD THICKNESS -nucal skin fold thickness is measured from outer skull table to outer skin surface -similar scan as that used to evaluate the cisterna magna -values > 6 mm between 15 and 21 weeks are considered abnormal and cause a flag for further investigation	-an abnormally thickened nucal skin fold measured between 15 and 21 weeks is highly associated with Down syndrome	calipers measured a thickened nucal skin fold at 8.5 mm (**) 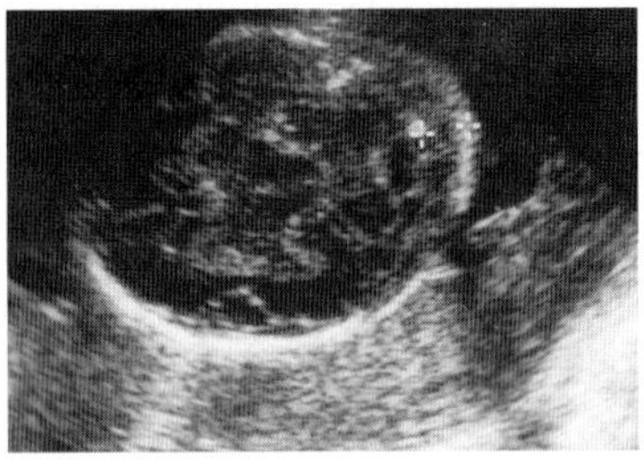
VENTRICLES -the axial diameter of ventricular atrium (trigone) remains stable throughout 2nd and 3rd trimester and therefore, is age independent -normal range is < 10 mm, with upper limits of normal from 10–12 mm -width of lateral ventricle in the atrium region is easily recognized by its choroid plexus and well defined walls -occipital horn is usually the first portion of the ventricular system to be dilated	-3 pathologic processes: 1. obstructive hydrocephaly 2. mal-development of ventricle or brain tissue 3. destruction of brain tissue -spina bifida (*Other methods of measurement include: bifrontal + bi-temporal measurements, ratio of lateral ventricular width to hemispheric width, ratio of lateral ventricle width to BPD)	transaxial scan of grossly enlarged lateral ventricles (between calipers) 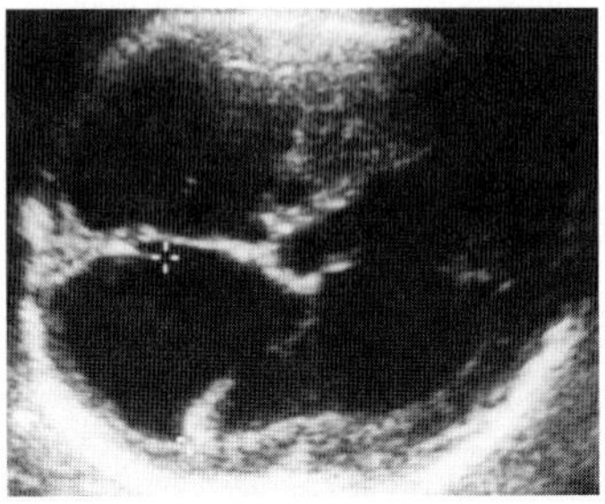 lateral ventricle, measuring 11 mm at upper limits of normal 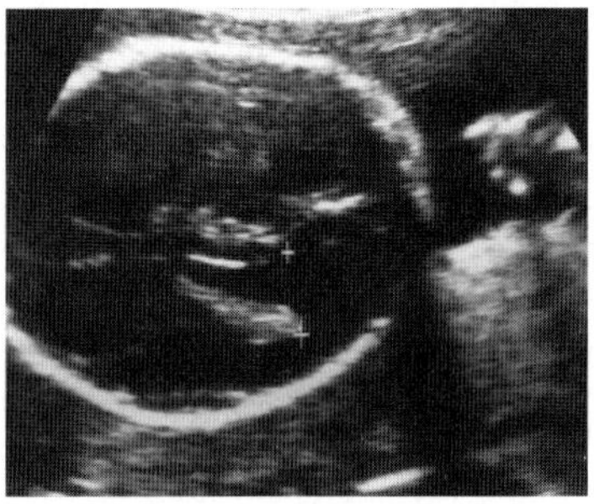

SECTION 4. HEART AND THORAX
A) NORMAL ANATOMY AND DEVELOPMENT

DEVELOPMENT OF FETAL THORAX AND HEART	
5 Weeks	-single heart tube forms and begins to contract -lung bud develops as outgrowth of primitive foregut
6-7 Weeks	-separation of the atria and ventricles begin
7 Weeks	-main stem bronchi of lung form and subdivide into secondary bronchi
10 Weeks	-heart is fully formed
26-40 Weeks	-lungs develop respiratory capability - mature alveoli form weeks 38–40

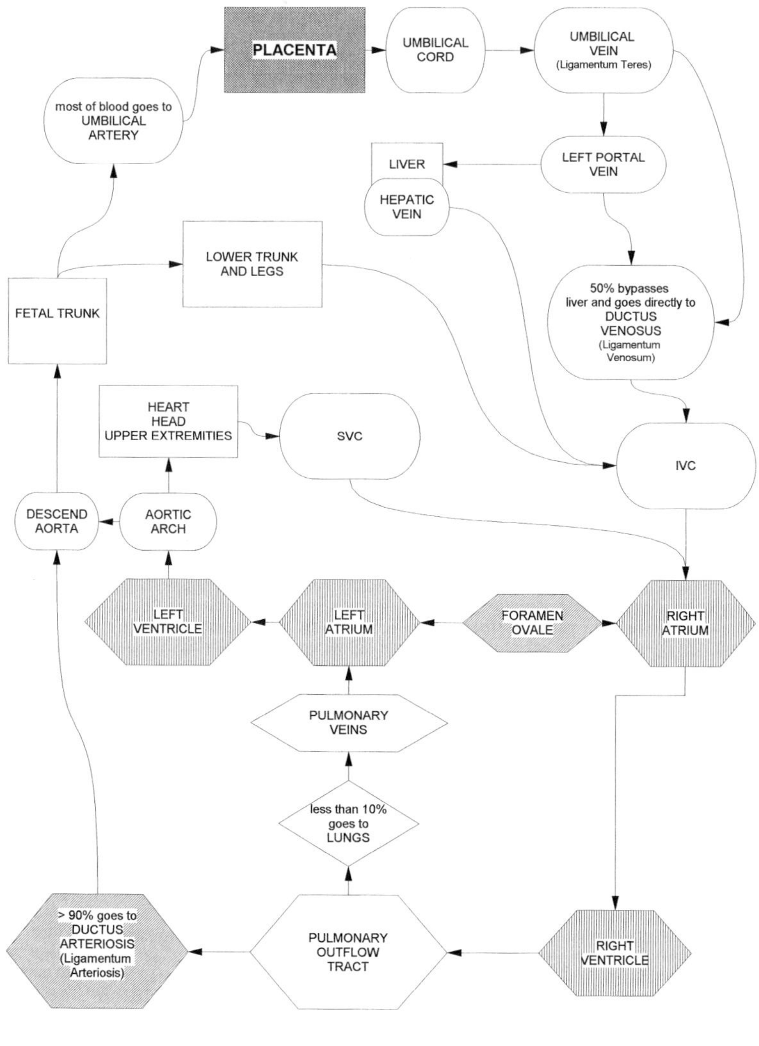

FETAL CIRCULATION SYSTEM

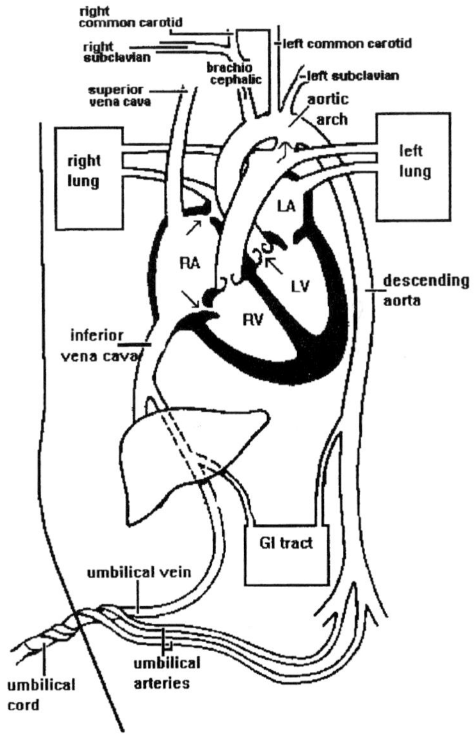

FETAL LUNGS

-factors important for normal lung development include:
1. fetal thorax large enough for growth
2. fetal breathing movements
3. adequate amniotic fluid volume to allow:
   a) normal balance of fluid volume and pressure in trachea and lung
   b) large enough sac space to allow for growth and movement of fetal thorax

-if severe oligohydramnios or a thoracic cavity restricted in size develops, pulmonary hypoplasia (absolute decrease in lung volume and weight for fetal age) could result
-fetal "breathing" is an airless thoracic mechanical movement which can occur anywhere between 12–60 times per minute and is noted as important part of biophysical profile
-pulmonary maturity cannot be accurately predicted by sonographic appearance

US appearance
-visualized mid second trimester
-homogenous, moderate echotexture with increasing echogenicity as gestation progresses
-separated from liver by the smooth hypoechoic diaphragm

sagittal scan of fetal body- the heart lies above the hypoechoic diaphragm (black arrows), with the stomach and liver lying below it

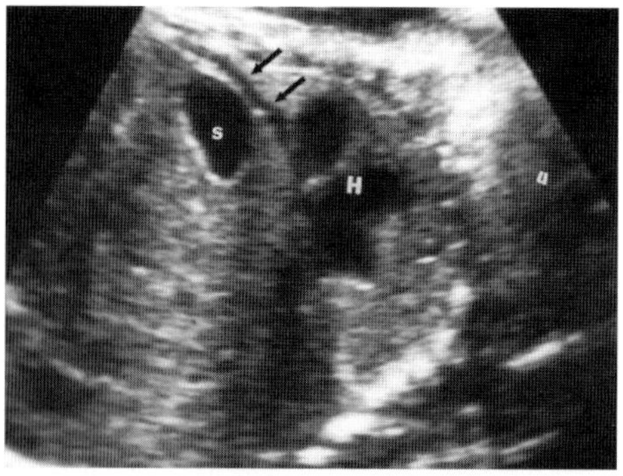

transverse oblique scan through fetal abdomen
-the liver (LIV) is hypoechoic to the lungs (L); the hepatic veins are emptying into the IVC adjacent to the heart

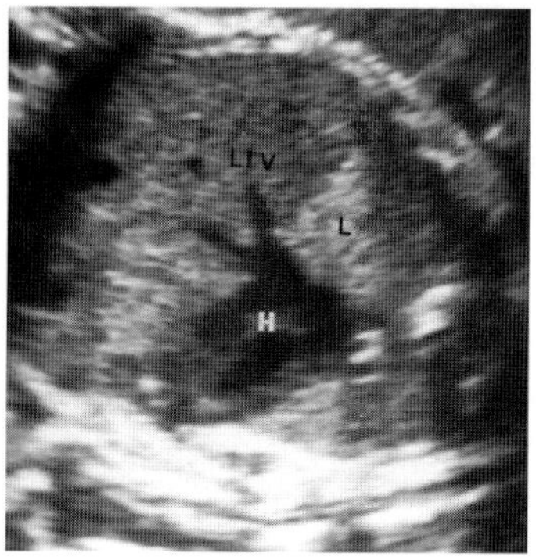

CARDIOVASCULAR SYSTEM	
FUNCTION	1. transport substances to and from body cells 2. exchange of substances between the various systems, organs and cells of the body 3. contributes to cellular metabolism, defense against micro-organisms, fluid volume, pH and temperature
1. HEART	-four chambered muscular organ that lies in mediastinum
2. PERICARDIUM	-3 layered sac investing entire heart and cardiac portion of great vessels Serous Pericardium (internal portion): -secretes serous fluid which allows the heart to move in its sac without creating friction a) Visceral (epicardium) - covers the heart and part of great vessels b) Parietal: - visceral pericardium turns outward at the origin of the aortic arch to line fibrous pericardium c) Fibrous Pericardium (external portion) -fibrous and fatty and strongly attached to sternum, great vessels, diaphragm -keeps heart in place
3. MYOCARDIUM	-muscular wall of heart
4. ENDOCARDIUM	-inner lining of heart
5. PERICARDIAL SAC	-potential space between visceral and parietal layers or pericardium -contains small amount of fluid for lubrication
6. MEDIASTINUM	-described as the portion of anatomy between the lungs -divided into subdivisions a) anterior mediastinum: thymus gland b) middle mediastinum: heart and pericardium c) posterior mediastinum: esophagus, descending aorta, thoracic duct, vagus nerve, paraspinal region also: -superior mediastinum: great vessels of heart (except IVC), trachea, esophagus, nerves -floor: diaphragm

TRANSVERSE CROSS SECTION OF HEART

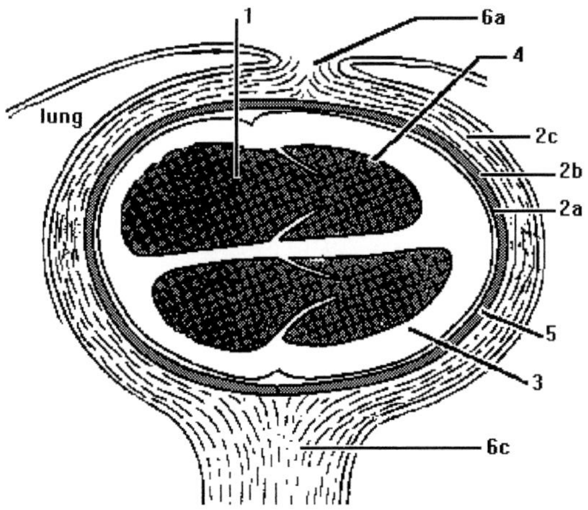

SONOGRAPHIC EVALUATION OF THE FETAL HEART

-sonographically the heart is evaluated for abnormalities of structure and rhythm
-most appropriate gestational age for sonographic evaluation is approximately 18–22 weeks
-majority of fetal cardiac malformations can be identified with the four chamber view
Documentation of:
1. position of heart within the body
-left anterior quadrant of chest with small portion of RV and RA right anterior quadrant
-horizontal position, due to large liver size in fetus
-axis of the heart is such that the apex points at a 45° angle toward the left anterior chest wall
2. identification of a 4 chamber heart
3. evaluation of atrioventricular and ventriculoarterial connections
4. symmetry of atria and ventricles
-atria are approximately equal size and the two ventricles are approximately the same size until later 3rd trimester when the right ventricle may appear slightly larger
5. cardiac size
6. septal integrity
7. normal endocardium, myocardium and pericardium

SCAN PLANES FOR FETAL HEART

Four Chamber Heart
-transverse view of thorax at level of lower sternum; should be seen routinely in all fetuses after second trimester
"Five" Chamber Heart
-direct beam more cephalad from 4 chamber to view aortic root ("5th" chamber) in center
Further Cardiac Evaluation
-other ways of examining the heart sonographically include views of the outflow tracts and the aortic arch and other techniques such as m-mode, pulsed doppler and color flow imaging

FETAL CARDIAC ARRHYTHMIAS

-cardiac rhythm is observed and recorded on an M-mode image, with awareness for sustained arrhythmias
-atria and ventricles evaluated separately on m-mode as arrhythmias may originate from either and occur independently
-arrhythmias can be associated with cardiac structural anomalies, maternal lupus erythematosus and rheumatoid arthritis
-normal heart rate baseline is 120-160 beats per minute (BPM)

TACHYCARDIA abnormally fast >80 BPM	**BRADYCARDIA** abnormally slow <100 BPM
SUPROVENTRICULAR TACHYCARDIA (SVT) -bulging of atrial septum -atrial rate of 180–300 BPM + ventricular response of 1:1 ATRIAL FLUTTER -atrial rate 300–460 BPM + ventricular rate of 60–200 BPM ATRIAL FIBRILLATION -atrial rate of 400–700 BPM + ventricular rate of 120–200 BPM	TRANSIENT BRADYCARDIA -commonly observed temporary arrhythmia caused by vasovagal reaction (ie. compressing fetus) ATRIOVENTRICULAR BLOCK- FIRST DEGREE -elongated PR interval on ECG SECOND DEGREE -a few atrial contractions are not followed by a ventricular contraction THIRD DEGREE-COMPLETE HEART BLOCK -atrial and ventricular contractions independent from each other -atrial rate of 120–140 BPM + ventricular rate of 40–60 BPM

NORMAL APPEARANCE AND ANATOMY OF THE FETAL FOUR CHAMBER HEART

1. RIGHT ATRIUM (RA)
-IVC and SVC empty into RA
-eustachian valve within IVC as it drains into right atrium
-foramen ovale is noted opening from right to left atrium

2. LEFT ATRIUM (LA)
-flap valve of foramen ovale (septum primum) seen within
-lies between left pulmonary artery and left ventricle
-most posterior chamber
-pulmonary veins empty into LA

3. ATRIOVENTRICULAR VALVES
-chordae tendinae attach to free edge and anchored at papillary muscles near apex
-prevent backflow from ventricles to atria during systole
a. TRICUSPID-RT. AV VALVE: inserted lower on the IVS than mitral valve
b. MITRAL (BICUSPID)-LT. AV VALVE

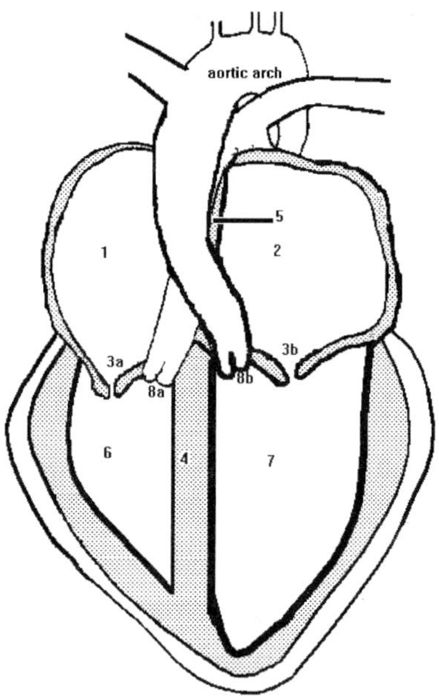

4. INTERVENTRICULAR SEPTA (IVS)
-separates ventricular chambers
-thickest at apex and tapers approaching the insertion of AV valves

5. INTERATRIAL SEPTA (IAS)
-thin, membranous-like structure
-seen as continuation of IVS
FORAMEN OVALE
-interruption of IAS

6. RIGHT VENTRICLE (RV)
-moderator band: septal attachment of tricuspid valve leaflets which can appear as a bright echogenic focus lying in apex
-anterior papillary muscle seen within
-RV appears larger than LV
-RV more anterior- touching inner aspect of left chest wall
-main pulmonary artery (MPA) arises from RV
-ductus arteriosus arises from distal MPA

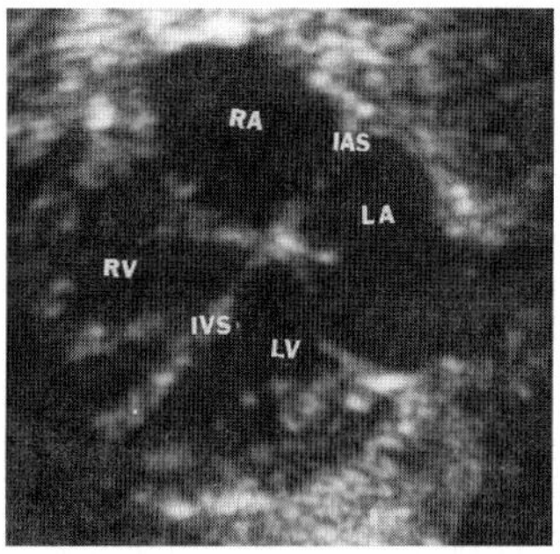

7. LEFT VENTRICLE (LV)
-papillary muscle within
-fluid-filled stomach lies inferior to LV
-ascending aorta (AAo) arises from LV
-chordae tendenae of AV valve (can be seen normally as hyperechoic focus on sonogram)

8. SEMILUNAR VALVES
-3 cup-like cusps attached to valve rings that separate ventricles from their arteries
-respond to pressure changes in ventricles and arteries
-prevent backflow from arteries into ventricles
a. Pulmonic: Rt. Ventricle + Pulmonary Artery
b. Aortic: Lt. Ventricle + Aorta

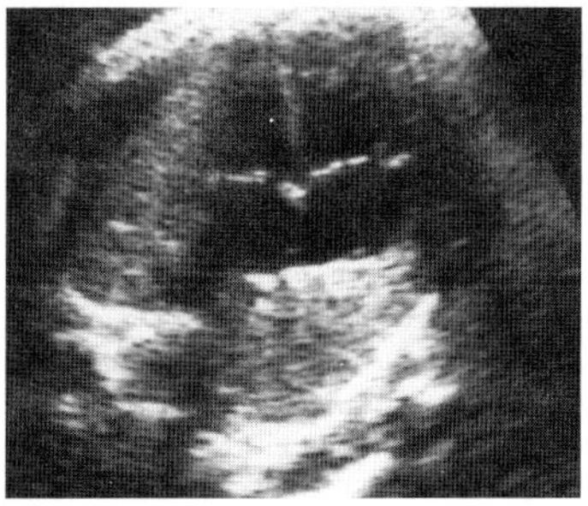

Associated Main Vasculature:
AORTA
PULMONARY ARTERY (Right and Left)
INFERIOR VENA CAVA (IVC)
SUPERIOR VENA CAVA (SVC)
DUCTUS ARTERIOSUS-channel communicating between main pulmonary artery and fetal aorta

AORTIC ARCH

1. AORTIC ARCH (A)
2. DESCENDING AORTA (DA)
3. HEAD AND NECK ARTERIES (arrows) innominate, left carotid, left subclavian
4. LEFT ATRIUM AND RT. PULMONARY ARTERY - seen in concavity of arch (H)

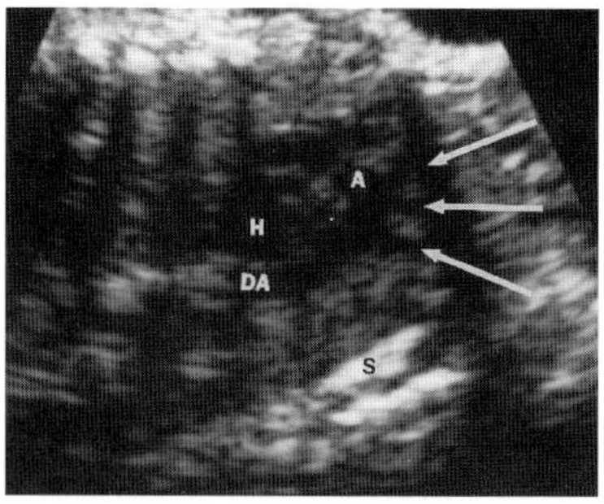

B) ABNORMAL DEVELOPMENT

SONOGRAPHIC APPEARANCES OF CHEST MASSES

congenital diaphragmatic hernia-transverse scan of fetal thorax; heart (H) in cross section with large irregular mass (M) adjacent (**)

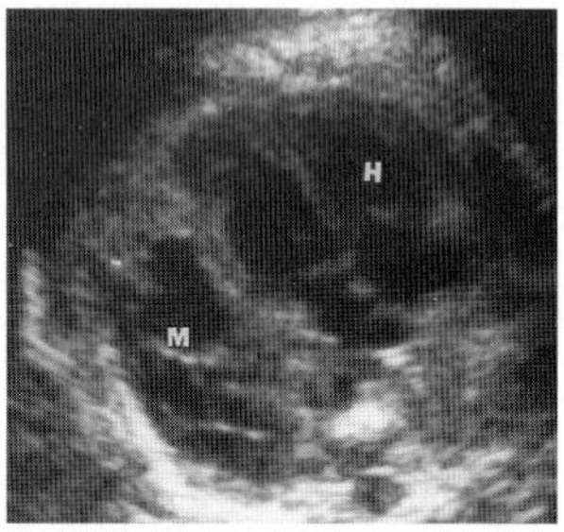

bronchogenic cyst-sagittal scan through thorax; large cystic (C) structure within lung (**)

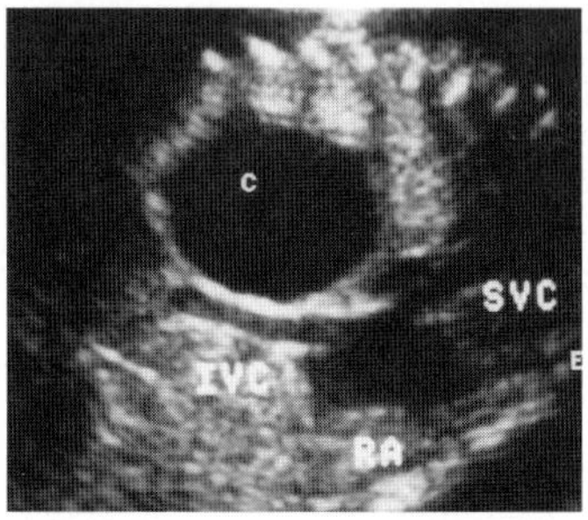

congenital cystic adenomatoid malformation of the Lung Type II- multicystic mass (**)

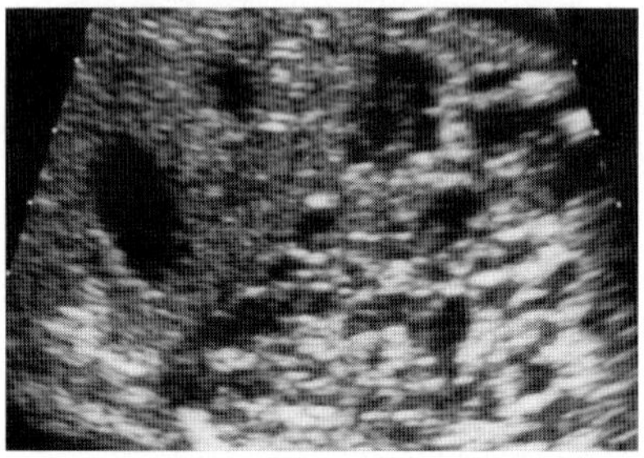

CAML Type III - solid echogenic mass (**)

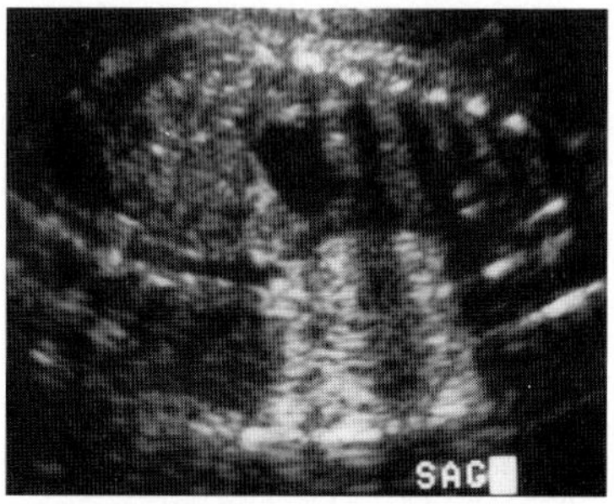

CHEST MASSES -survival correlates with degree of pulmonary hypoplastic and associated anomalies	**US FINDINGS**
BRONCHOGENIC CYSTS -abnormal development in tracheobronchial tree	-mediastinal or pulmonary unilocular or multilocular cystic masses that can cause mass effect -not commonly diagnosed
BRONCHOPULMONARY SEQUESTRATION -ectopic lung tissue which can occasionally be located in abdomen -no communication with normal bronchial tree and receives its arterial blood supply from aorta	-well defined, homogenous, highly-echogenic mass in thorax or upper abdomen -solid or may contain cysts -associated with fetal hydrops and polyhydramnios -colour doppler may detect vessel feeding it
CARDIAC TUMOURS -rare -most common type is rhabdomyoma	-must not be mistaken as chordae tendinae or papillary muscles -one or more solid masses that originate in myocardium
CONGENITAL CYSTIC ADENOMATOID MALFORMATION OF THE LUNGS (CAML) -early arrested cellular development producing abnormal alveolar differentiation, ie. adenomatoid proliferation of alveoli resulting in multiple cyst formation -cystic masses replace normal lung tissue -solitary lobar involvement is common, but multiple lobes can be affected (upper more commonly than lower lobes) -3 classifications	-multicystic (types I,II) or solid echogenic (type III) lung mass -usually diagnosed after 20 weeks -unilateral usually -inverted diaphragm CLASSIFICATIONS: Type I -small number of large cysts (most common and has the best prognosis) Type II -numerous cysts smaller than 1 cm Type III -large solid echogenic mass which occupies the entire lobe
CONGENITAL DIAPHRAGMATIC HERNIA -fusion formation defect of diaphragm resulting in herniation of abdominal contents into chest -classified according to location -most common form is Bockdalek hernia which occurs most frequently posterolaterally on the left -usually unilateral -creates mass effect which results in lung compression and reduction in fetal lung tissue and possible pulmonary hypoplasia -associated malformations: cardiac defects, neural tube defects, chromosomal abnormalities and multiple syndromes	-polyhydramnios -visualization of abdominal organs (peristalsing bowel) in thorax -displacement of the heart -fluid-filled mass behind left heart in lower thorax -absence of stomach's normal position -shift of mediastinum -small abdominal circumference
ECTOPIC CORDIS -any part of the heart outside thoracic cavity -fusion defect of anterior thoracic wall, sternum prior to 9th week LMP -several types depending on location of defect eg. thoracic/ abdominal/cervical -associated with facial, skeletal, CNS, cardiac anomalies and amniotic band syndrome	-mass (heart) outside thoracic cavity protruding through defect in either sternum, diaphragm etc.
PERICARDIAL EFFUSION -heart surrounded by fluid within pericardium -occurs with fetal hydrops from CHF or with generalized lumphedema associated with a posterior cystic hygroma	-fluid surrounding heart within pericardium
PLEURAL EFFUSION -fluid accumulated in the pleural space -associated with fetal hydrops, chest mass, fetal ascites, cardiac anomaly, chromosomal anomaly	-anechoic fluid collections in fetal chest -conform usually to chest size -large effusions can invert diaphragm

CONGENITAL CARDIAC ANOMALIES -associated with maternal conditions such as diabetes mellitus, alcoholism, TORCH	
ANOMALY	**DIAGRAM**
COARCTATION OF THE AORTA Type 1 - Juxtaductal (adult type) -focal narrowing at or just distal to ductus -most common type Type 2 - Preductal (infantile type) -area of narrowing is proximal to ductus -long segment of narrowing (associated with VSD) -always associated with a patent ductus arteriosus so that blood gets to the lower body	TYPE 1 COARCTATION OF THE AORTA 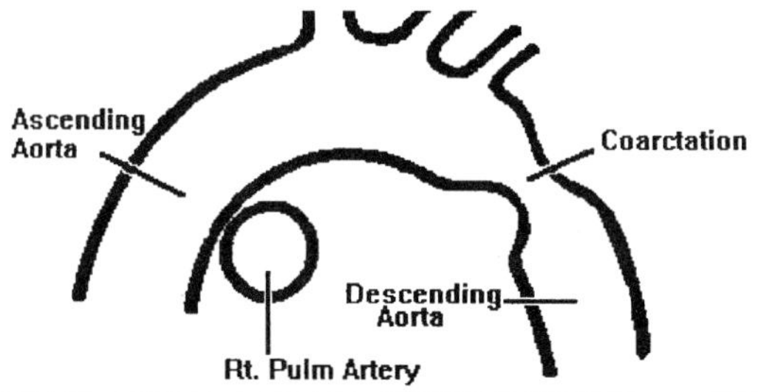
EBSTEIN'S ANOMALY -malformation of tricuspid valve where the septal tricuspid leaflet is foreshortened while the anterior leaflet is elongated -both leaflets are displaced inferiorly to create an atrialized right ventricle -causes functional obstruction to right atrial emptying resulting in increased right atrial pressure and right to left atrial shunting -causes gross tricuspid regurgitation -grossly enlarged right atrium with the atrial septum deviated to the left -associated with ASDs, tetralogy of fallot, coarctation of Aorta, Transposition of great vessels	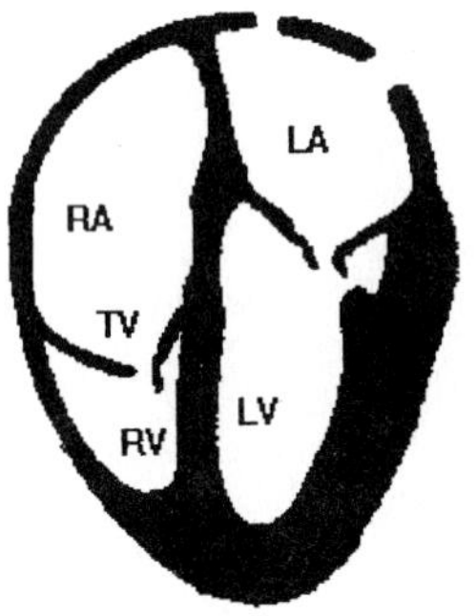

ANOMALY	DIAGRAM
HYPOPLASTIC LEFT HEART SYNDROME -left ventricle is underdeveloped and diminutive -left ventricle varies in size from slit-like to smaller than normal depending on the amount of hypoplasia of the mitral valve -enlarged right ventricle -left atrium small to normal in size -small aorta and aortic arch and may be difficult to visualize -aortic valve atresia -mitral valve is absent or hypoplastic -associated with coarctation of the aorta and aortic atresia	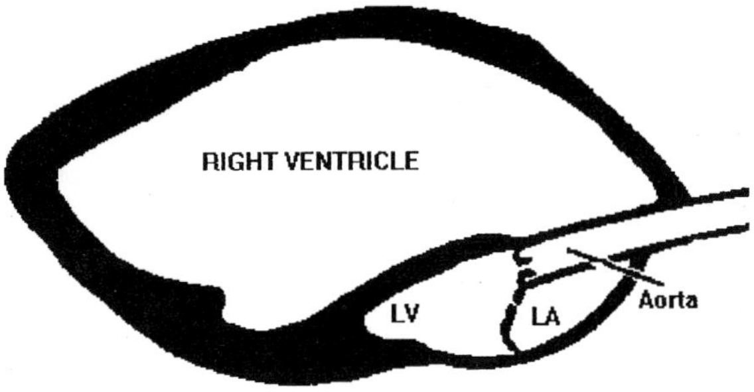
SEPTAL DEFECTS -defect or discontinuity within the septum <u>ATRIAL SEPTAL DEFECT (ASD)</u> 3 types: 1. Ostium Primum -5% of all ASDs -defect in lower part of septum adjacent to AV valves and associated with deformity of AV valve (cleft in valve) and VSD (endocardial cushion defect) -common in Down syndrome 2. Ostium Secundum -90% of ASDs -most common kind is a defect in the center or middle third of the atrial septum in area of foramen ovale -associated with patent ductus arteriosis, VSD, pulmonary stenosis, transposition of great vessels and tetrology of fallot 3. Sinus Venosus -located high in atrial septum near superior vena cava -associated with anomalous pulmonary venous return <u>VENTRICULAR SEPTAL DEFECT (VSD)</u> -interruption of the interventricular septum -can be muscular or membranous and large or small <u>Pitfalls:</u> -membranous portion of the ventricular septum may appear quite hypoechoic and should not be misinterpreted as septal defects -blood flows rapidly between the right and left atrium through the foramen ovale and should not be misinterpreted as an atrial defect	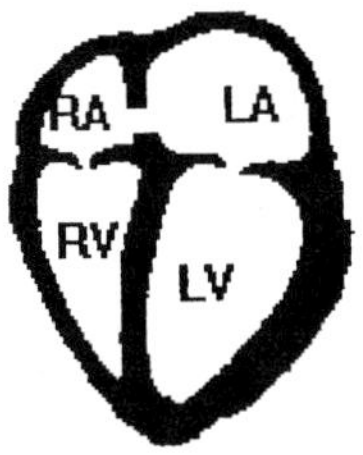 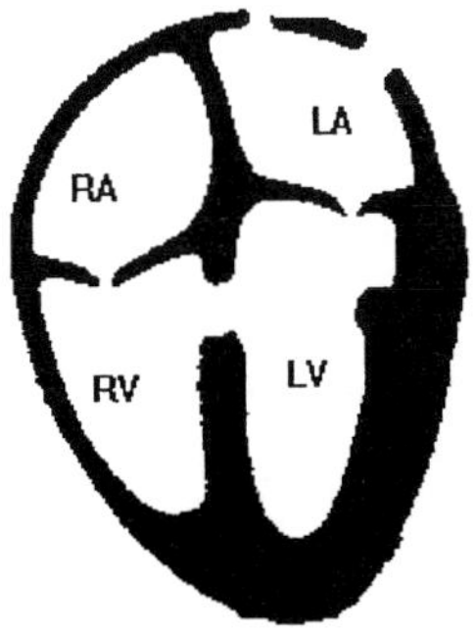

ANOMALY	DIAGRAM
SINGLE VENTRICLE -single ventricular chamber due to absent ventricular septum -however, usually refers to 2 ventricles where one is rudimentary and one is dominant -transposition is often present but of little functional significance -two varieties: 1. both mitral and tricuspid valves present 2. mitral or tricuspid valve absent	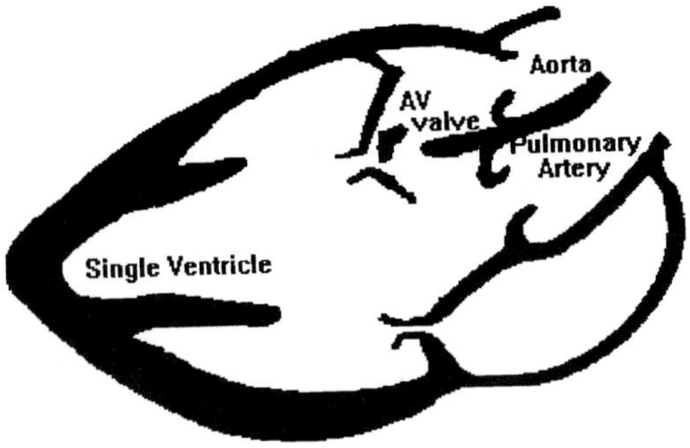
TETROLOGY OF FALLOT -right ventricle hypertrophy (in utero the ventricles may be symmetrical) -ventricular septal defect (VSD) -some form of pulmonary artery stenosis; pulmonary valve or artery or both -absent pulmonary (RV) outflow tract with pulmonary atresia -overriding aorta; dilated aorta overrides a VSD	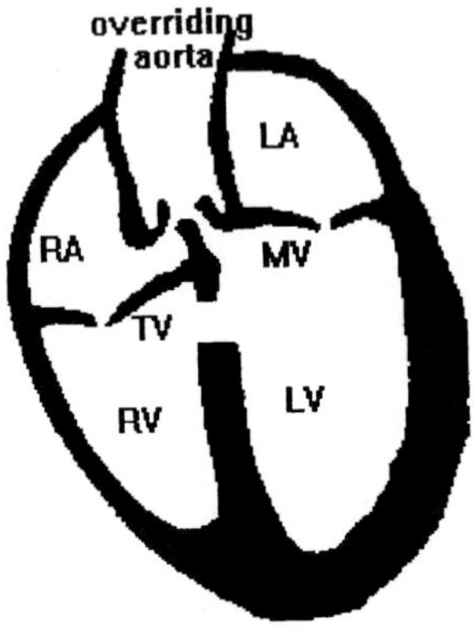
TRANSPOSITION OF THE GREAT ARTERIES -aorta arises from right ventricle and supplies systemic circulation -pulmonary artery arises from left ventricle and supplies the lungs -anterior rightward origin of the aorta -posterior leftward origin of the pulmonary artery -associated anomalies: pulmonic stenosis, VSD, underdevelopment of right or left ventricles, coarctation of the aorta	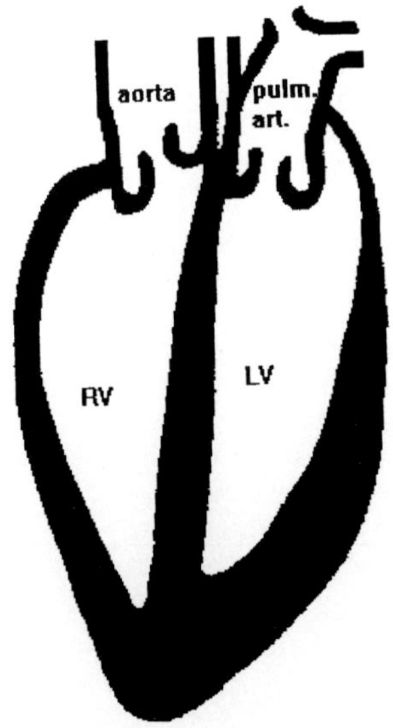

ANOMALY	DIAGRAM
TRUNCUS ARTERIOSIS -single large truncal artery arising from the base of the heart which supplies the coronary, pulmonary and systemic arterial circulations -absent right ventricular outflow tract -associated anomalies: VSD, ASD, situs inversus, GU anomalies, asplenia	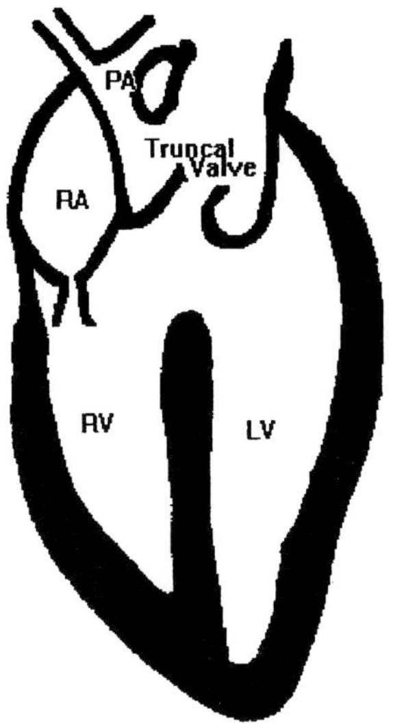

DIFFERENTIAL FOR ABNORMAL HEART CHAMBER SIZE	
SMALL LEFT VENTRICLE	hypoplastic left heart syndrome coarctation or hypoplasia of the aortic arch
SMALL RIGHT VENTRICLE	pulmonary atresia (with or without ventricular septal defect) tricuspid atresia (with or without ventricular septal defect) aortic stenosis or insufficiency
ENLARGED RIGHT ATRIUM	ebsteins anomaly tricuspid dysplasia tricuspid regurgitation without inferior displacement of valve

SECTION 5. SKELETAL (APPENDICULAR AND AXIAL) SYSTEM

A) NORMAL ANATOMY AND DEVELOPMENT

SKELETAL SYSTEM EMBRYOLOGY		
MESODERM Mesenchyme Proliferation ⇓		
INTRACARTILAGINOUS OSSIFICATION bone formed where the pre-existing cartilage was		INTRAMEMBRANOUS OSSIFICATION bone formed in mesenchyme without cartilage formation
LONG BONES (eg. femur, humerus)	**VERTEBRAL COLUMN**	**FLAT BONES (eg. clavicle, mandible)**
Ossification Process	3 Primary Ossification Centres	Ossification Process
1. begins in middle of shaft at diaphysis 2. progresses outward toward ends of bone or epiphyses 3. near birth ossification centers form in epiphyses 4. metaphysis is the area of cartilage that persists between epiphyses and diaphysis, where growth takes place	1. CENTRUM (body) -ossified first at thoraco-lumbar region then progresses toward both ends of spine from there 2 & 3. NEURAL -located on each side of posterior neural arch -ossifies first at base of transverse process then proceeds to ossify anterior to pedicles and posterior to laminae	mesenchymal cells differentiate into ↓ osteoblasts create ↓ osteoid which forms primary center of ossification where new bony trabeculae are formed

FIRST APPEARANCE OF OSSIFICATION CENTRES OF APPENDICULAR SKELETON	
7-8 weeks	clavicles, mandible, palate
9 weeks	frontal bones, zygomatic arch, femur
10-11 weeks	occipital, parietal bone, ribs, scapula, ileum, long bones, phalanges
by 16 weeks	metacarpals, metatarsals, ishium
22-24 weeks	talus, calcaneus
32 weeks	secondary ossification centres of distal femoral epiphysis
35 weeks	secondary ossification centres of proximal tibial epiphysis

SONOGRAPHIC APPEARANCES OF SKELETAL SYSTEM

sagittal fetal mandible, maxilla (1st trimester)

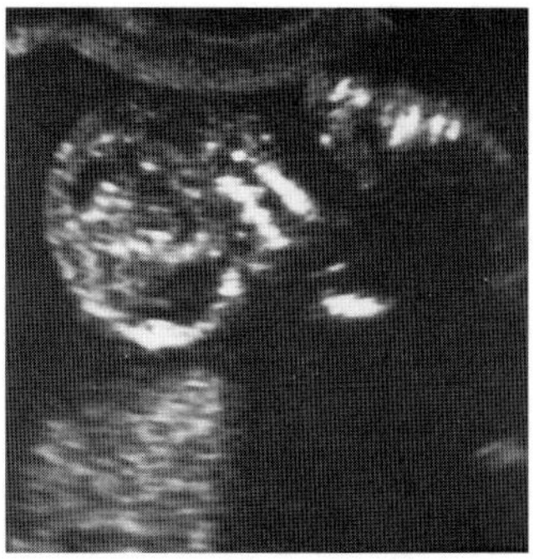

humerus (3rd trimester)

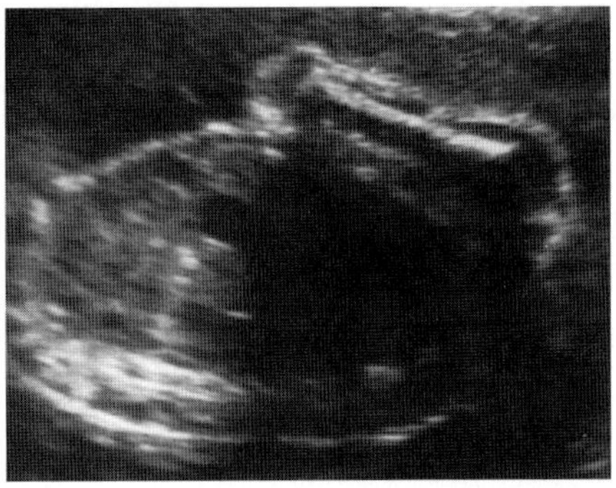

femur (1st trimester)

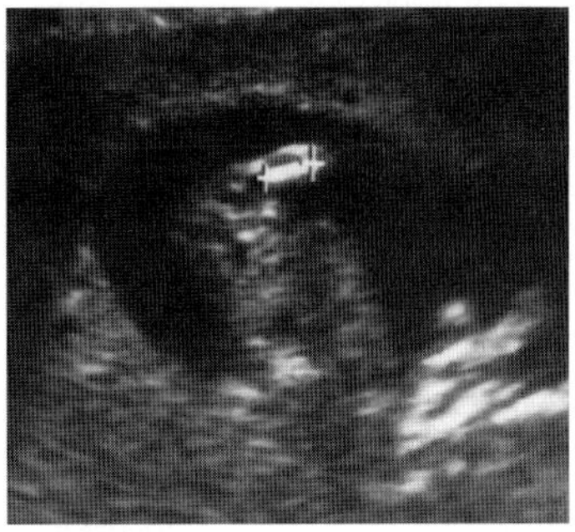

arm (with fingers) and head (1st trimester)

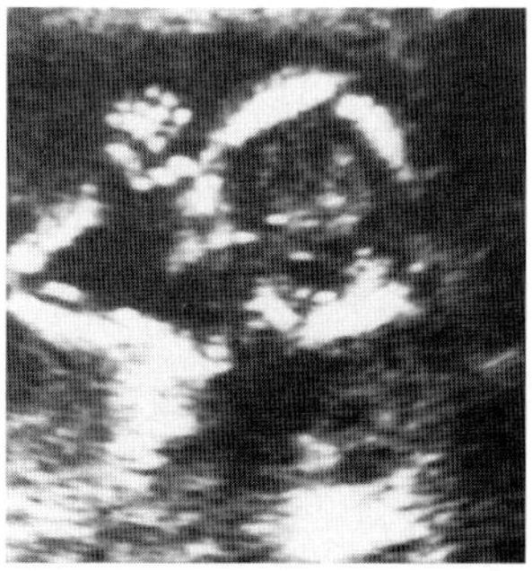

both forearms and hands (2nd trimester)

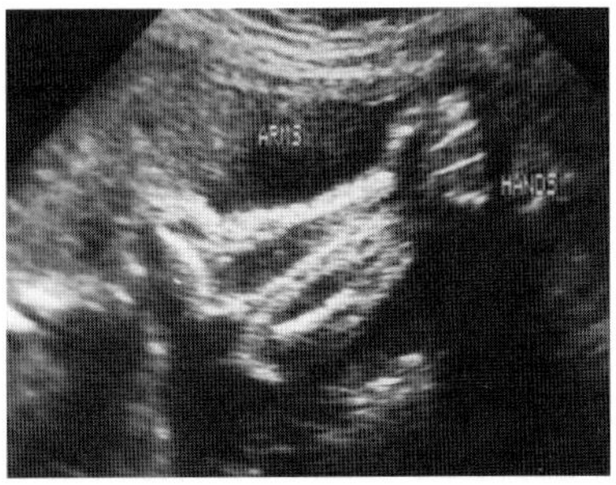

both legs within amniotic sac (1st trimester)

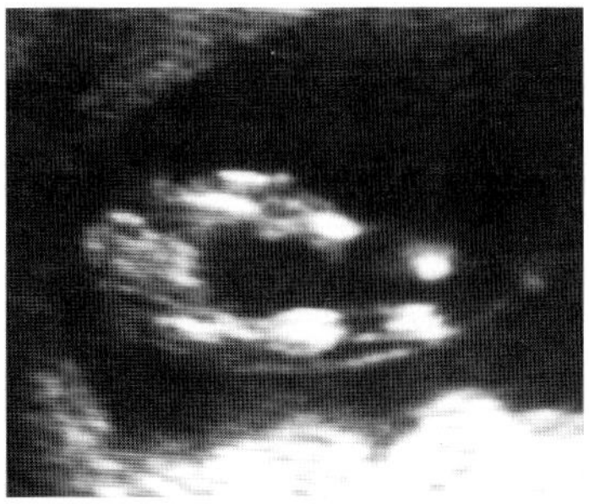

fingers (3rd trimester)

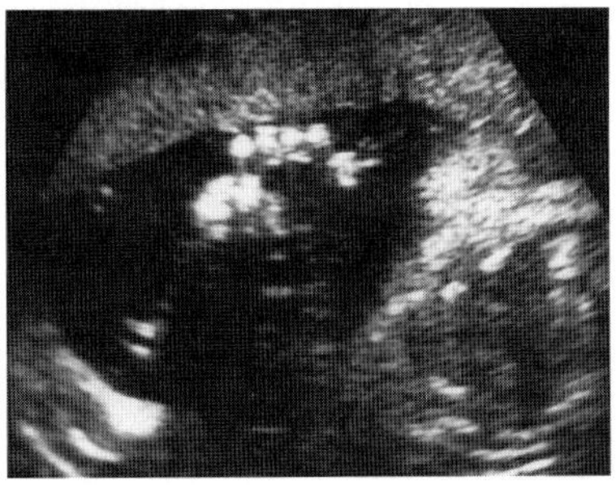

foot (3rd trimester)

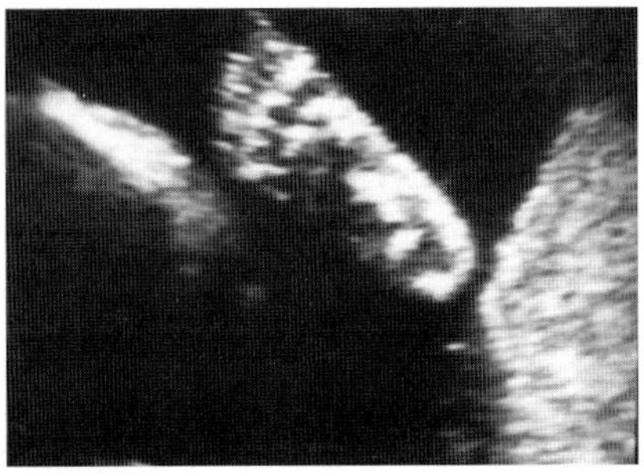

femur (on left) and tibia-fibula (on right) (2nd trimester)

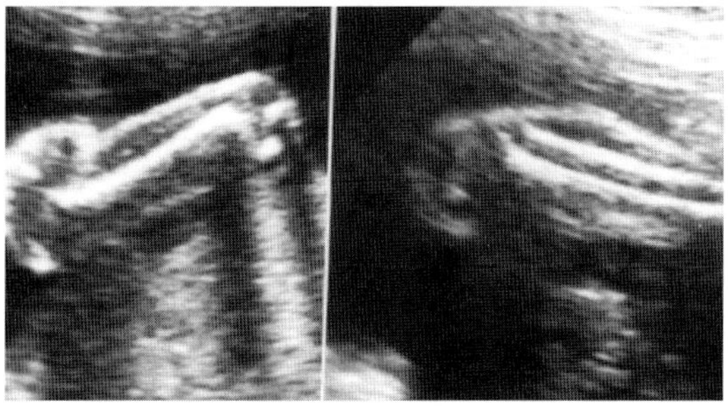

FIRST APPEARANCE OF LAMINAE OSSIFICATION IN THE AXIAL SKELETON

-imaged best in transverse axial scan plane to show normal inward angulation of laminae of the posterior neural arch
-longitudinal scan plane shows posterior elements as parallel echos with a normal flair at upper cervical spine, slight widening at lumbar region and convergence at sacrum
-primary centers of ossification of vertebral bodies and neural arches begin to from at 9 weeks
cervical spine: best seen at 18–19 weeks
thoracic spine: best seen at 20–22 weeks
lumbar spine: best seen at 22–24 weeks
sacrum: best seen at 25 weeks

Spine in first trimester	transvaginal coronal scan of fetal lumbar spine at 10 weeks 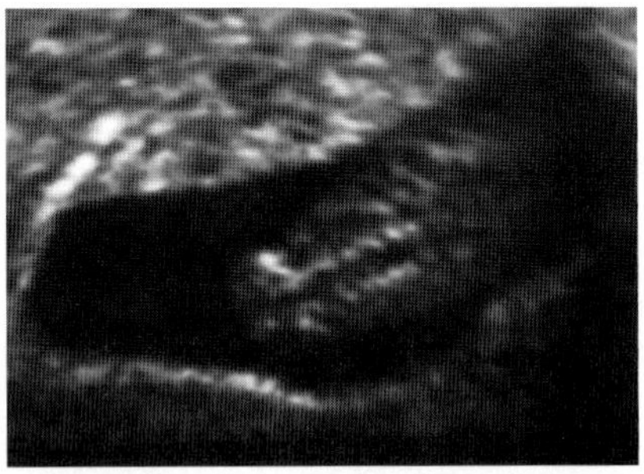	spine in first trimester 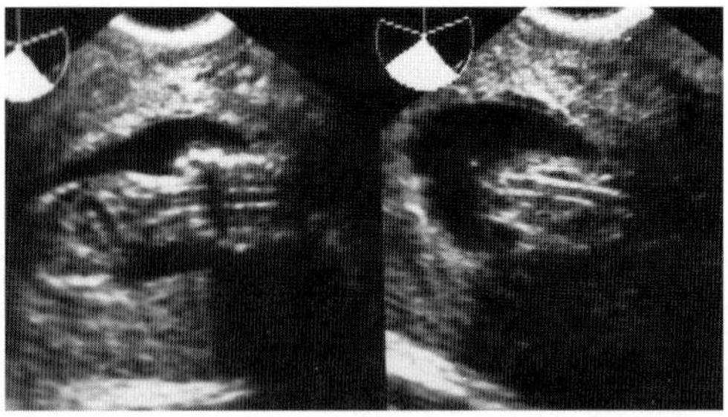
Spine in second trimester	transverse view of spine; three ossification centres (arrows) 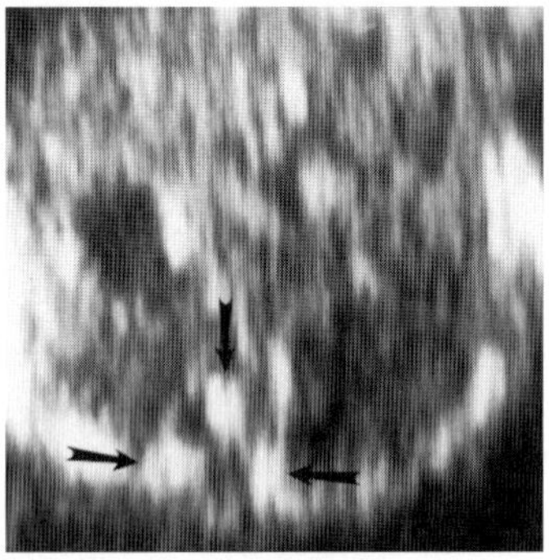	coronal view of length of spine 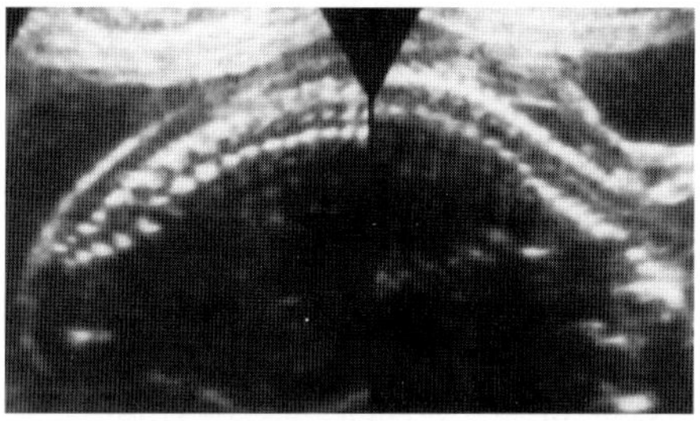
	transverse view of sacral spine 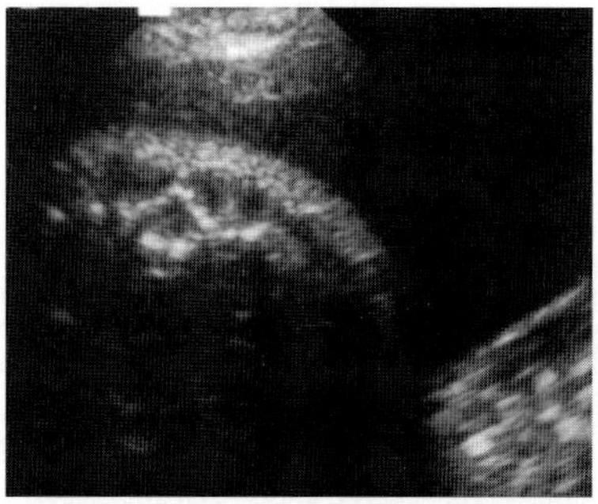	coronal view of lumbar spine and sacrum 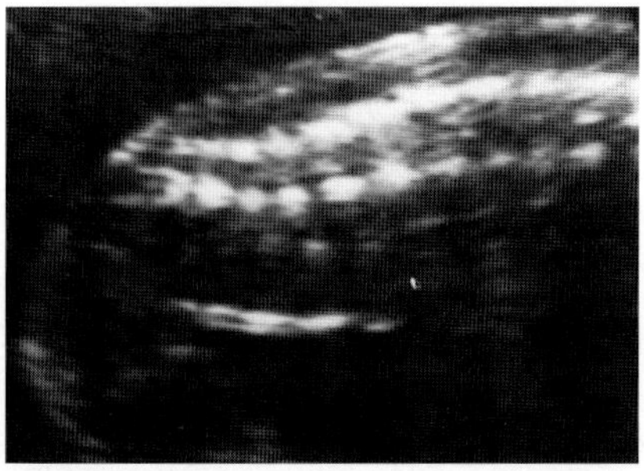

B) ABNORMAL DEVELOPMENT AND ANOMALIES

LIMB ANOMALIES -TERMINOLOGY		
BONE SHORTENING	Acromelia	-shortening of distal segments ie. hand
	Mesomelia	-shortening of middle segments ie. forearm, tib/fib
	Micromelia	-shortening involves entire limb ie. humerus, radius + ulna, hand
	Platyspondylisis	-flatness of vertebral bodies
	Rhizomelia	-shortening of proximal segments ie. humerus, femur
ABSENCE DEFORMITIES	Acheiria	-absence of hand
	Acheiropodia	-absence of hand and foot
	Adactyly	-absence of fingers or toes
	Amelia	-absence of an extremity
	Dystoses	-absence or malformation of individual bones
	Extrodactyly	-absence of fingers or toes
	Hemimelia	-absence of extremity below knee or elbow
	Phocomelia (Tetra....)	-absence of middle segment with preservation of proximal and distal segments
FUSION ANOMALIES	Lobster Claw	-abnormal cleft between 2nd & 4th metacarpals and absence of 3rd and fusion of 1+2, 3+4
	Sirenomelia	-fusion of legs "mermaid syndrome", severe manifestation of caudal regression syndrome
	Syndactyly	-fusion of fingers or toes

SOME MORE COMMONLY REFERRED TO APPENDICULAR ANOMALIES VISUALIZED SONOGRAPHICALLY	ASSOCIATED WITH
Amputation of limbs -congenital absence of limbs	Amniotic Band Syndrome limb body wall complex isolated entity
Clinodactyly -overlapping digits	trisomy 13,18 various syndromes
Clubfoot / Talipes Equinovarus -sole of foot is turned inward and foot is adducted and plantar flexed	isolated entity trisomy 18
Hitchhiker's thumb -abnormal flexion of thumb	diastrophic dysplasia
Polydactyly -more than the normal number of fingers or toes	trisomy 13, 18 skeletal dysplasias isolated entity various syndromes
"Rockerbottom" feet -foot deformity which includes short 1st digit, hammer toes and hypoplastic distal phalanges	trisomy 13, 18
Splayed first and second toes	trisomy 21

ULTRASOUND APPEARANCE

club foot (**)

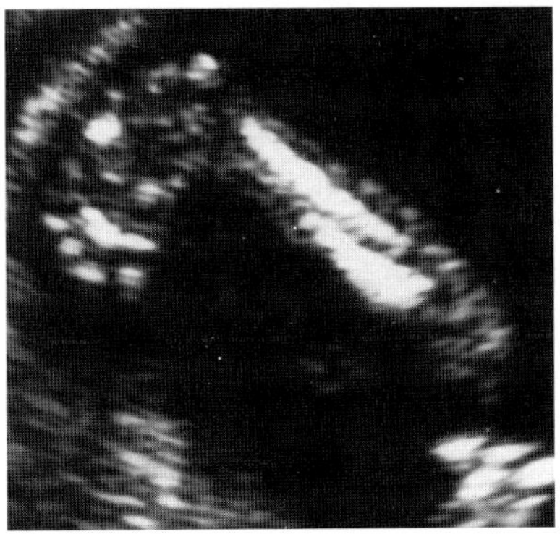

polydactyl

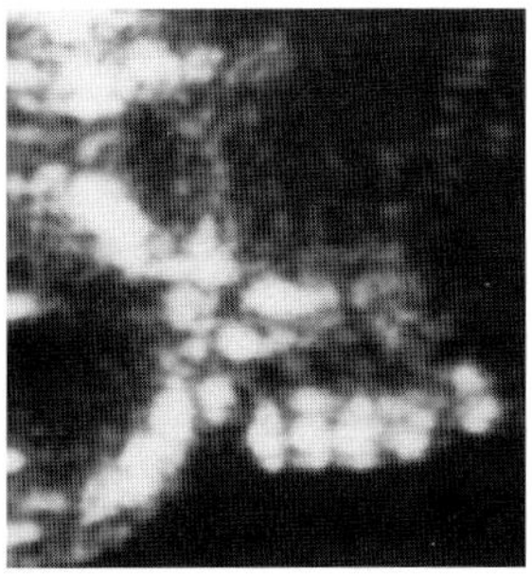

splayed 1st and 2nd toe (arrow)

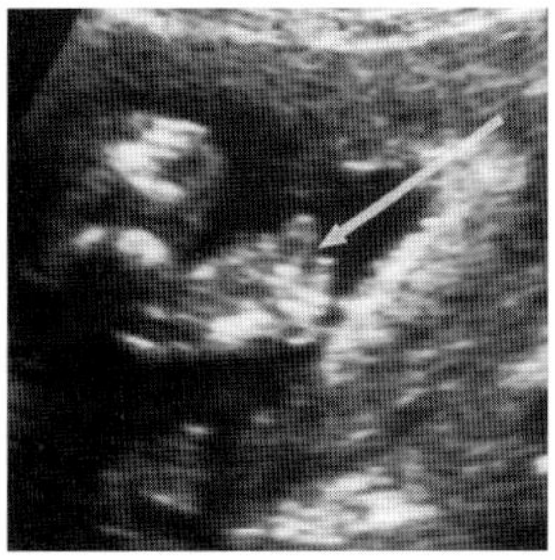

SPINAL ANOMALIES	US FINDINGS	US APPEARANCES
CAUDAL REGRESSION & SACRAL AGENESIS -sacrum and coccyx are absent -with caudal regression- hypoplasia, reduction or fusion (sirenomelia) of pelvis and lower extremities -associated with uncontrolled maternal diabetes mellitus	-flexed lower extremities immediately inferior to liver -spine ending near level of liver -lower limb anomalies (hypoplasia, reduction or fusion)	posterior sagittal image of thorax and abdomen shows spine (S) ending near level of liver (Li); fetal head is lying toward right 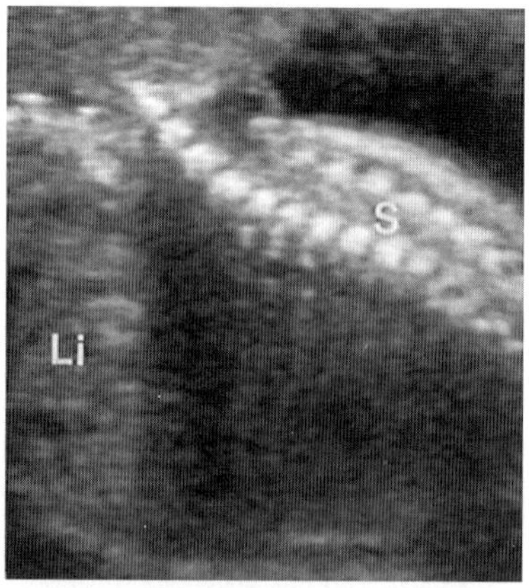
CURVATURE ABNORMALITIES KYPHOSIS -abnormal anterior curvature of spine caused by failure of formation or failure of segmentation of the spine SCOLIOSIS -abnormal lateral curvature of spine -seen with hemivertebra or as part of a group of anomalies	-marked abnormal bending of spine	spina bifida with marked lumbar kyphosis 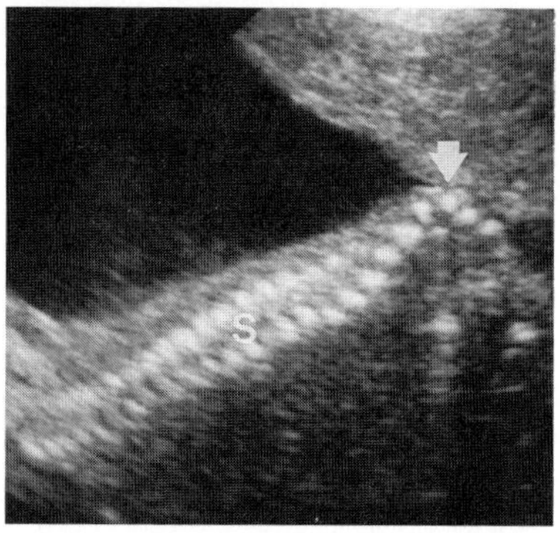
		coronal scan of lumbar spine shows splaying of posterior elements 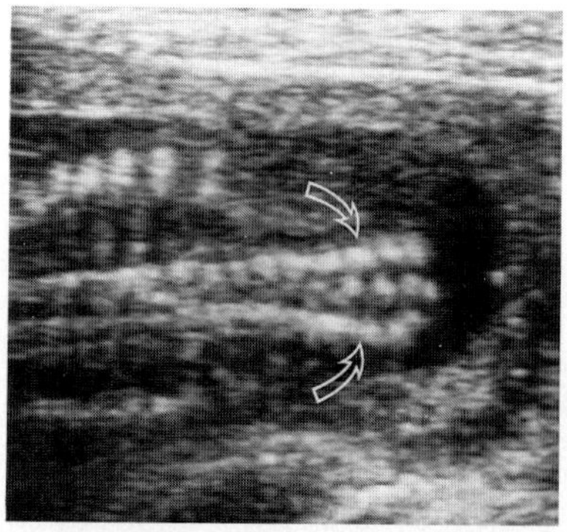

SPINAL ANOMALIES	US FINDINGS	US APPEARANCES
SPINA BIFIDA -abnormal or incomplete fusion of laminae neural arch with varying degree of central nervous system involvement -can occur anywhere along spinal axis Classified as: <u>1. Open</u>: (80%) -defect is uncovered or covered with a thin translucent membrane <u>2. Closed</u>: (20%) -defect is covered with skin or thick opaque membrane <u>SPINA BIFIDA OCCULTA</u> -failure of vertebrae to close **without** hernial protrusion -often is asymptomatic and not visualized prenatally <u>SPINA BIFIDA CYSTICA</u> -failure of vertebrae to close **with** sacular protrusion through the spinal defect -further subdivided: 1. Meningocele: sac + CSF only 2. Myelomeningocele: sac + CSF + neural elements <u>SPINAL DYSRAPHIA</u> -bony spina bifida + caudal displacement of spinal cord	-separation and splaying outward of laminae which varies with location and size of defect -seen as separation of the posterior ossification centers -deviated posterior elements of spine best seen with transverse scan plane -detected optimally at 17–18 weeks -soft tissue findings with spinal bifida cystica are associated with cranial findings (Chiari malformations)	coronal scan of spine with splaying of the neural arch (**) 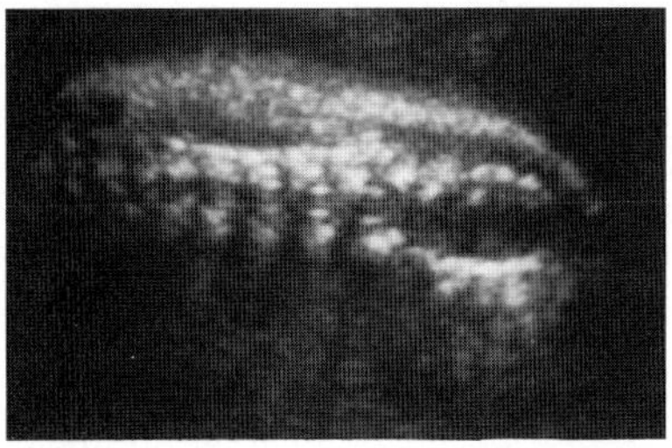 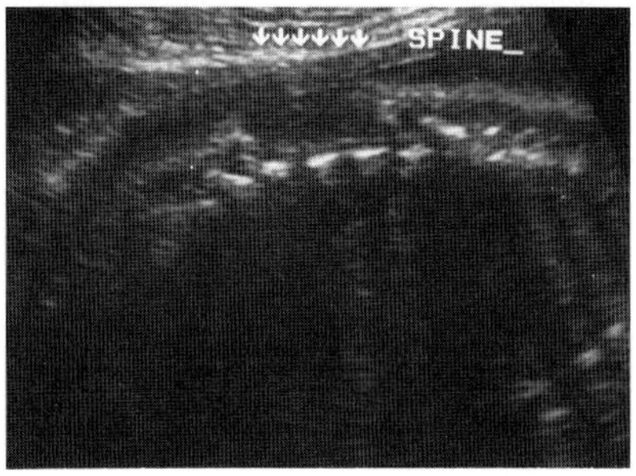 transverse scan of spine with splaying of the neural arch and soft tissue protrusion 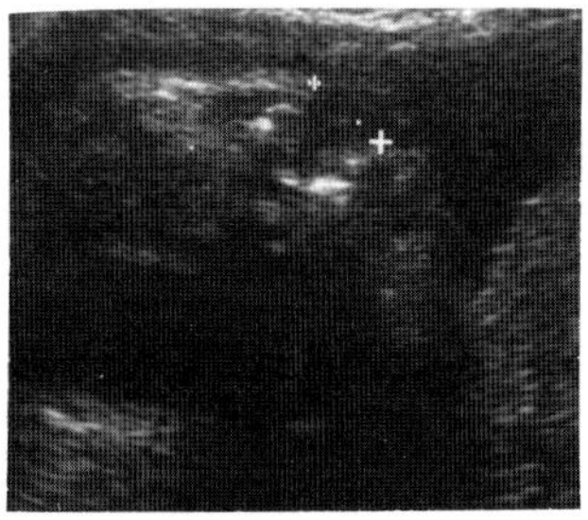 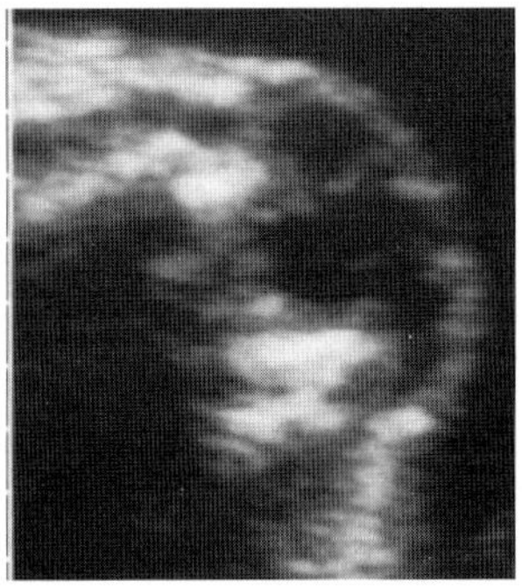 sagittal scan of spine with herniation of some spinal elements through the bony defect 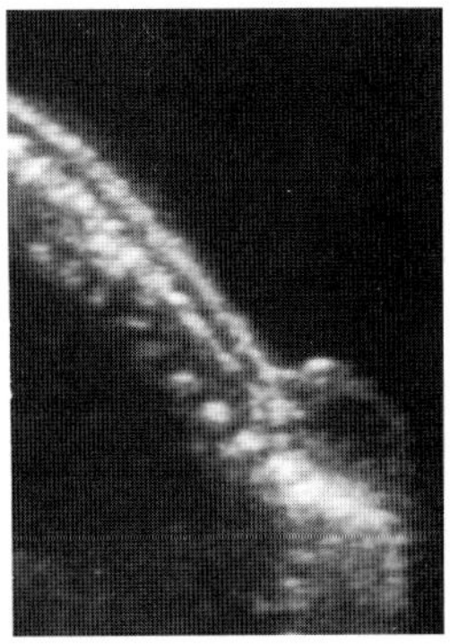 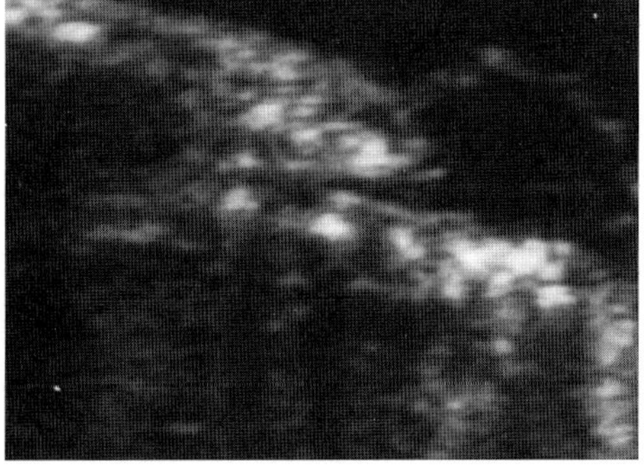

LETHAL SKELETAL DYSPLASIA

ABNORMALITY	BONE LENGTH	BONE SHAPE/MINERALIZATION	COMMENTS
ACHONDROGENESIS	-severe micromelia -diffuse shortening	-focal hypomineralization: spine and sacrum are demineralized with normal ossified skull -bone bowing, fractures	-autosomal recessive
CAMPOLMELIC DYSPLASIA	-mild micromelia -limbs short due to bowing	-anterior bowing of femur, tib + fib but all have normal length -scoliosis: spine anomalies -hypoplastic scapulae -narrow chest	-autosomal recessive or sporadic
HOMOZYGOUS ACHONDROPLASTIC -resembles Thanatophoric Dysplasia	-rhizomelia	-bowing -cloverleaf skull/large head -rib fractures -narrow thorax	-parent(s) have heterozygous achondroplasia -autosomal dominant
HYPOPHOSPHATASIA	-normal	-bowed long bones -hypomineralization, thin delicate bones -bone fractures but no rib fractures	-autosomal recessive
OSTEOGENESIS IMPERFECTA TYPE II	-extreme micromelia -diffuse shortening	-curved or bowed long bones -hypomineralization -multiple bone and rib fractures -long bones "thickened" and angulated	-autosomal recessive or sporadic
SHORT RIB POLYDACTYLY	-severe micromelia -short ribs, tibias	-narrow thorax -polydactyly	-autosomal recessive -possible cleft lip, renal cysts
THANATOPHORIC DYSPLASIA	-extreme micromelia -diffuse shortening	-cloverleaf skull (Kleeblattschadel) -bowed long bones -narrow thorax -narrow spine with flattened vertebral bodies -large head /hydrocephalus	-parents of normal stature (sporadic inheritance) -most common lethal dwarfism -polyhydramnios
NON-LETHAL BONE DYSPLASIA			
HETEROZYGOUS ACHONDROPLASIA	-rhizomelia (mild to moderate shortening)	-femoral and humeral lengths drop off after 20 weeks, therefore head size and femur length discrepancy becomes more apparent in 3rd trimester	-most common nonlethal bone dysplasia -autosomal dominant -good prognosis
OSTEOGENESIS IMPERFECTA TYPE I +IV	-overall normal limb length	-extreme bone bowing with fractures may occur in 3rd trimester	-autosomal dominant -rarely spontaneous -Type I produces deafness

Thanatophoric Dysplasia: coronal image of the thorax and abdomen at 24 weeks shows a "bell"-shaped or narrow thorax (white arrows) with larger abdomen (black arrows)

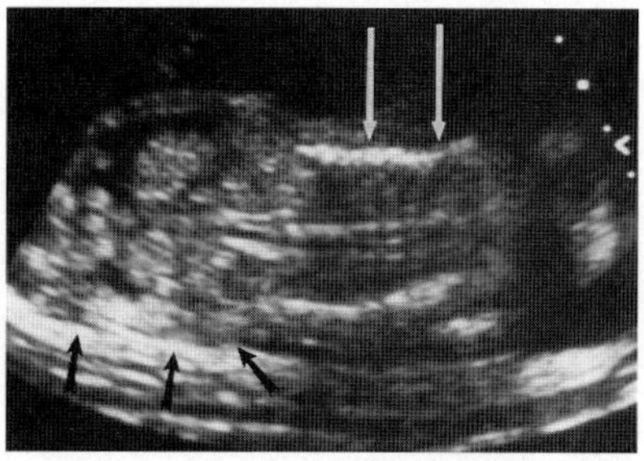

Dwarf with shortening of humerus (H), radius and ulna (R) and hand (H) of unknown nature

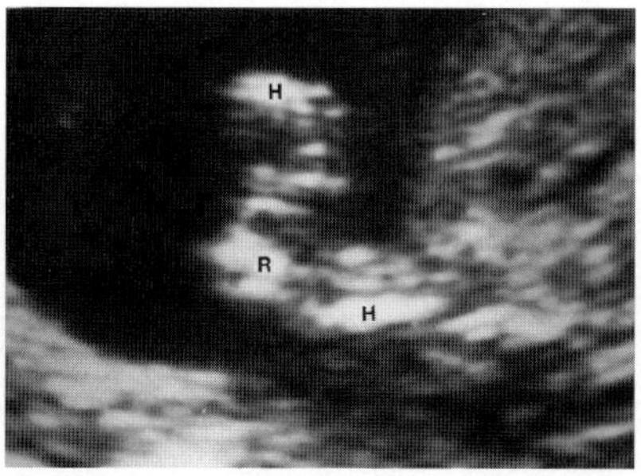

CHAPTER 9
SEQUENCES, SYNDROMES, ASSOCIATIONS AND CHROMOSOMAL ABNORMALITIES

Sequence: occurs when a single defect leads to the development of one or more abnormalities
Syndrome: two or more embryonically unrelated anomalies occur together at a relatively high occurrence. Two or more different body areas must be involved
Association: nonrandom occurrence of two or more structural defects that occur together more frequently than by chance alone; they are not the result of a sequence
Chromosomal Abnormalities: as the number of sonographically detectable defects increase, the likelihood of chromosome abnormality also increases
-this chapter lists some more commonly found sequences, syndromes, associations and chromosomal abnormalities in sonography

CONDITION	US FINDINGS
AMNIOTIC BAND SYNDROME -early rupture of amnion results in amniotic bands that stick, entangle and disrupt fetal parts resulting in congenital malformations	-abnormal sheet or band that attaches to fetus or flaps with fetal movement -restriction of fetal mobility due to entrapment by amniotic bands -fetal deformities and malformations: extremity amputation, edema, postural and body wall defects, facial clefts, etc.
BECKWITH–WEIDEMANN SYNDROME -autosomal dominant -placental endocrine dysfuntion leading to increased level of growth hormone causing viseromegaly -early viseromegaly leads to omphalocele, malrotation anomalies and diaphragmatic hernia	-omphalocele -macroglossia -gigantism -hepatosplenomegaly -nephromegaly -cardiac anomalies
CAUDAL REGRESSION SYNDROME or SIRENOMELIA SEQUENCE -associated with poorly controlled maternal diabetes mellitus -defect of primitive streak which causes incomplete development of the caudal portion of the embryo -variable absence of structures derived from caudal axis	-absent lower spine and sacrum -hemivertebra -no bladder -single umbilical artery -genital defects -renal agenesis and oligohydramnios sequence -fusion of lower extremities -imperforate anus, absent rectum
CLOACAL EXSTROPHY -rare and fatal -nondevelopment of the urorectal septum which leads to other congenital abnormalities	-omphalocele -exstrophy of bladder with resulting nonvisualization of bladder -imperforate anus -spinal defects (meningomyelocele) -single umbilical artery
LIMB–BODY WALL COMPLEX -shortened umbilical cord caused by the peritoneal cavity and chorionic cavity's failure to separate -abdominal contents remain in the chorionic cavity	-scoliosis -limb defects -large body wall defects -neural tube defects
MECKEL–GRUBER SYNDROME -autosomal recessive -midtrimester onset -pulmonary hypoplasia from severe oligohydramnios	-occipital encephalocele -polycystic kidneys -microcephaly -polydactyly -facial clefts -oligohydramnios
PENTALOGY OF CANTRELL -associated with 2 major defects: omphalocele and ectopic heart -defect in sternum, anterior diaphragm and diaphragmatic pericardium	-omphalocele -ectopic heart (complete or partial through defect sternum) -pleural / cardiac effusion
POTTERS SEQUENCE -single malformation - renal agenesis that gives rise to multiple deformations such as Potter facies rounded forehead, hypoplastic ears, micrognathia	-oligohydramnios -no kidneys -urinary bladder not seen
PRUNE BELLY SYNDROME -series of pathological events related to bladder outlet obstruction -enlarged fetal bladder prevents testicular descent, distends the abdominal wall and stretches its musculature	-bladder outlet obstruction - huge bladder -abdominal wall laxity -cryptorchidism -oligohydramnios -bilateral hydronephrosis

CONDITION	US FINDINGS
ROBERT SYNDROME -autosomal recessive inheritance	-microcephaly -limb reduction -IUGR -atrial septal defect -facial clefts
TORCH -mnemonic for congenital infections toxoplasmosis, rubella, cytomegalovirus, herpes simplex virus, syphilis	-microcephaly -hydocephaly, hydranencephaly -Dandy–Walker Syndrome -periventricular calcification -cardiac anomalies -liver calcifications
TRIPLOIDY SYNDROME -complete extra set of chromosomes (2 sperm fertilize 1 egg) -most miscarry, therefore, live births rare	-IUGR -renal anomalies (multicystic renal dysplasia, hydronephrosis) -ambiguous genitalia -congenital heart disease -omphalocele -facial clefts -central nervous system malformations (holoprosencephaly, agenesis of corpus callosum, hydrocephalus, meningocele)
TRISOMY 13 - PATAU SYNDROME -mental retardation, seizures, failure to thrive -very high infant mortality	-IUGR -polyhydramnios -congenital heart disease (VSD, ASD, dextrocardia) -midline defects-central nervous system malformations (holoprosencephaly, agenesis of corpus callosum) -craniofacial malformations (micrognathia, facial clefts) -extremity anomalies (polydactyly, rocker bottom feet) -renal malformations (cysts, hydronephrosis, horseshoe kidneys) -omphalocele
TRISOMY 18 - EDWARD SYNDROME -second most common cytogenetic abnormality -severe mental retardation, failure to thrive -extremely high infant mortality	-IUGR -polyhydramnios -congenital heart disease -diaphragmatic hernia -omphalocele -esophageal atresia (VACTERL) -renal anomalies (hydronephrosis, horseshoe kidney) -extremity abnormalities (clubfoot, rocker bottom feet, clenched hands) -craniofacial malformations (micrognathia, dolichocephaly) -intracranial malformations (large cisterna magna, choroid plexus cysts)
TRISOMY 21 - DOWN SYNDROME -most common cytogenetic abnormality -moderate retardation - can range from mild to severe -high mortality during first year of life from congestive heart failure or leukemia	-thickened nucal skin fold -cystic hygroma -mildly dilated cerebral ventricles -congenital heart disease -esophageal / duodenal atresia -diaphragmatic hernia -nonimmune hydrops -renal pyelectasis -short femur and humerus -clinodactyly of 5th digit -wide space between first and second toes
TURNER SYNDROME - 45X0 -short stature, webbed neck, hearing loss, renal malformations, congenital heart disease -low IQ, but mental retardation is rare -abnormal sex chromosomes and sexual development	-cystic hygroma -nonimmune hydrops -renal anomalies -cardiac malformations (coarctation of aorta)
VACTERL(S) ASSOCIATION -combination of associated anomalies V - vertebral A - anal atresia C - cardiac TE - tracheoesophageal fistula R - renal L - limb S - single umbilical artery	-fetuses with one anomaly should be screened for associated other anomalies -anomaly number and type relate to prognosis -IUGR

CHAPTER 10 - MULTIPLE GESTATION

MULTIPLE GESTATIONS	
FREQUENCY	1:90 for twin pregnancy 1:90 x 90 for triplets 1:90 x 90 x 90 for quadruplets
PREDISPOSING FACTORS	-advanced maternal age -multiparas -post-pill pregnancies -ovulation-inducing agents -maternal history of twinning
CLINICAL SIGNS	-hyperemesis gravidarum ($\uparrow\uparrow$ hCG) -large for dates -more than 1 heart beat
RISKS AND COMPLICATIONS	-higher rates of mortality than singleton pregnancies with triplets and quads have an even higher mortality -prematurity -growth retardation -placental insufficiency

US APPEARANCE OF MULTIPLE GESTATIONS

-may be diagnosed from 6 weeks
-care must be used in order to exclude artifacts and uterine anomalies that could result in a false diagnosis (rare split image artifact; collection of fluid adjacent to gestational sac, uterine septum)

transvaginal axial scan of uterus at 5 weeks gestation; two gestation sacs, each with their own yolk sac is demonstrated; separating membrane seen	transvaginal axial scan of uterus with two gestational sacs with fetal poles and a very thick separating membrane-dichorionic diamniotic	three fetuses are visualized within their own gestational sac; this was actually quadruplets, the 4th not in this scan plane
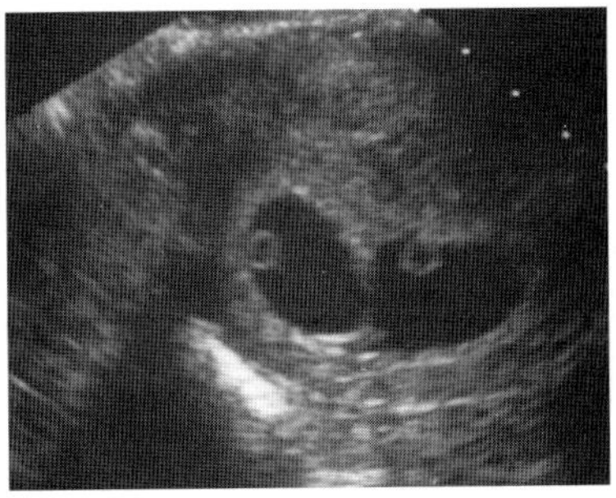	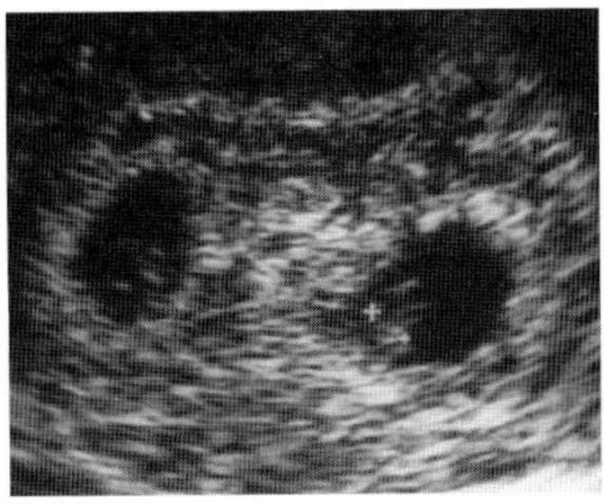	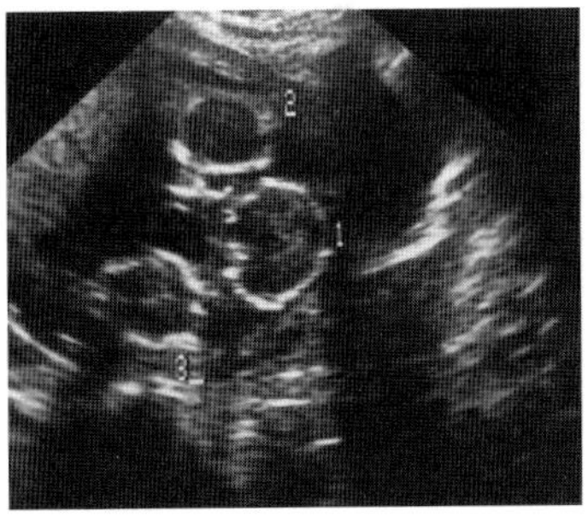

TYPE OF TWINNING - EMBRYOLOGY	MEMBRANES BETWEEN FETUSES	NUMBER OF PLACENTAS
DIZYGOTIC TWINS (70%) - FRATERNAL -most common type of twins; incidence related to heredity -genetically different - male:female pair indicates dizygotic twins -simultaneous shedding of two oocytes and the fertilization by two different spermatozoa -blastocysts implant separately and develop own placenta, amnion and chorionic sac -least risk of complications in twin pregnancy	4 LAYERS 2 layers of chorion 2 layers of amnion	2 PLACENTAS -may be separate but can fuse -rarely anastomose circulations

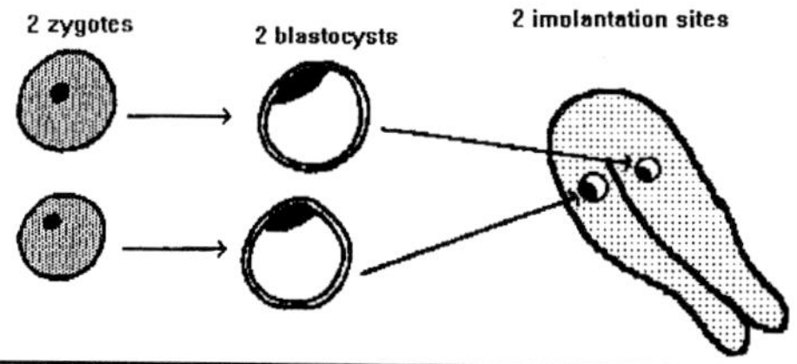

MONOZYGOTIC TWINS (30% OF TWINS) - 3 TYPES
-incidence not related to heredity
-division of single fertilized ovum; same sex and identical genetic makeup
-3 patterns of chorionicity and amnionicity depend on the stage at which the fertilized ovum splits

1-DICHORIONIC DIAMNIOTIC (25% of monozygotic twins) -early separation at 2 cell stage (3rd day), which results in two separate zygotes -both blastocysts implant separately -each embryo has its own placenta and chorionic sac -membranes resembles dizygotic twins	4 LAYERS 2 layers of chorion 2 layers of amnion	2 PLACENTAS can fuse and appear as one

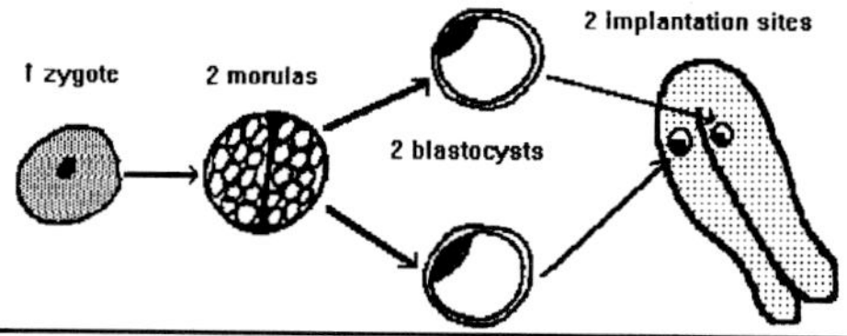

2-MONCHORIONIC DIAMNIOTIC (75% of monozygotic twins) -most common type of monozygotic twinning -divides at inner cell mass stage, days 4–8; chorion already developed -one blastocyst, therefore, one implantation site and one placenta -risk for twin-to-twin transfusion -greater mortality than dichorionic twins	2 LAYERS -2 layers of amnion -one chorionic sac, two amniotic sacs	1 PLACENTA

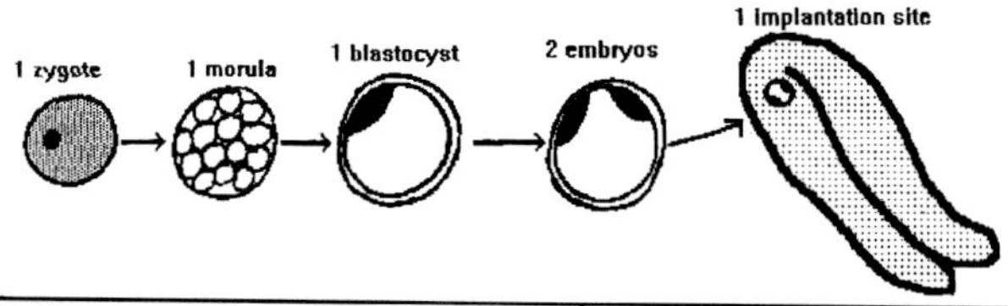

3-MONCHORIONIC MONOAMNIOTIC (2% of monozygotic twins- rare) -division of bilaminar disc just before appearance of primitive streak but after formation of the amniotic cavity; between day 8 and 13 -high association of addition risks: entanglement of cord, twin-to-twin transfusion -division occurring after embryonic disc formation results in co-joined twins -high fetal mortality	0 LAYERS -no separating membrane -one chorionic sac, one amniotic sac	1 PLACENTA

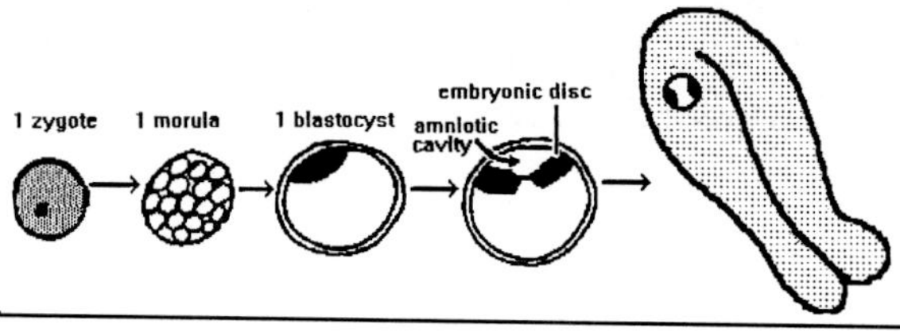

FETAL PRESENTATION	-presenting fetus is Twin A -sometimes difficult to determine, but must describe as accurately as possible	
VERTEX + VERTEX (45%)	VERTEX + BREECH (37%)	BREECH + BREECH (10%)
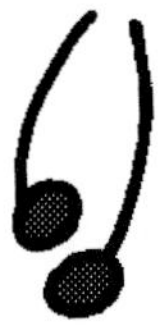	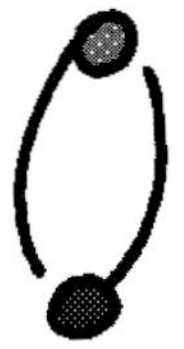	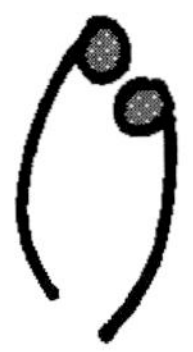
VERTEX + TRANSVERSE (5%)	BREECH + TRANSVERSE (2%)	TRANS. + TRANS. (0.5%)
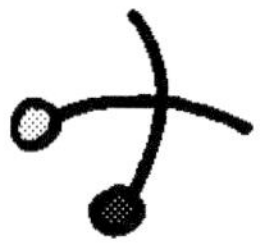	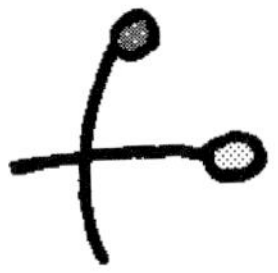	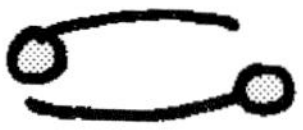

SONOGRAPHIC DETERMINATION OF CHORIONICITY

DICHORIONIC PLACENTA	MONOCHORIONIC PLACENTA
dichorion-diamnion - 4-layer-thick separating membrane proliferating chorionic villi -triangular projection of placental tissue extending between the layers of the membranes in dichorionic placenta creating the twin peak sign <u>"TWIN (CHORIONIC) PEAK" SIGN</u> -only occurs in dichorionic pregnancy -can be useful sign but absence does not exclude dichorionicity nor implies monochorionicity	-monochorionic diamniotic twinning results in a thinner membrane composed of only two amniotic layers <u>NO "TWIN PEAK" SIGN</u> -the chorion is a single layer surrounding both amniotic sacs, therefore, prevents placental tissue from extending up between the two sacs as it does in a dichorionic pregnancy

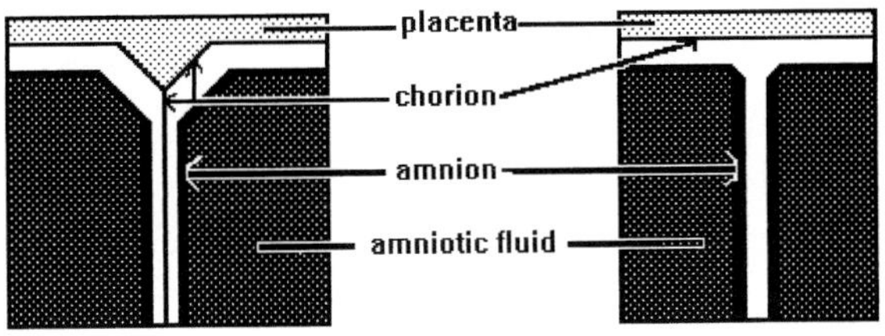

DICHRONIC MONOCHORIONIC

scan demonstrating "twin peak" sign (arrow)	no "twin peak" sign demonstrated; thin membrane seen dividing two sacs
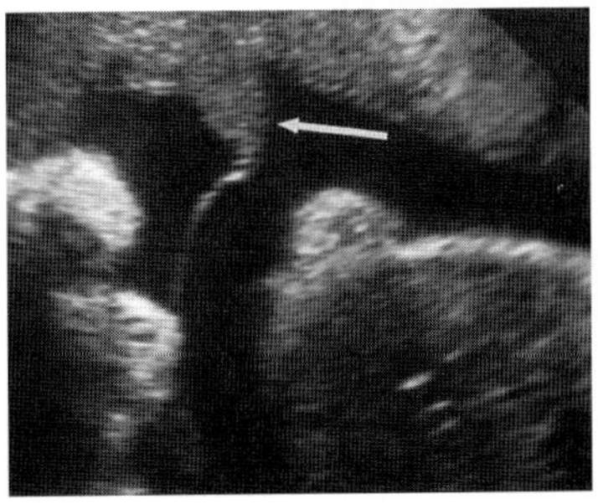	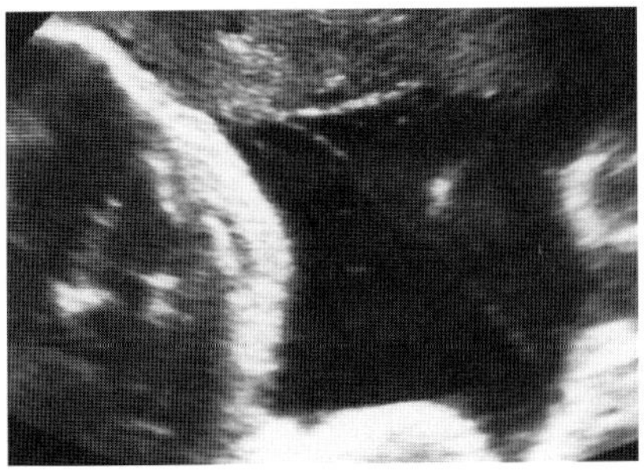

ANOMALIES	US APPEARANCE
ACARDIAC TWINS -TRAP -*T*WIN *R*EVERSED *A*RTERIAL *P*ERFUSION SEQUENCE -rare complication of monozygotic twinning -monochorionic twins develop abnormal placental vascular anastomoses -used deoxygenated blood of pump twin enters perfused twin by an artery-to-artery anastomosis in placenta -blood shunted from "pump" twin to "perfused" twin's lower body first, where any extra oxygen is used -now completely depleted of oxygen, the blood flows in a retrograde direction to the perfused twin's upper body resulting in severe abnormalities	-fused placentas, polyhydramnios 1. pump twin - morphologically normal but with cardiac overload (hydrops, IUGR, hypertrophy of right ventricle, hepatosplenomegaly, ascites) 2. perfused twin - acardiac monster, absent or rudimentary heart, unidentifiable head, trunk, extremities
CONJOINED TWINS -rare, sporadic event resulting from late and incomplete division of embryonic disk -mortality is high and dependent on pattern of fusion -ultrasound has a role in determining the extent to which organs are shared	<u>craniopagus</u> -joined at skull <u>omphalopagus</u> -joined at abdomen <u>thoracopagus</u> - joined at thorax <u>xiphopagus</u> - joined at the xiphoid process
TWIN-TO-TWIN TRANSFUSION SYNDROME (TTTS) -abnormal arterial to venous anastomoses between the two circulations in monchorionic twinning resulting in shunting of blood from one twin (donor) to the other (recipient) -donor twin: growth retardation, oligohydramnios -recipient twin: increased size and polyhydramnios <u>Stuck Twin:</u> -diamniotic twin -interamniotic membrane is closely applied to donor twin causing twin to remain confined to a fixed, possibly nondependent position against the uterine wall **monoamniotic pregnancy: can have twin-to-twin transfusion but since donor shares sac with recipient, there will be no "stuck" twin	-diminished/absent fetal movement and absence of intermingling fetal parts between twins -weight discordance -polyhydramnios
VANISHING TWIN PHENOMENON -early spontaneous twin death resulting is resorption or shrinkage to a nondetectable size over a short period -may be clinically silent or accompanied by first trimester bleeding	-smaller, empty sac (eventually resorbs) adjacent to sac that contains living fetus -if death occurs later on, twin may persist as an irregular structure along the placental or uterine margin

<table>
<tr><th colspan="2">US APPEARANCE OF TWIN ANOMALIES</th></tr>
<tr>
<td>Conjoined twins: scan through thorax of twins shows thoracopaqus and fusion of their hearts (arrow); twins marked A & B
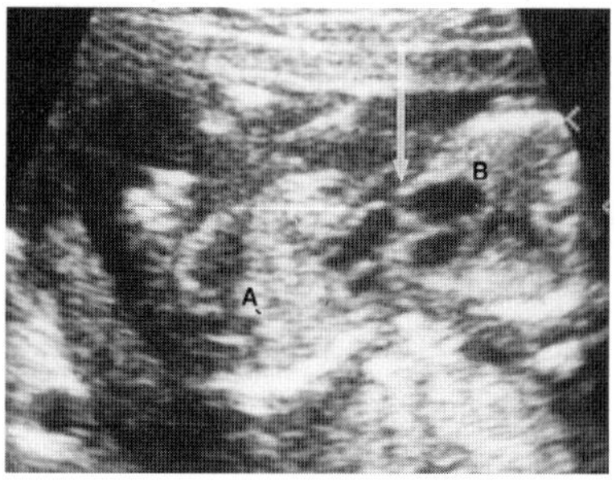
</td>
<td>Conjoined twins: transverse oblique scan through abdomens of twins shows omphalopaqus; twins marked A & B
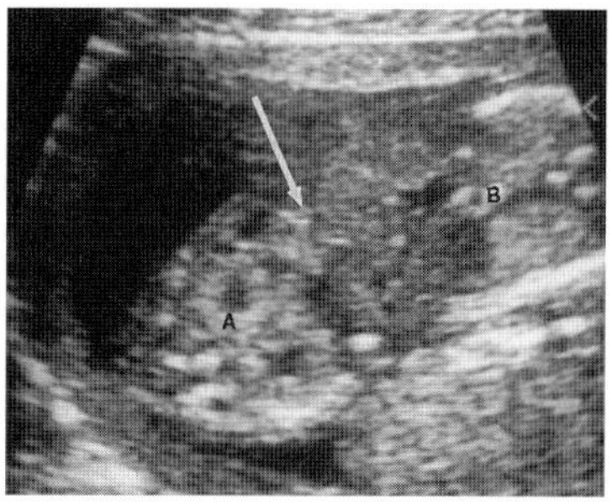
</td>
</tr>
<tr>
<td>Twin to Twin Transfusion: an image through portions of the abdomens of both fetuses at 20 weeks shows the smaller twin in a fixed non dependent position against the anterior uterine wall and the larger twin in a dependent position
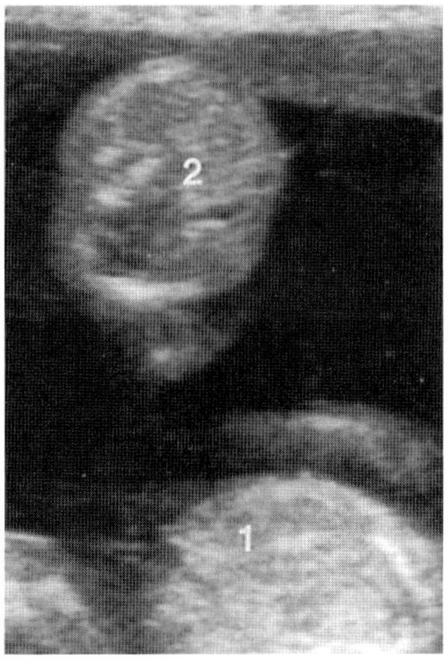
</td>
<td>Twin to Twin Transfusion: A transverse image of both twins at 25 weeks shows markedly discordant size of the two abdomens and ascites (A) in the larger twin from early hydrops.
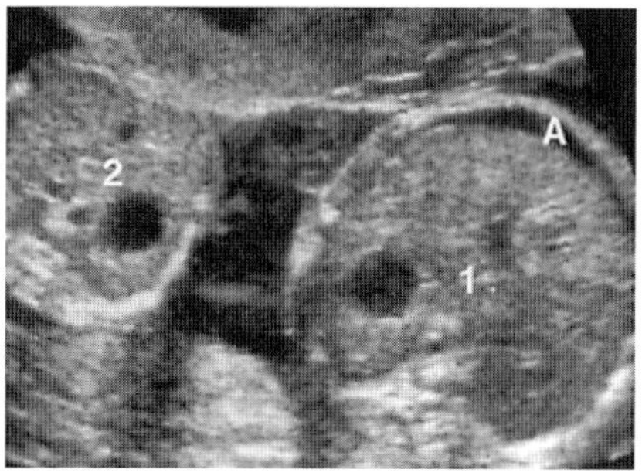
</td>
</tr>
</table>

CHAPTER 11 - PLACENTA AND MEMBRANES
A) NORMAL ANATOMY AND DEVELOPMENT

PLACENTA EMBRYOLOGY & STRUCTURE

-trophoblast cells are from the extraembryonic peripheral cells of the blastocyst
-trophoblast cells invade endometrial epithelium and differentiates into 2 layers: cytotrophoblast and syncytiotrophoblast

Cytotrophoblast
-inner layer of the trophoblast that generally forms the chorion
-in early stages, folds into finger-like projection (primary villi) that surround the entire gestation sac and extend into the forming lacunar network
-at about 10 weeks, the villi associated with the decidua capsularis become compressed and degenerate into the smooth (laeve) chorion
-the villi associated with decidua basalis persist to form villous chorion frondosum and eventually the placenta

Syncytiotrophoblast
-outer layer of trophoblast that envades and erodes epithelium to and from lacunae spaces
-lacunae become filled with blood from ruptured capillaries and secretions from eroded endometrial glands
-embryotrophe: nutritive which passes to embryo by simple diffusion
-at about 4 weeks, lacunae spaces fuse into lacunar network, a primitive utero-placental circulation
-as the lacunae further enlarge they become the intervillous spaces

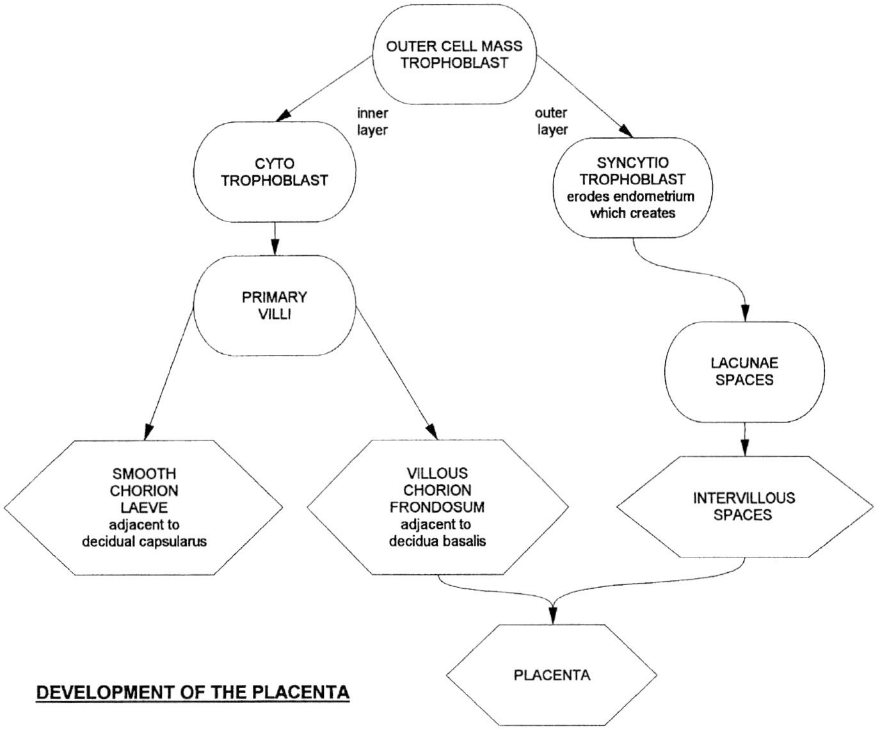

DEVELOPMENT OF THE PLACENTA

FIRST TRIMESTER PLACENTA

-by 8 weeks the placenta is recognized sonographically as an area of localized thickening within the endometrium which represents the chorion frondosum and decidua basalis
-placental flow is a relatively high velocity, low impedance signal localized to the site of implantation of the placenta either in the uterus or in the adnexa with ectopic pregnancies

1. MYOMETRIUM

DECIDUA -functional layer of endometrium
2. DECIDUA BASALIS
-thick decidua under embryo at implantation site between chorion frondosum and myometrium
-forms maternal component of placenta
3. DECIDUA VERA (decidua perietalis)
-the rest of the decidua along uterine cavity
4. DECIDUA CAPSULARIS
-superficial part overlying conceptus which protrudes into uterine cavity

CHORION = trophoblast + fetal mesenchyme with villous stems protruding into decidua
5. CHORION FRONDOSUM
-part adjacent to decidua basalis
-forms primitive placenta
6. CHORION LAEVE
-smooth portion of chorion with atrophied villi
7. AMNIOTIC CAVITY
8. ENDOMETRIAL CANAL
-between decidual layers
9. EMBRYO

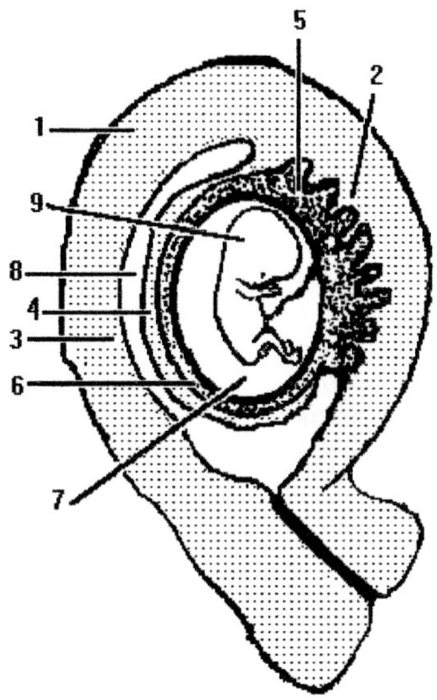

SECOND TRIMESTER PLACENTA

-by the 4th month the placenta has a maternal (decidua basalis) and fetal (chorion frondosum) component
Maternal Portion - Decidua Basalis
-convex and irregular surface bordered by decidual plate
-during erosion of decidual basalis by syncytiotrophoblast, parts of decidua remain as solid projections called the placental septa
- septi divide the placenta into about 12 compartments, lobes or cotyledons that each contain 2 or more main stem villi arising from chorionic plate region
-the septi do not reach the chorionic plate, therefore, the intervillous spaces in the various cotyledons are continuous with each other
-erosion of decidual basalis creates intervillous spaces which bathe the villi that extend into them in maternal arteriole blood
-chorionic villi are anchored to decidual basalis by a covering over the villi and decidual plate called the cytotrophoblastic shell

Fetal Portion - Chorion Frondosum
-smooth, concave surface covered by amniochorionic membrane
-umbilical cord is attached to center of this surface
-placenta bordered by chorionic plate on fetal side

1. ENDOMETRIAL VEINS
2. ENDOMETRIAL ARTERIES
3. SPIRAL ARTERIES
4. INTERVILLOUS SPACES/LAKES
5. PLACENTAL SEPTA
6. CHORIONIC PLATE
7. DECIDUAL PLATE
8. MYOMETRIUM
9. UMBILICAL CORD
10. UMBILICAL VEIN
11. UMBILICAL ARTERIES
12. MAIN STEM CHORIONIC VILLI
   a) cytotrophoblastic shell
   b) anchoring villus
13. DECIDUAL BASALIS
14. AMNION/CHORION
15. AMNIOTIC FLUID

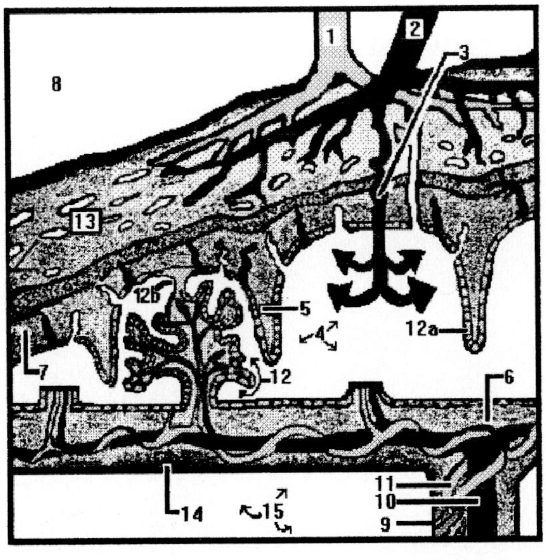

SIZE	
NORMAL	ABNORMAL
-thickness measured perpendicular to the plane of the placenta -grows most rapidly during first half of pregnancy -up to 32 weeks gestation, thickness increases linearly with pregnancy, after which decreases gradually -thickness (mm) = menstrual age (weeks) -normally < 4.5 cm thick -500–600 grams at term	TOO THICK> 5.0 cm -associated with diabetes, Rh immunization factor, chronic intrauterine infections, hydrops, maternal anemia, multiple gestation TOO THIN< 3.0 cm -may appear in cases of polyhydramnios, IUGR, preeclampsia, long-standing diabetes, placental insufficiency PSEUDOTHICKENING- retroplacental or intraplacental hematoma

UTEROPLACENTAL CIRCULATION	
OXYGENATED MATERNAL BLOOD	DEOXYGENATED FETAL BLOOD
spiral arteries in endometrium ↓ through holes in decidual plate (basalis) into intervillous spaces ↓ forced toward chorionic plate under pulsatile pressure ↓ circulates in intervillous spaces over surface of villi ↓ exchange of material through placental barrier (membrane) into thin-walled veins in villi ↓ smaller veins converge into one umbilical vein ↓ fetus	two umbilical arteries in umbilical cord to placenta ↓ arteries divide and branch into main stem villi ↓ cross dividing membrane - placental barrier ↓ intervillous spaces/lakes ↓ during a drop in pressure in intervillous spaces, blood can move toward decidual plate ↓ enters endometrial veins in endometrium ↓ maternal circulation

FUNCTION OF PLACENTA

1. Exchange of metabolic and gaseous produces between maternal and fetal circulations (respiration, nutrition, excretion, protection, storage)
2. Production of hormones needed to maintain pregnancy

protein hormones - human chorionic gonadotropin, human chorionic somatomammotropin, relaxin
steroid hormones - progesterone, estrogens
-early pregnancy: secretes chorionic gonadotropin which maintains estrogen and progesterone secretion by corpus luteum
-later pregnancy: produces estrogen, progesterone and other steroids

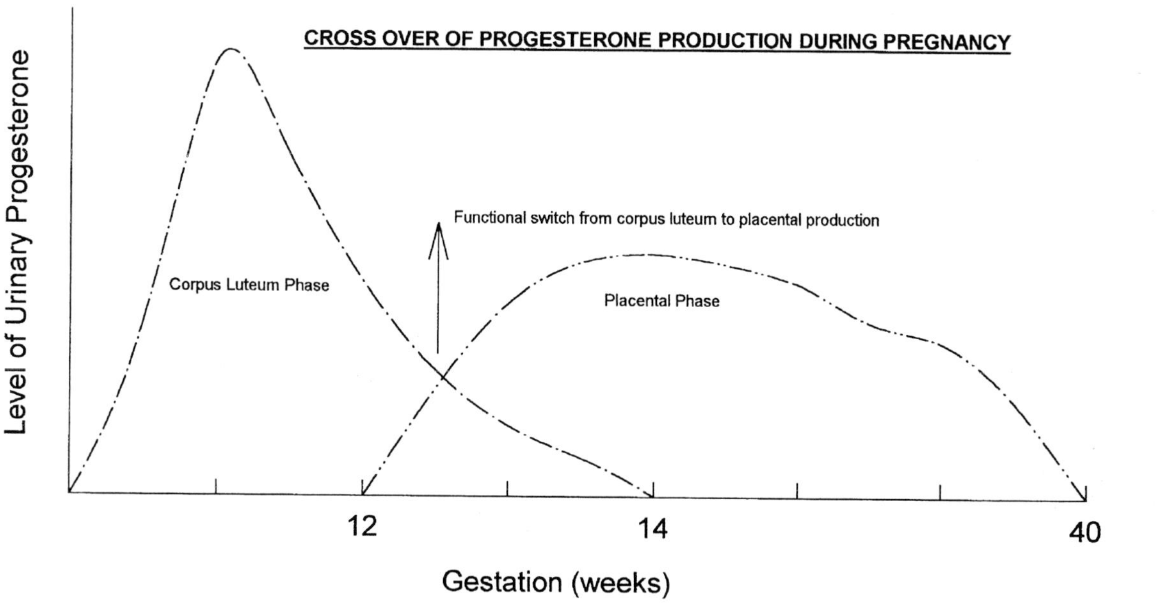

LOCATION

-first seen sonographically at 9–10 weeks in a general region known as chorionic frondosum

CLASSIFICATION OF PLACENTAL POSITION

-placenta may develop anywhere along the uterine endometrial lining
-placenta can develop and grow outside uterine cavity in cases of ectopics
-placental location can be described by stating on which side of uterus it mainly lies and by indicating how far it lies from the internal os
-uterine wall: placenta can be anterior, posterior, right lateral, left lateral
-placental height: placenta can be located at the fundus, mid way, low lying or previa

PLACENTAL MIGRATION

-the apparent change in placental location during the course of a pregnancy on serial scans
-it is the internal os of the cervix that moves, not placenta
-is a result of the differential growth of the lower uterine segment relative to the rest of the uterus causing a low lying placenta in early 1st and 2nd trimester scans to appear to "move" up

GRADING

-calcium deposits occur normally in placenta
-appear sonographically in 3rd trimester as echogenic intraplacenta echos with or without acoustic shadowing
-some authors assign a grade based on appearance of calcium in placenta

CLINICAL SIGNIFICANCE

-there have been attempts to associate grading the placenta with fetal lung maturity, IUGR, fetal distress
-there is overlap of placenta gradings in normal and abnormal pregnancies, therefore there is no conclusive evidence that grading is a clinically useful predictor of outcome
-early maturation (grade 3 seen in gestation < 34 weeks) can be seen with maternal hypertension, diabetes mellitus, IUGR

Postmaturity Syndrome

-inability of aging placenta to support fetal demands

GRADE 0	GRADE I	GRADE II	GRADE III
appears early pregnancy -all 1st + 2nd trimester	appears 31 weeks -40% will stay at this grade until term	can appear at 36 weeks -45% will stay at this grade until term	can appear at 38 weeks -rarely seen < 34 weeks
CHORIONIC PLATE -specular reflector at the fetal surface of placenta			
-straight, smooth and well defined	-subtle undulations	-indentations extending into placenta but not to basal layer	-calcified intercotylidonary septa reach basal plate, often surrounding sonolucent center
PLACENTAL SUBSTANCE -homogenously echogenic -no calcifications	-few scattered echogenic echos representing calcification	-more pronounced foci -linear, "comma-shaped" echogenic densities	-circular densities with echosparse (fallout) areas in centre -large irregular densities that can shadow
BASAL LAYER no echogenic foci	unchanged	linear arrangement of small echogenic foci known as basal stippling	large and more continuous echogenic areas which can shadow
a 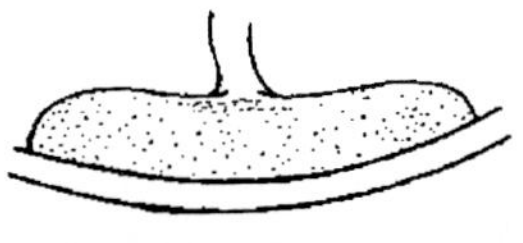	b 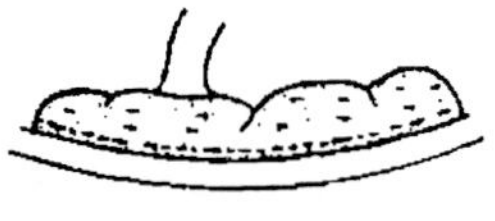	c 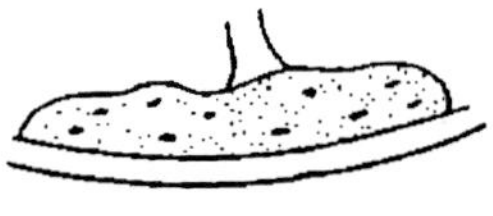	d 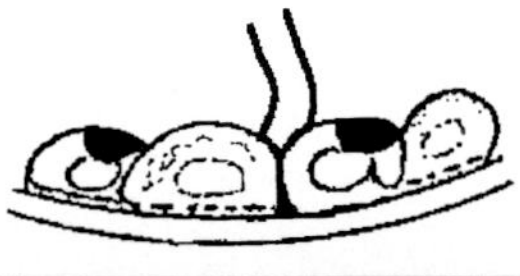
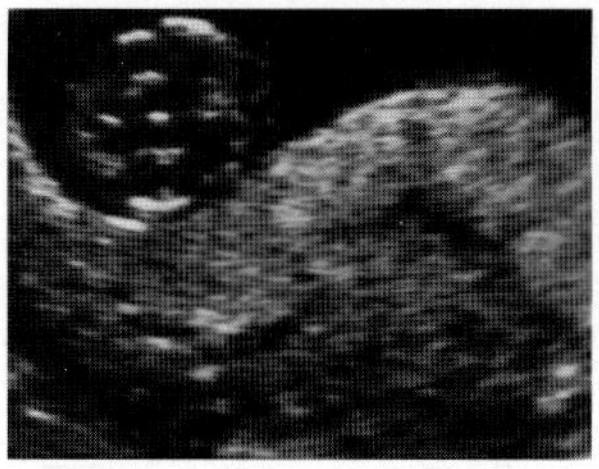	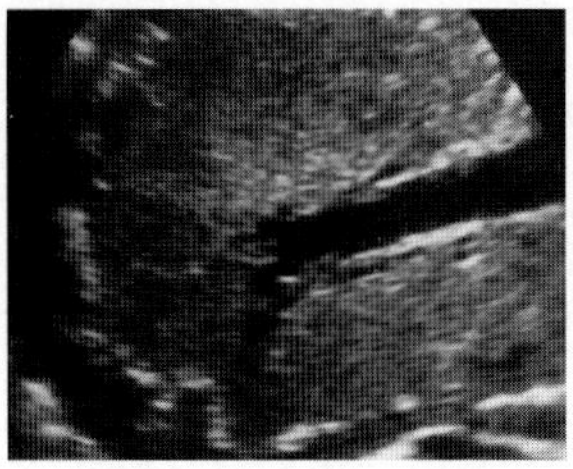	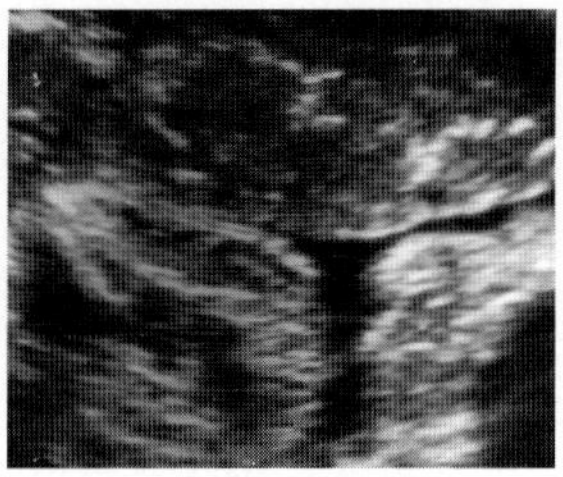	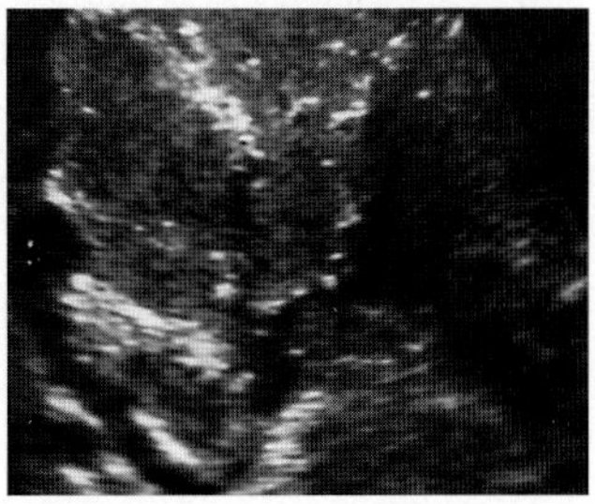

B) ABNORMAL DEVELOPMENT

ABNORMALITIES

ABRUPTION, PERIPLACENTAL HEMORRHAGE, PLACENTA ABRUPTIO

-premature separation of the normally implanted placenta between 20 weeks and birth
-abruptions have several sonographic appearances
-separated into types by their primary area of detachment

RETROPLACENTAL HEMATOMA
-high pressure bleeding under placenta which separates basal plate from uterine wall
-related to spiral artery hemorrhage
-etiology: maternal hypertension, substance abuse

SUBCHORIONIC (MARGINAL) HEMATOMA
-usually associated with a marginal separation of placenta, therefore commonly referred to as marginal hematoma
-low pressure bleeding seen at periphery of placenta which separates the chorionic membrane from decidua with accumulation of blood in subchorionic space
-related to hemorrhage of marginal veins which elevate edge of placenta
-must not confuse with normal marginal veins
-increased incidence with cigarette smoking
-associated with lower fetal mortality than retroplacental hematomas

SUBAMNIOTIC HEMORRHAGES
-seen on fetal surface of placenta
-most likely caused by rupture of fetal vessels on placental surface

CLINICAL SIGNIFICANCE
-vaginal bleeding
-amount of pain depends on severity of abruption
-larger hematoma volumes associated with poorer outcomes/fetal demise

US
-depends on site, age of hematoma, amount of bleeding, gestational age
-sonogram can be normal
Retroplacental
-hypoechoic area (hematoma) separating placenta from underlying myometrium (retroplacental clot and extra membranous clot)
-rounded placental margins

Subchorionic (Marginal)
-marginal separations of the placenta
-hematoma contiguous with placental margin
-membrane elevations will end at the placenta

Differential should include:
1. Basal Veins
-decidual and uterine veins at basal plate region are normal variant
-these do not form mass effects and have flow within them
-on ultrasound have lacy appearing network of veins under placenta
2. Retroplacental Contraction Or Fibroid
-can mimic retroplacental hematoma

retroplacental hematoma (arrows)

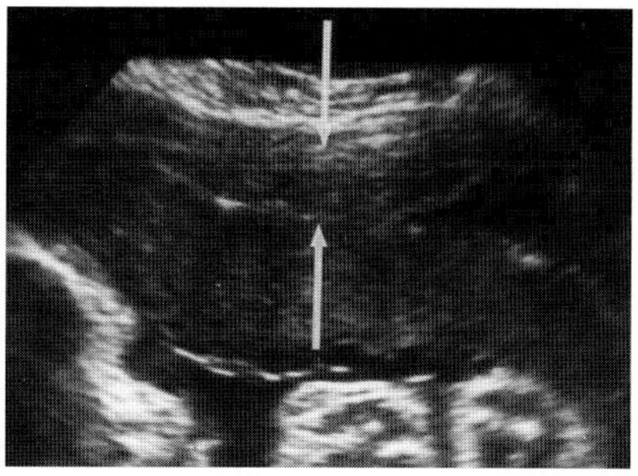

basal veins (arrows) beneath placenta (P) : differential for retroplacental hematoma

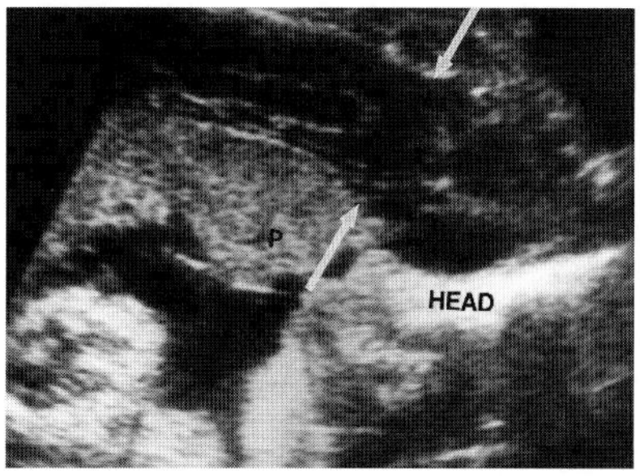

large extrachorionic hematoma (arrows) reaches margin of placenta (P) and elevates the fused chorion and amnion membrane

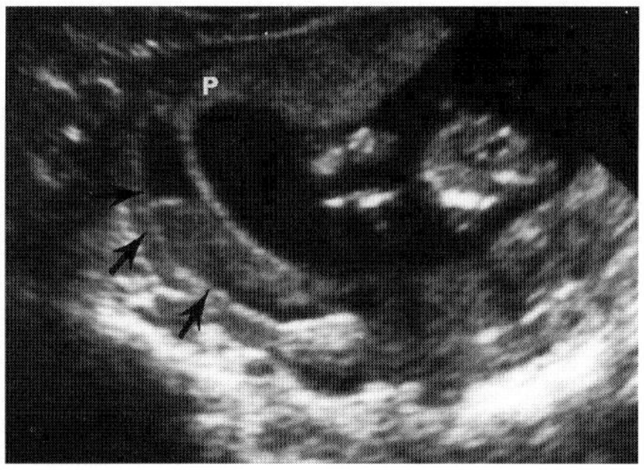

transvaginal scan at 6 weeks displays a small subchorionic hematoma

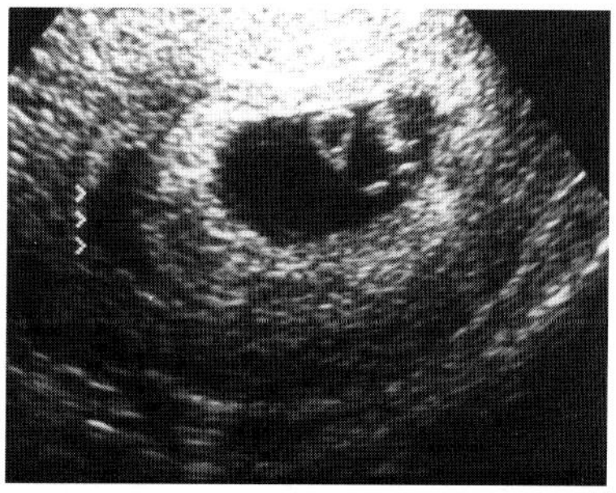

ABNORMALITIES	US APPEARANCE
ABRUPTION, PERIPLACENTAL HEMORRHAGE, PLACENTA ABRUPTIO contd. PERIPLACENTAL AND PLACENTAL HEMATOMAS 1. MARGINAL 2. RETROPLACENTAL 3. SUBCHORIONIC 4. SUBAMNIOTIC 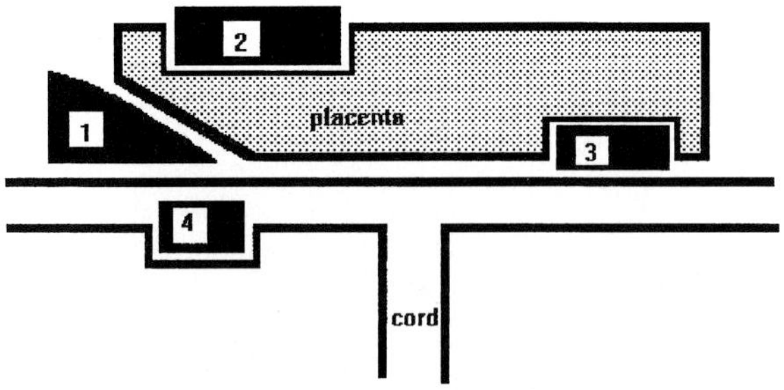	The following three scans are of a 15 weeks pregnancy with placental hemorrhage (calipers, arrows). The hematoma is anterior and left of the gestational sac. It measured less than 60 cc. Hematoma was seen to diminish during pregnancy which ended successfully at 39 weeks 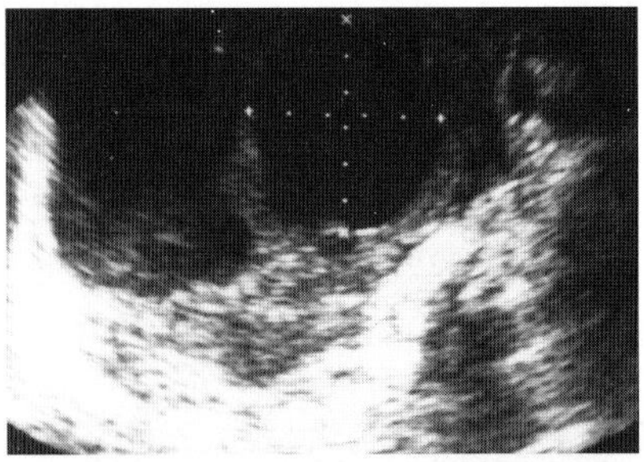 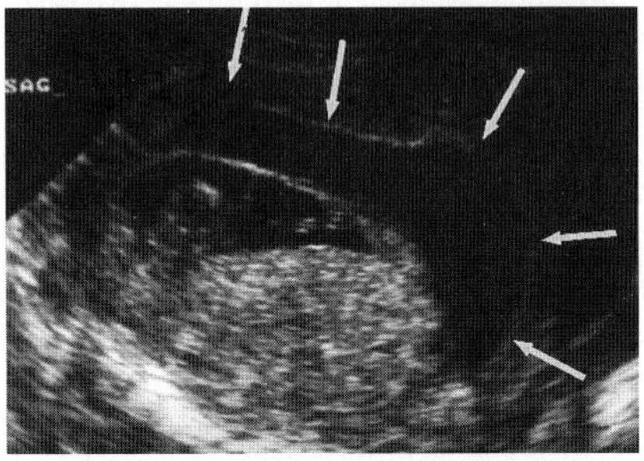 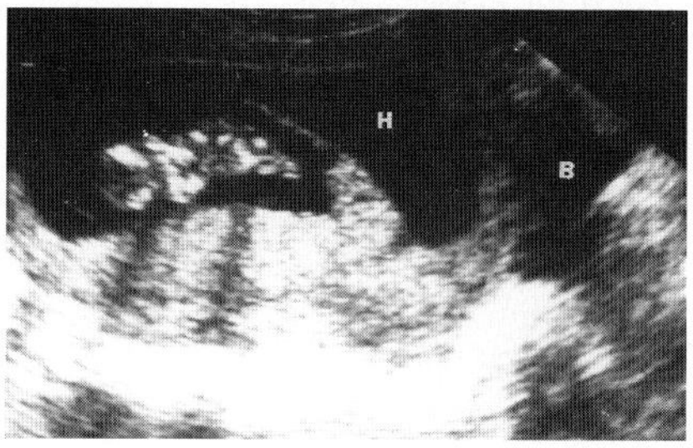

<table>
<tr><th>ABNORMALITIES</th><th>US APPEARANCE</th></tr>
<tr><td>CHORIOAMNIOTIC SEPARATION
-normally seen < 16 weeks due to incomplete fusion of amniotic membrane with chorionic plate
-separation > 17 weeks is usually secondary to hemorrhage or resulting from a tear in the amnion with fluid leaking between the amnion and chorion membranes
-pathological causes are rare and, therefore, rarely seen in 2nd and 3rd trimesters

CLINICAL SIGNIFICANCE
-intact amnion has little effect, but ruptured amnion and intact chorion can give rise to amniotic band syndrome

US
-thin mobile echogenic amniotic membrane identified which is separate from chorion
-elevated amnion over top of placenta which stops at origin of umbilical cord</td><td>normal transvaginal scan at 9 weeks shows the amnion (arrow) not yet fused with the chorion
-amnion surrounding the fetus (F) in amniotic sac (A) with chorionic sac (C) is still visualized
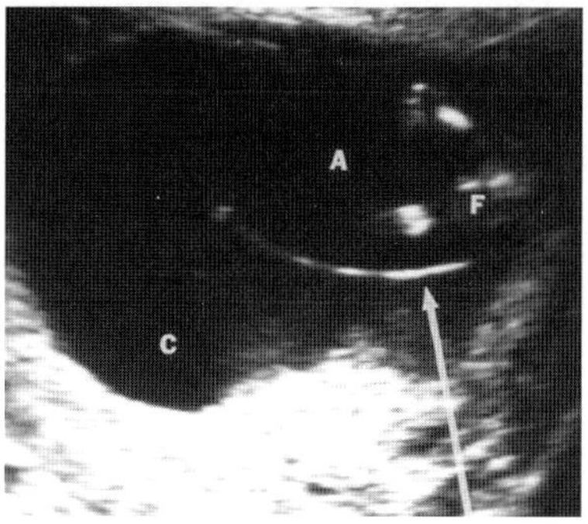
</td></tr>
<tr><td>CHORIOANGIOMA
(HEMANGIOMA / HAMARTOMA / HEMANGIOMATA)
-benign tumor arising from the placental capillaries
-most common placental tumor
-usually grows as a lobulated, solitary nodule within the placenta

CLINICAL SIGNIFICANCE
-if large, can obstruct fetal circulation causing IUGR, hydrops, fetal anoxia

US
-single or multiple discrete, solid masses with complex echo pattern on fetal surface of the placenta
-can vary in echogenicity
-smaller masses are isoechoic to placenta
-arterial signal on Doppler in angiomatous chorioangioma
-associated with polyhydramnios and other fetal anomalies</td><td>small circular hypoechoic mass (M) representing a chorioangioma within the base of the placenta (P)
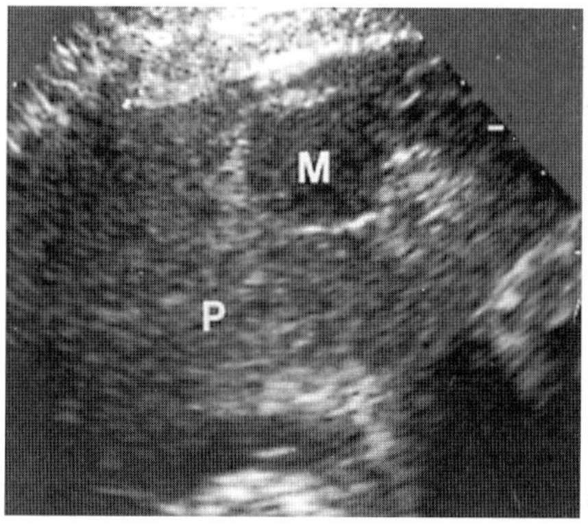
</td></tr>
</table>

ABNORMALITIES	US APPEARANCE
INTRAPLACENTAL SONOLUCENCIES <u>DECIDUAL / CHORIONIC SEPTAL CYSTS</u> -seen at the top of the septa and are probably from obstructed venous drainage -these insignificant hypoechoic areas occur later in pregnancy <u>INTERVILLOUS THROMBOSIS</u> -caused by fetal bleeding into intervillous spaces -associated with elevated maternal serum alpha-fetoprotein related to Rh isoimmunization -new lesion may have flow within <u>MATERNAL VENOUS LAKES</u> -prominent collections of venous blood seen under chorion on fetal side of placenta -clinically insignificant -has whirlpool motion of flowing blood on real time or venous flow on doppler <u>PERIVILLOUS FIBRIN DEPOSITS</u> -result of turbulence and stasis of maternal blood in intervillous spaces and deposition of fibrin <u>PLACENTAL INFARCT</u> -avascular triangular-shaped areas of varying size based on the maternal side of the placenta -occurs when maternal circulation is interrupted <u>SUBCHORIONIC FIBRIN DEPOSITS</u> -result of pooling and stasis of blood in subchorionic space leading to thrombosis and deposition of fibrin -flow can be seen within US -hypoechoic lesions within placental substance, free of placental tissue varying in size from 1– 10 cm	transabdominal scans of third trimester placentas with several intraplacental sonolucencies 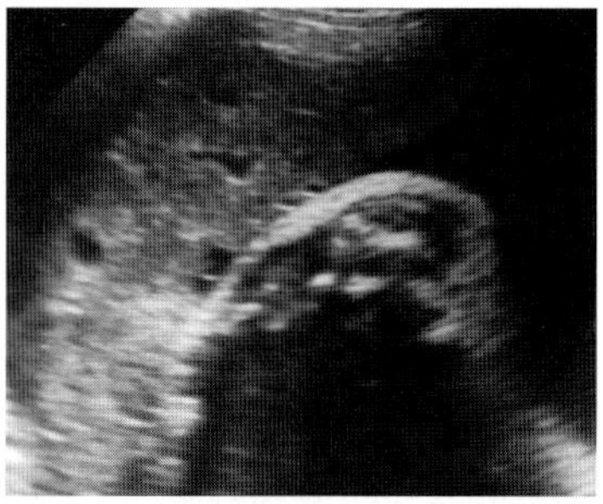 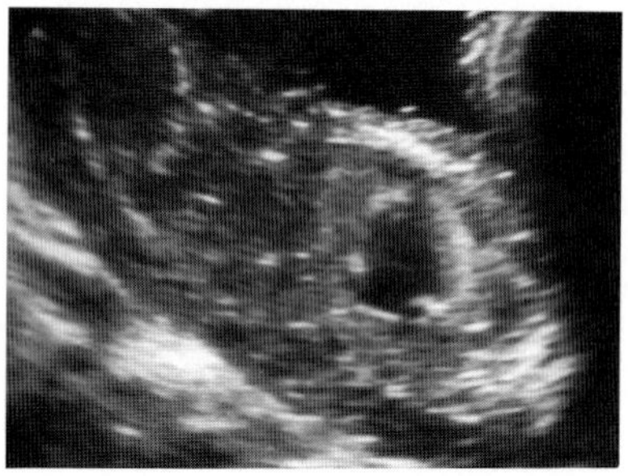 thick inhomogenous anterior placenta (arrows): differential includes fibrin deposition or intervillous thrombosis within placenta 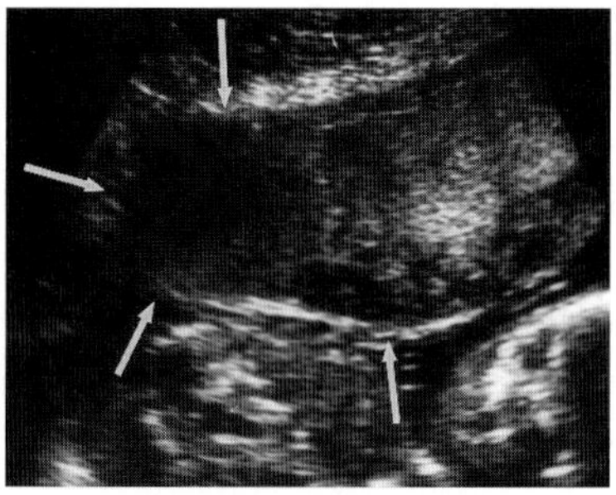

ABNORMALITIES	US APPEARANCE

PLACENTA PREVIA

-most common cause of painless 2nd and 3rd trimester bleeding
-abnormally low implantation of ovum with the placenta covering part or all of internal os
-incidence increases with multigravidas, previous c-sections and therapeutic abortions
-classifications determined by the relationship of the placental margin to the internal cervical os are obstetrical, not sonographic definitions

1. Symmetrical Complete Previa

-placenta implanted on both anterior and posterior walls and centered over os

2. Asymmetrical Complete Previa

-most of placenta is implanted on one side of os but some implantation on opposite side

3. Partial Previa**

-placenta implanted on only one side of os but partially covers it

4. Marginal Placenta Previa** LOW LYING PLACENTA

-placenta ends at edge (< 2 cm) of internal os without covering it
**the difference between a partial and marginal placenta previas usually cannot be distinguished sonographically

CLINICAL SIGNIFICANCE
-most common cause of bleeding in second and third trimester
-recurrent, painless bleeding as early as 20 weeks
-massive bleeding in vaginal delivery resulting in maternal and fetal death
-Marginal Previas -can be still significant, especially with bleeding but not as severe as previa

US
-diagnosis made after 15 weeks by demonstrating the whole surface of the internal os, undistorted by bladder pressure or contractions
-transvaginal and transperineal sonography are alternate methods
-fetal shadowing can sometimes obscure good visualization of the placenta's position relative the internal os

False Positive Placenta Previas
1. Placental "migration" - differential growth rates between lower uterine segment and placenta
2. Over distended bladder compresses anterior myometrium against posterior myometrium
3. Lower uterine contractions can compress anterior and posterior uterine walls together simulating previa

False Negative Placenta Previas
1. Internal os obscured by fetal head
2. Placenta on lateral uterine wall
3. Blood in region of internal os which looks like amniotic fluid

US APPEARANCE

transabdominal midline sagittal scan showing a posterior placenta (P) covering the internal os of cervix (white arrow) creating a complete placenta previa (maternal bladder = B)

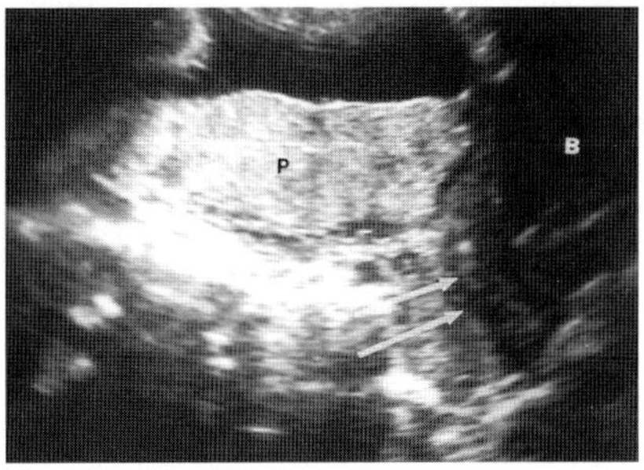

transabdominal midline sagittal scan showing a contracture (C) on the posterior uterine wall which is "pushing" the posterior placenta (P) toward the anterior surface creating the illusion of covering the internal os (arrow)

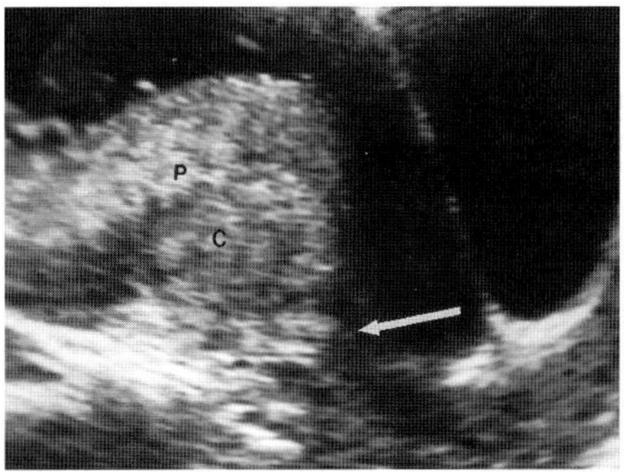

marginal placenta previa: transvaginal scan of posterior placenta (P) covering the posterior aspect of the internal cervical os but does not cover the sonolucent endocervical canal (arrow)

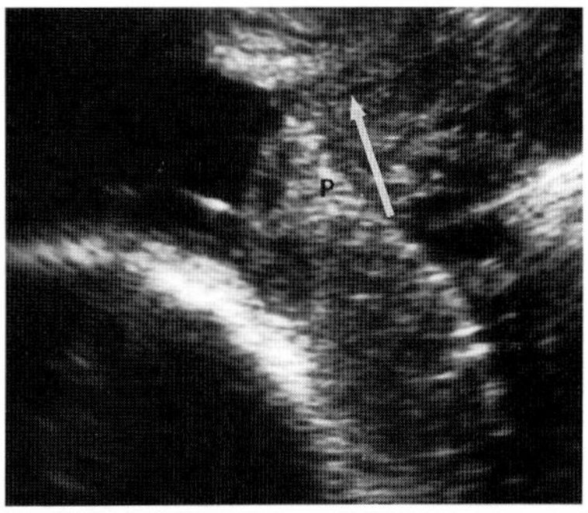

PREMATURE / PRETERM RUPTURE OF MEMBRANES (PROM)

-spontaneous rupture of chorioamniotic membranes before the normal onset of labour
-rupture is spontaneous and for unknown reasons

CLINICAL SIGNIFICANCE
-infection, chorioamnionitis
-increased possibility of cord prolapse and compression
-respiratory distress syndrome (RDS) in neonate
-stillbirth

US
-oligohydramnios

US APPEARANCE

severe oligohydramnios: transverse fetal body at 24 weeks with no surrounding fluid

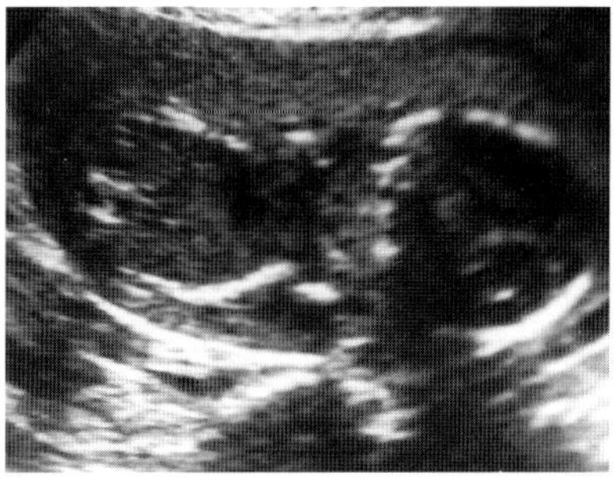

ABNORMALITIES	US APPEARANCE
TROPHOBLASTIC DISEASE -gestational -neoplasms based on changes in trophoblast within uterus -persistent proliferation and hydropic swelling of the lining of the chorionic villi trophoblast in a missed abortion -peak incidence related to advanced maternal age, previous molar pregnancy, Asian population, nutritional factors, genetic predisposition Formation -fertilization of an ovum without any active chromosomal material -karyotype of a complete mole = 46XX, but all chromosomes are of paternal origin -pronucleus fails to develop properly and disappears -fertilization of empty ovum by haploid 23x sperm which duplicates its chromosomes without cell division SS -1st trimester vaginal bleeding, hyperemesis gravidarum, large for dates, severe eclampsia < 20 weeks -abnormal elevation of beta-hCG levels that returns to normal after removal of GTD in 10–12 weeks US 1st Trimester -can be difficult to assess as appearance is variable (hydropic villi cannot be recognized until second trimester) -mimics blighted ovum, miscarriage 2nd Trimester -vesicular sonographic texture (formerly called "snowstorm appearance") -echogenic central soft tissue mass containing multiple small cysts (3–5 mm) within uterine cavity (hydropic villi) -anembryonic pregnancy, no fetal heart -bilateral theca lutein cysts which regress 2–4 months after removal of GTD Doppler of mass - low impedance, high flow state with high systolic and diastolic frequencies	classic appearance of hydatidiform mole -multiple sonolucent areas corresponding to the hydropic grape-like villi (**) 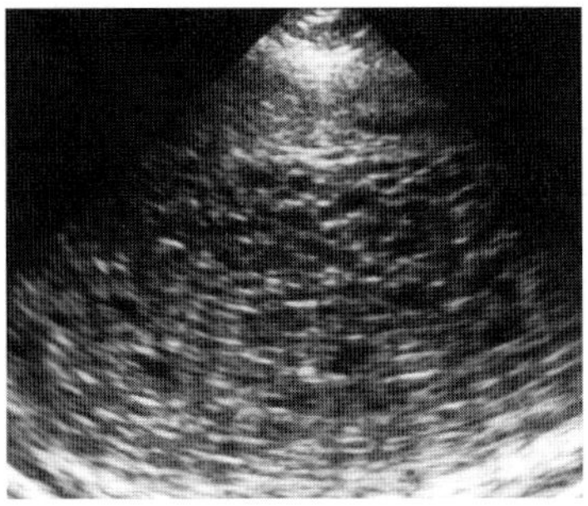 transverse scan through gestational sac shows a co-existing mole (M) with a live fetus (F) (**) 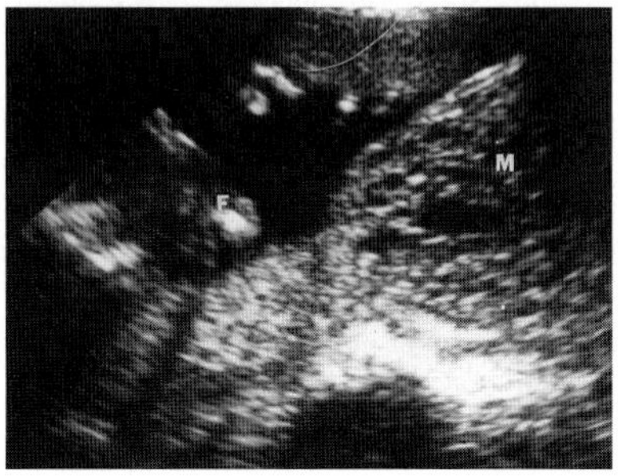

HYDATIDIFORM MOLE BENIGN		CHORIOADENOMA DESTRUENS	CHORIOCARCINOMA MALIGNANT AND METASTATIC
COMPLETE MOLE -benign proliferation of trophoblast -most benign and common (90%) GTD -chorionic villi are grossly swollen -"bunch of grapes"	INCOMPLETE MOLE (PARTIAL MOLE) -some fetal tissue present -triploid karyotype -placenta: 2 areas of villi; some normal and some typical grape like appearance -embryo sometimes present but doesn't survive co-existent with normal twin -rare; molar transformation of a two ovum twin placenta -same malignancy potential as true GTD	INVASIVE TRUE -malignant potential -locally invasive into myometrium and associated blood vessels -there is preservation of villous structure -uterine perforation may occur -treatment: hysterectomy and chemotherapy	-5% GTD, rare -most malignant form -GTD that extends outside uterus and can metastasize to liver, lungs, GI tract, pelvis, brain -3–20% arise from trophoblastic disease -22% arise after normal pregnancy -25% arise after abortions -3% arise after ectopic pregnancies SS: ↑↑ βhCG 6 weeks post pregnancy, irregular bleeding, hemoptysis -treatment: hysterectomy, chemotherapy, weekly βHCG, CXR, R/O mets

ABNORMAL FORMS OF PLACENTA

ACCRETA, INCRETA, PERCRETA

-abnormal adherence of placenta to the myometrium such that separation does not occur after delivery
-predisposed to areas of uterine scarring, and associated with placenta previa
Three Types:
<u>1. Accreta</u> - placenta villi attach but do not invade myometrium
-more common than invasive types
<u>2. Increta</u> - villi invade myometrium
<u>3. Percreta</u> - villi penetrate completely through the myometrium to the serosal surface of uterus

CLINICAL SIGNIFICANCE
-morbidity related to the extraction of placenta after delivery
-persistent postpartum bleeding, infection, hysterectomy may be necessary
US
-rarely diagnosed sonographically
-lack of visualization of hypoechoic myometrium and sonolucent venous complex underneath placenta
-with invasive types, tissue seen extending into adjacent organs and bladder

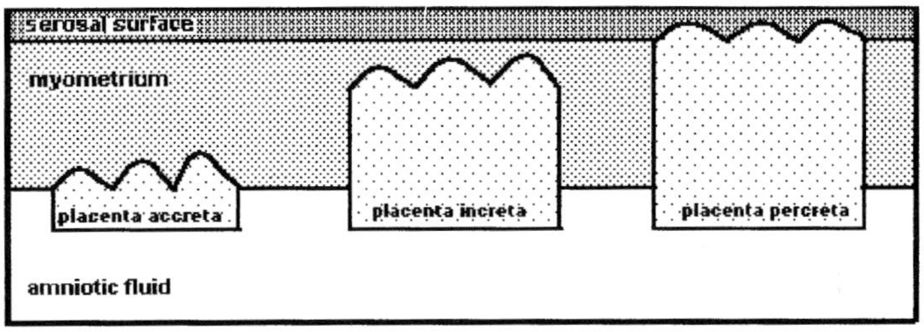

ANNULAR PLACENTA

-placenta that extends like a belt around interior of uterus

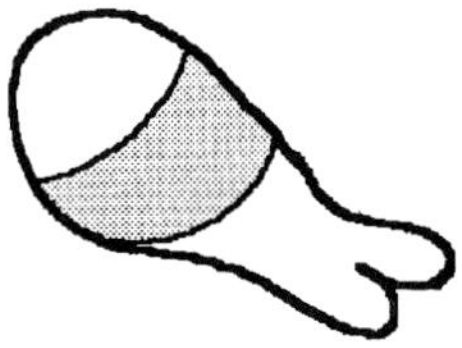

BATTLEDORE PLACENTA

-cord inserts laterally on placenta, also known as <u>MARGINAL INSERTION</u>

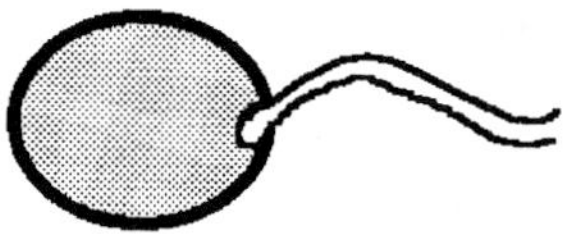

PLACENTA EXTRACHORIALIS

-chorionic plate of placenta is smaller than the basal plate
-this small chorionic plate is surrounded by a thick pale ring composed of a double fold of amnion, chorion, fibrin and degenerated decidua in between

<u>1. CIRCUMMARGINATE</u>
-interface between thick whitish ring and placenta remains flat
-no clinical significance and usually not detected sonographically

<u>2. CIRCUMVALLATE</u>
-thick whitish ring has a rolled edge
-can result in vaginal bleeding, preterm labor
-on ultrasound visualize in folding of fetal membranes and placenta on the fetal surface of the placenta
-not normally seen sonographically after second trimester

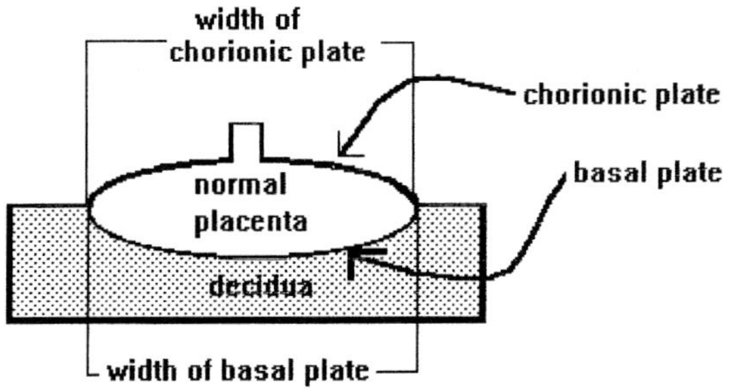

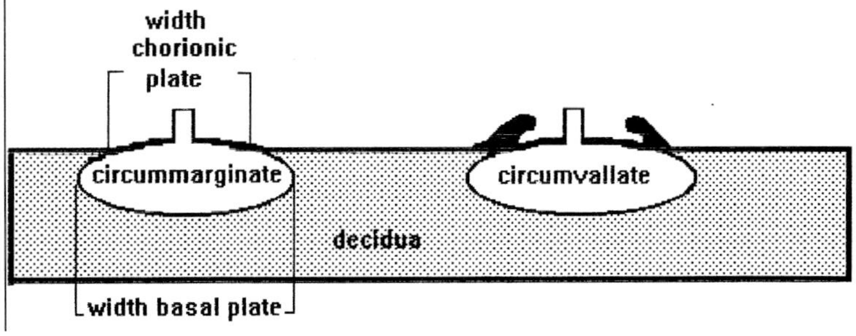

ABNORMAL PLACENTAS	DIAGRAM
PLACENTA MEMBRANACEA -placenta that covers entire gestational sac rather than forming at specific location -thinning of placenta from atrophy -rare but serious condition	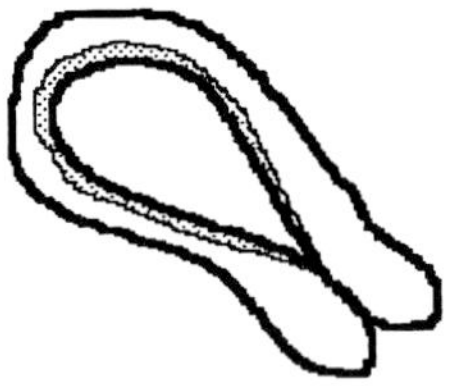
SUCCENTURIATE (ACCESSORY LOBES) -failure of chorionic villi to fully compress which causes development of some placental tissue separate from the main body of the placenta -separate mass of placenta connected to primary placenta by vessels within membrane <u>Bilobate Placenta</u>: two lobes of nearly equal size and cord inserts on bridging tissue -can result in retained placenta which causes postpartum bleeding and infection -on ultrasound, visualize a small island of placental tissue away from placenta	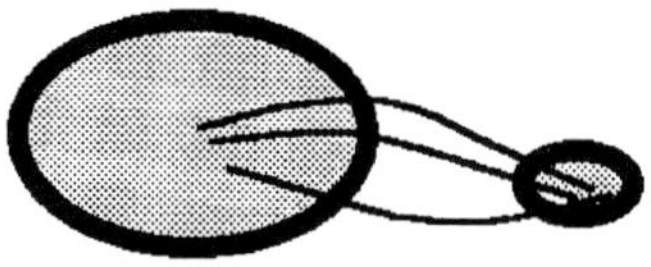
VASA PREVIA -fetal vessels within a membrane lie over the internal os of the cervix -can occur in cases of succenturiate placenta and velamentous insertion of cord -rupture of these vessels can cause fetal demise -colour Doppler flow imaging valuable in detection	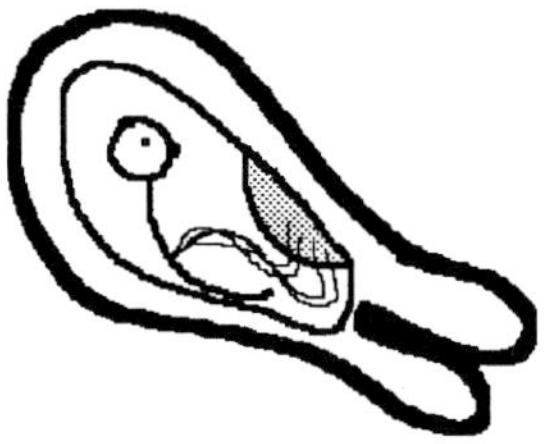
VELAMENTOUS INSERTION OF CORD -high-risk pregnancy -umbilical cord inserts into the chorion laeve membrane rather than into the placental mass -membranes unfold and can lie over cervix causing vasa previa -on ultrasound, must demonstrate the relationship between the cord and its insertion on the placenta	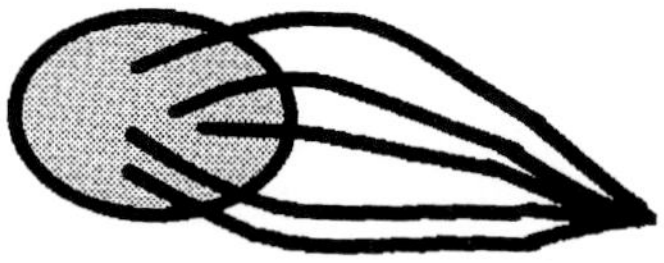

CHAPTER 12-UMBILICAL CORD

ANATOMY

-inserts near middle of placenta
-consists of three vessels - 2 arteries, 1 vein
-usually 5–6 cm in length, 1–2 cm in diameter
-cord contains mucoid substance called Wharton's jelly surrounds the vessels which help prevent compression of vessels
-outside surface covered by amnion

cross section image of normal three vessel cord; two smaller umbilical arteries (arrows) with the large umbilical vein (v)

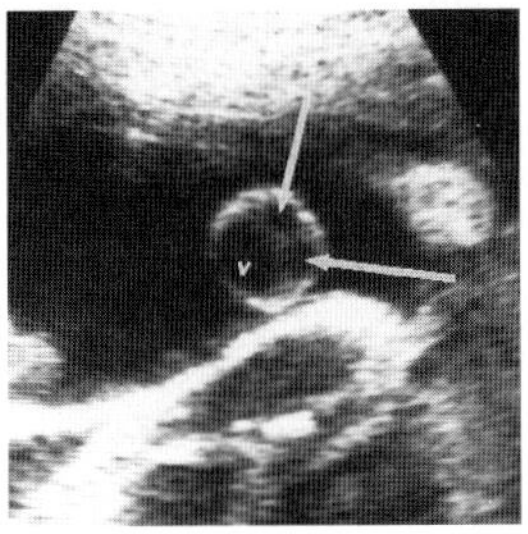

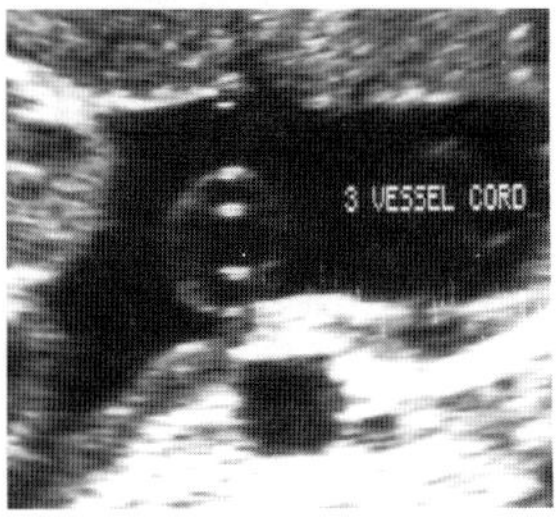

longitudinal image of abnormal 3 vessel cord

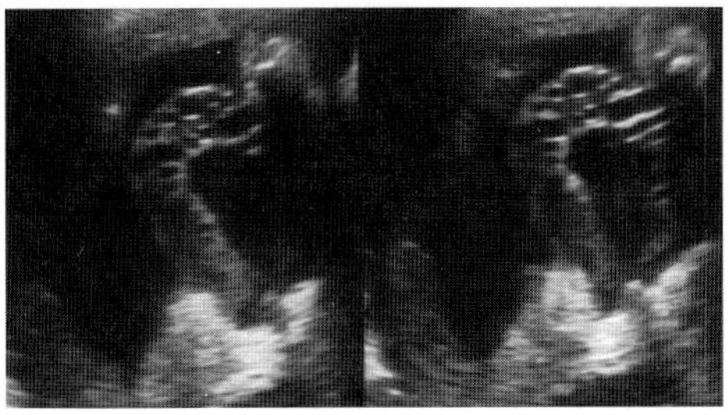

FUNCTION

-conduit for oxygen, nutrients and wastes between fetus and mother

NORMAL DEVELOPMENT

-by the end of the 4th week, the embryo is attached to its trophoblastic shell by a narrow connecting stalk
-primitive umbilical cord is formed by fusion of yolk sac stalk (containing vitelline vessels) and connecting stalk (containing allantois and umbilical vessels)
-allantois and vitelline duct are obliterated leaving only the umbilical vessels and surrounding jelly of Wharton in the cord

<u>PHYSIOLOGICAL UMBILICAL HERNIA</u>:
-fetal abdominal cavity is too small for rapidly developing intestinal loops and some are pushed into umbilical cord
-at end of 3rd month, the bowel withdraws back into abdomen of fetus

1. chorionic cavity
2. yolk sac
3. vitelline duct
4. amniotic sac
5. fetus
6. connecting stalk
7. trophoblast

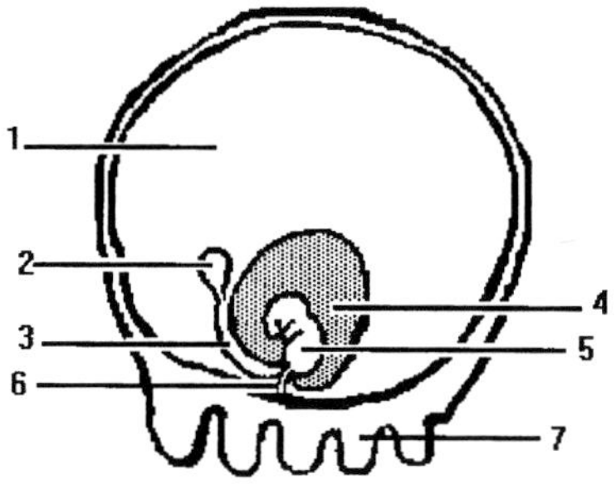

transvaginal scan of 6-week gestation; fetal pole with connecting stalk and yolk sac

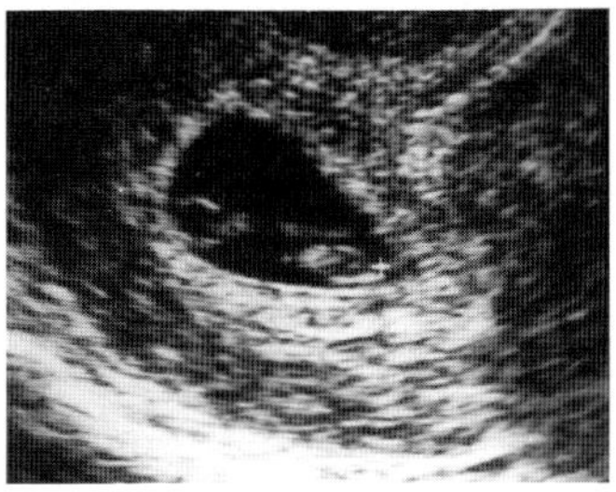

transvaginal scan at 11 weeks showing normal cord insertion

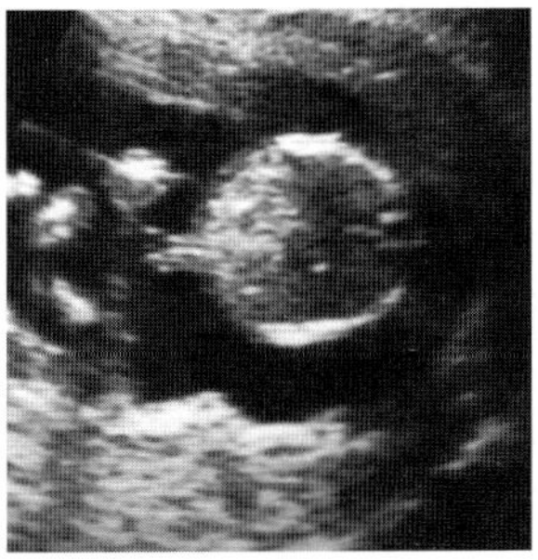

transverse scan of 24-week fetus, showing normal cord insertion

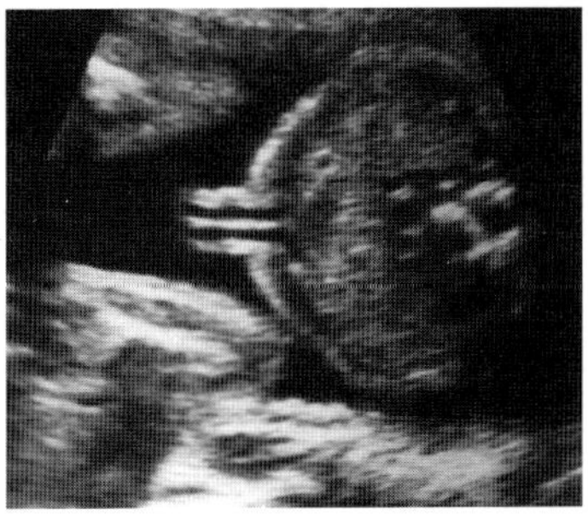

ANOMALIES	US APPEARANCE
NUCHAL CORD -umbilical cord is wrapped around fetal neck -etiology of variable heart rate decelerations may be related to nuchal cord -can simulate cystic hygroma	sagittal scan of fetus with cord adjacent to neck 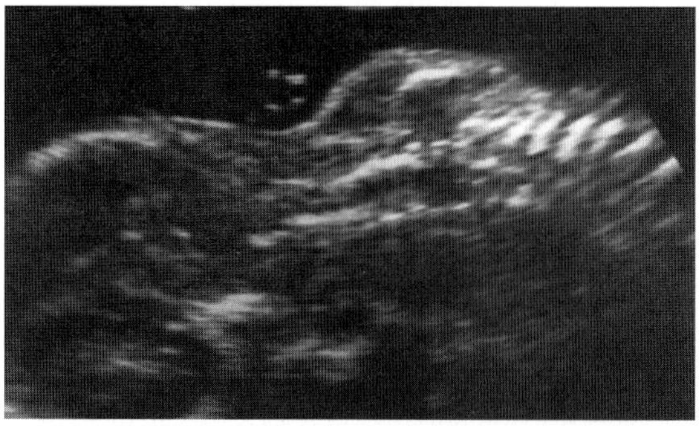
SINGLE UMBILICAL ARTERY (SUA) TWO VESSEL CORD -most common anomaly of umbilical cord -etiology: atrophy of one umbilical artery or persistence of the normal embryological phase of the SUA in body stalk CLINICAL SIGNIFICANCE -high association (25–50%) with congenital anomalies such as cardiac (most frequent), CNS, GU, ventral wall defect, diaphragmatic hernia -IUGR -prematurity, perinatal mortality, stillbirth -chromosomal anomalies US- -transverse view of cord shows two vessels -colour flow Doppler of single blue vein and single red artery -umbilical artery normally bifurcates into right and left common iliac artery -with a single umbilical artery, there will only be a common iliac artery on one side with a hypoplastic ipsilateral common iliac artery	scan of 2 vessel umbilical cord 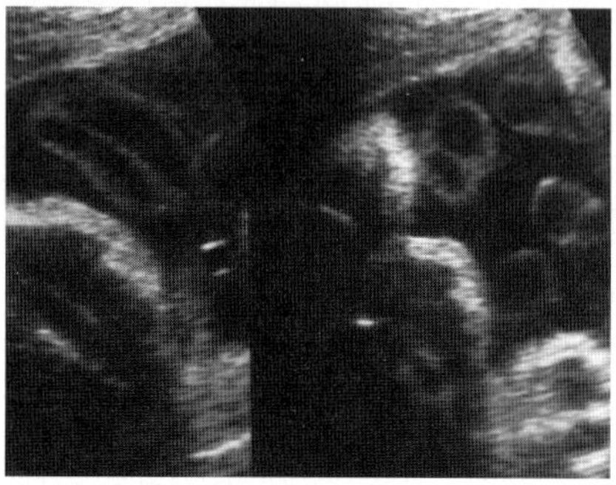

UMBILICAL CORD MASSES

ALLANTOIC DUCT CYST	-true: remnant of allantoise located close to fetus -false: liquefaction of Wharton's jelly
FALSE KNOT	-varix of umbilical vessel which appears as irregular protrusion in cord
HEMATOMA	-rupture of wall of umbilical vein secondary to trauma or congenital weakness of vessel wall
NEOPLASM	-include angiomyxoma, hemangioma, myxosarcoma
OMPHALOCELE	-malformation of cord whereby abdominal contents herniate into base of umbilical cord
OMPHALO MESENTERIC CYST	-persistence and dilatation of a segment of the omphalomesenteric duct joining the embryonic gut and the yolk sac
TRUE KNOT	-caused by excessive fetal movement which appears as localized distention of umbilical vein with tortuosity of cord at level of knot

transvaginal scan of 10-week fetus with umbilical cord cyst (arrow)

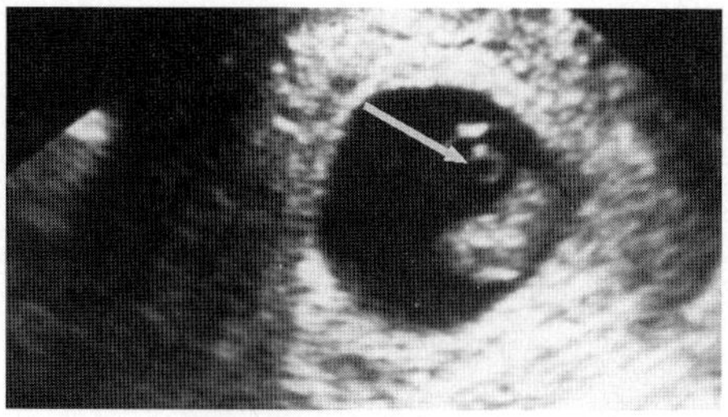

sagittal scan of fetal abdomen with omphalocele (arrow)

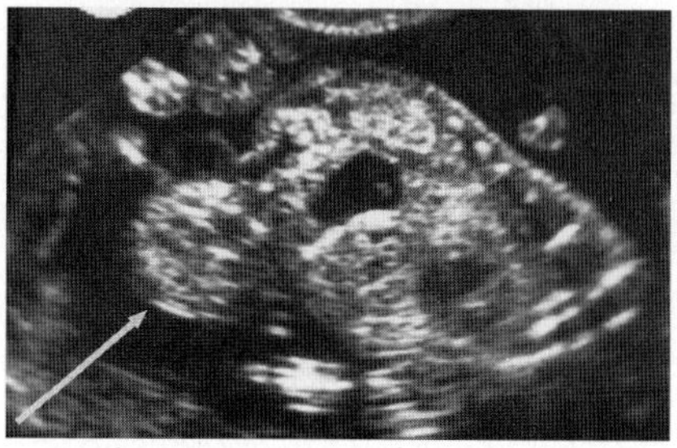

CHAPTER 13 - AMNIOTIC FLUID AND AMNION

AMNION DEVELOPMENT

amnion- smooth membrane that forms the walls of amniotic cavity
- first appears 2nd week gestation
- eventually enlarges to surround embryo and umbilical cord
- completely fills chorionic cavity and fuses with chorion to form amniochorionic membrane at about 3 months

transvaginal scan of fetus (F) surrounded by amnion (arrows) adjacent to echogenic fluid of chorionic sac (C)

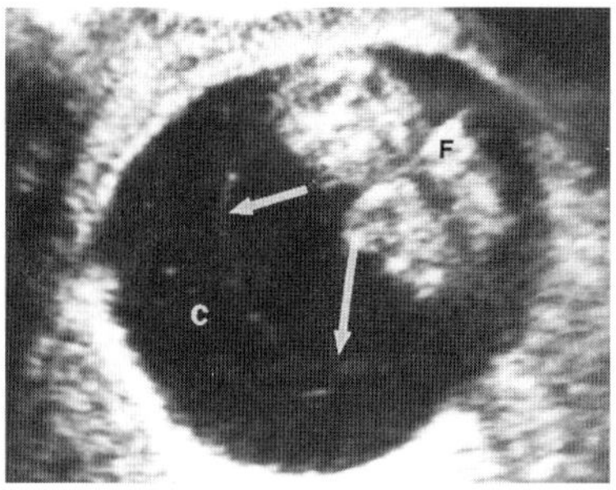

transvaginal scan of early pregnancy showing physiological separation of amnion (arrow) and chorion fetus (F)

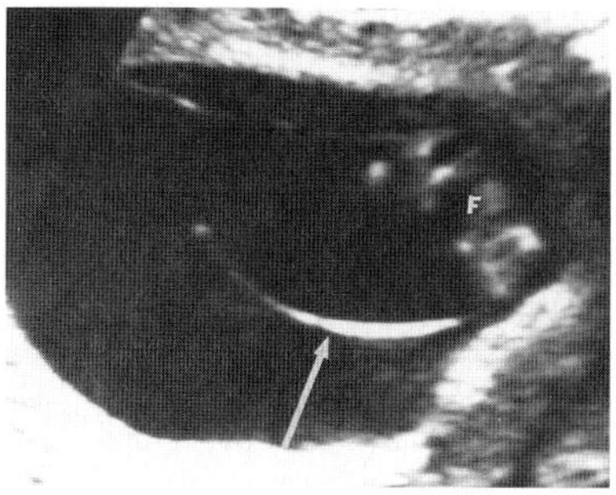

Things To Look For When Examining The Amniotic Fluid

1. Membranes
-between multiple fetuses
-abruption
-amniotic bands
-septations
-chorioamniotic separation

2. Particles
-vernix
-meconium
-blood
-cellular debris

fine echogenic particulate matter within the amniotic fluid

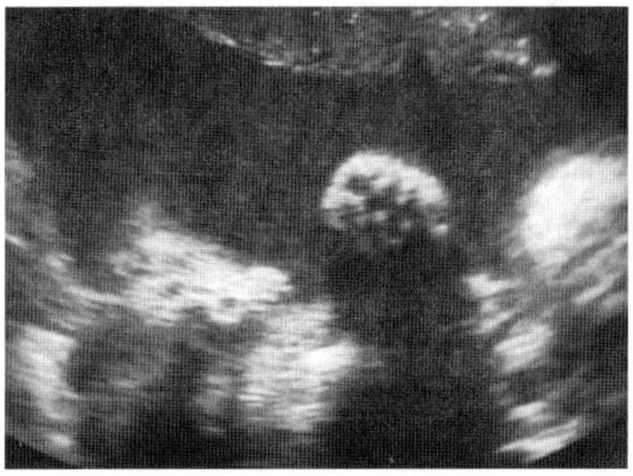

AMNIOTIC FLUID SOURCE

< 15 weeks : from the amnion, diffusion of maternal plasma infiltrate through chorionic plate, exchange of fluids through fetal maternal circulation
15-30 weeks: renal glomeruli filter (500 ml/day), skin diffusion
>30 weeks: decrease in skin diffusion with concurrent increase in renal function and urine output

FUNCTION

1. protection, acts as shock absorber by cushioning jolts
2. prevents adherence of embryo to amnion
3. allows for fetal movements
4. temperature control
5. allows fetal lung development

PHYSIOLOGY

-water in amniotic fluid changes every 3 hours indicating the extensive exchange between the maternal circulation and the amniotic cavity

COMPOSITION

-98% water, 2% inorganic and organic solids
-alpha-fetoprotein present up to 15 weeks then decreases
-vernix (caseosa) - sebaceous covering on fetus from skin gland secretions which is seen in late 3rd trimester "floating" in amniotic fluid

REGULATION

1) Maternal–fetal circulation: exchange via umbilical arteries and veins
2) Fetal renal filtration: urine output into amniotic cavity
3) Fetal absorption: in GI tract, through skin, lungs
FLUID PRODUCTION - function of fetal kidneys, membranes and cord, lungs, skin

AMNIOTIC FLUID VOLUME

NORMAL AMNIOTIC FLUID VOLUMES

10 weeks - 30 ml.
20 weeks - 300 ml.
30 weeks - 600 ml.
36 weeks - 1000 ml
38-42 weeks - 600 ml.

QUANTITATION BY ULTRASOUND

AMNIOTIC FLUID INDEX (AFI)

-sum of the largest amniotic fluid pockets without fetal parts or umbilical cord in each quadrant of uterus expressed in cm.
-using chart below, find age of fetus and read across to find the sum of the four quadrants and the corresponding percentile
-for example: a 37 week gestation having the total sum depth of amniotic fluid in each quadrant equaling 75 cm. would be in the 5th percentile for amniotic fluid volume

Ultrasound image of 4 quadrants of uterus. Calipers are measuring the largest pocket in each quadrant.

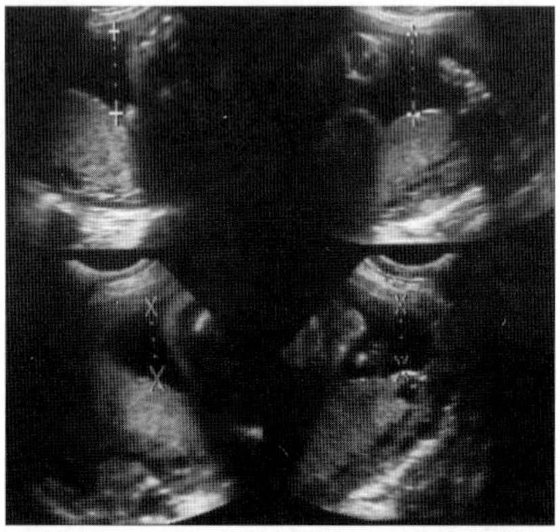

LARGEST VERTICAL POCKET

-measurement of the single largest pocket of AFV without fetal parts or umbilical cord is reported
-this method for measurement does not correlate amount with gestation age
Polyhydramnios = pocket > 8 cm.
Mild Oligohydramnios = pocket between 1 and 2 cm.
Oligohydramnios = pocket <1 cm.

Ultrasound image showing measurement of single largest pocket of fluid.

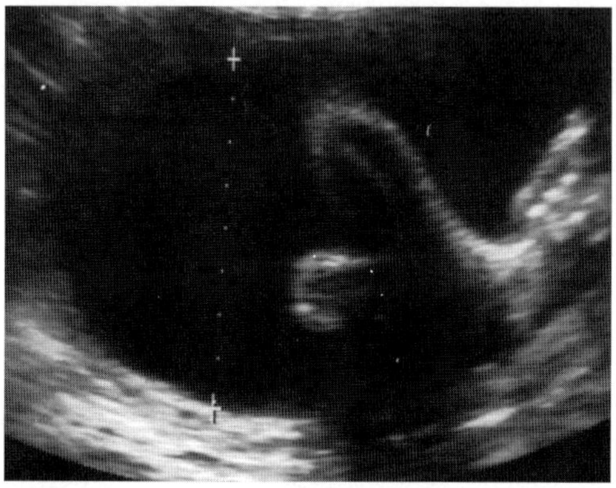

AMNIOTIC FLUID INDEX (PERCENTILE)

WEEKS GESTATION	SUM OF LARGEST POCKET OF AMNIOTIC FLUID IN EACH QUADRANT IN CM				
	2.5th PERCENTILE	5th PERCENTILE	50th PERCENTILE	95th PERCENTILE	97.5th PERCENTILE
25 - 27	85 - 89	95 - 97	146 - 147	221 - 226	240 - 245
28 - 29	84 - 86	92 - 94	145 - 146	228 - 231	249 - 254
30	82	90	145	234	258
31-32	77 - 79	86 - 88	144	238 - 242	263 - 269
33	74	83	143	245	274
34 - 35	70	79- 81	140- 142	248 - 249	278 - 279
36	68	77	148	249	279
37	66	75	135	244	275
38	65	73	132	239	269
39	64	72	127	226	255
40	63	71	123	214	240
41	63	70	116	194	216
42	63	69	110	175	192

ABNORMAL AMNIOTIC FLUID VOLUMES

-abnormal amniotic fluid volume is associated with adverse perinatal outcome, fetal anomalies and obstetrical and neonatal complications

	POLYHYDRAMNIOS / HYDRAMNIOS	**OLIGOHYDRAMNIOS**
DEFINITION	-an excess of amniotic fluid 1. Amniotic Fluid Index > 97TH percentile 2. largest pocket of fluid > 8 cm 3. more than 2000 ml of fluid at term	-an abnormally small amount of amniotic fluid defined as 1. Amniotic Fluid Index <5TH percentile 2. mild oligohydramnios = pocket <2 and >1 cm. oligohydramnios = pocket < 1 cm. 3. less than 400–500 ml of fluid at term
ETIOLOGY	-increased secretion of amniotic fluid by large placenta or fetal malformation which prevents swallowing or absorption -diabetes (maternal or gestational) -idiopathic - most cases fall into this category -fetal anomalies (neural tube, GI, cardiac, chest, chromosomal) -Rh incompatibility -twins	-demise of fetus -iUGR -placental vascular insufficiency (pre-eclampsia, placental infarcts, post maturity) -premature rupture of membranes -renal anomalies (IPKD, MCDK, potters, posterior urethral valves)
CLINICAL FINDINGS	-sudden maternal weight gain -large for dates (LFD) -edema of lower limbs -"distant fetal parts and heart tones"	-lack of normal maternal weight gain -small for dates (SFD) or small for gestational age (SGA)
SONOGRAPHIC FINDINGS	-large amount of amniotic fluid (AFI, pocket, subjective) -fetal parts well-defined, with good image quality -placenta can appear thin -potential loss of contact between fetus and uterine wall	-reduced amount of amniotic fluid (AFI, pocket, subjective) -poor scan quality secondary to lack of tissue–fluid interfaces -crowding of fetal parts -decrease in number of pockets of fluid
SONOGRAM	example of polyhydramnios with a large amount of fluid surrounding the fetus creating exceptional visualization 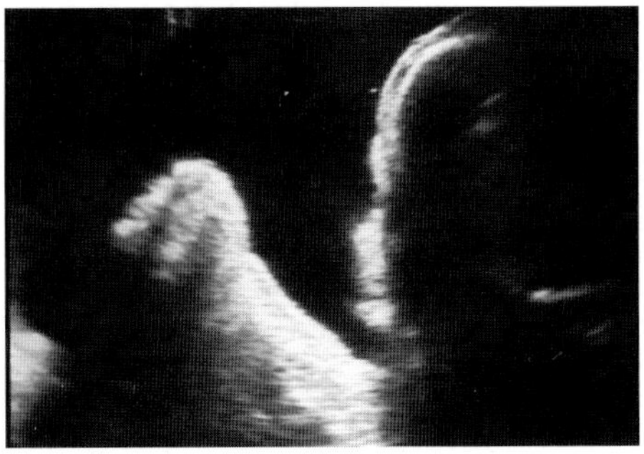	example of oligohydramnios with no amniotic fluid surrounding fetus creating poor sonographic visualization 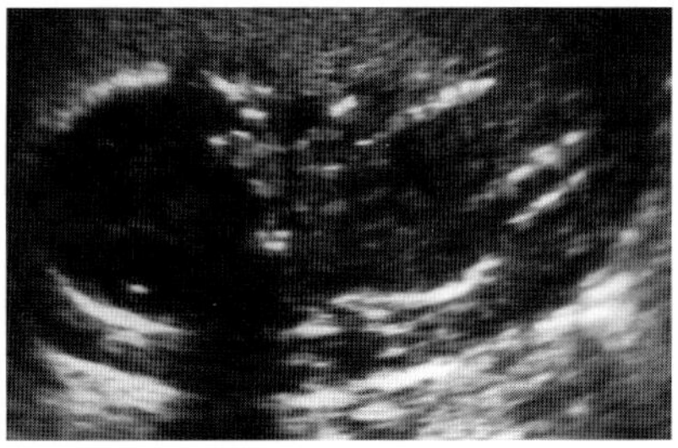

CHAPTER 14 - MEASURING AND DOCUMENTING FETAL GROWTH AND POSITION

MEASURING THE FETUS CLINICALLY	
CONCEPTUAL or GESTATIONAL AGE	-used by embryologists -fetal age from day of fertilization
MENSTRUAL AGE	-used by obstetricians, sonologists and sonographers -fetal age since the last normal menstrual period (LMP) began, projecting the estimated due date or estimated date of confinement (EDC) -average duration of pregnancy is 280 days or 40 weeks or 9 calendar months or 10 lunar months -if LMP unknown, date when it would have been if regular 28-day cycles were occurring, and pregnancy began in mid cycle -LMP uncertain in many cases due to oligomenorrhea, metrorrhagia, implantation bleeding, pregnancy following post-partum amenorrhea
UTERINE SIZE	-tape measurement distance from symphysis to fundus -gestational age (weeks) = fundal height in inches + 1/2 week -can be unreliable due to many reasons such as maternal body build, retroverted uterus, amniotic fluid volume, fibroids

DOCUMENTING THE FETUS SONOGRAPHICALLY

-documenting the pregnancy is a careful, well thought out process that considers historical, clinical and sonographic information

PARAMETER	METHOD	US APPEARANCE
FIRST TRIMESTER		
GESTATIONAL SAC SIZE & GROWTH -used mainly when no embryo is seen in diagnosis of early pregnancy, blighted ovum and suspected ectopic -used from 5–7 weeks accuracy +/- 1 week	-measure sac diameters in three dimensions; length (L), width (W) and AP diameter (H = height) Mean Sac Diameter (MSD) $= \frac{L \times W \times H}{3}$ Gestational Age (days) = MSD (mm) +30 normal growth = 1 mm per day abnormal growth < .6 mm per day	transvaginal scans, coronal and transverse uterus measuring early gestation sac 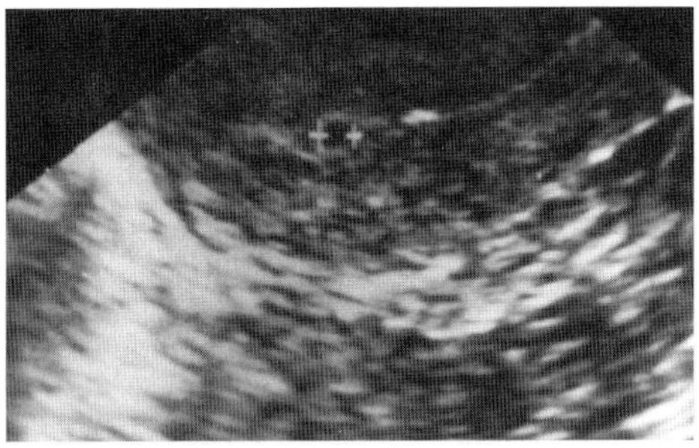 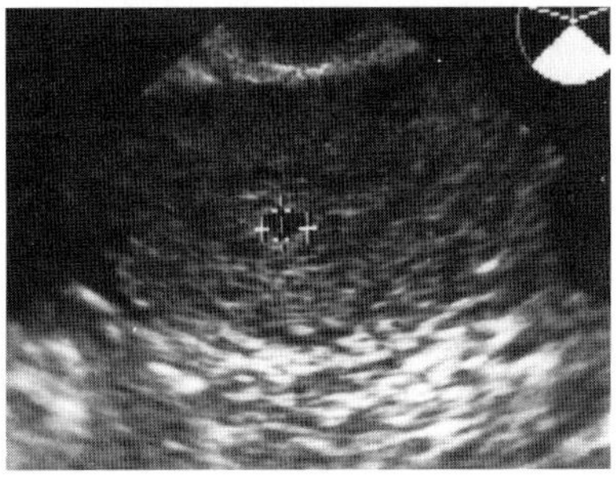
FETAL HEART -using heart rate from 6–9.5 weeks as dating method under investigation -heart rate is documented in all obstetrical exams	-fetal heartbeat recorded by m-mode -heart rate directly traced on ultrasound screen and calculated by formulas programmed into machine Gestational age (days) = heart rate x 0.3 + 7	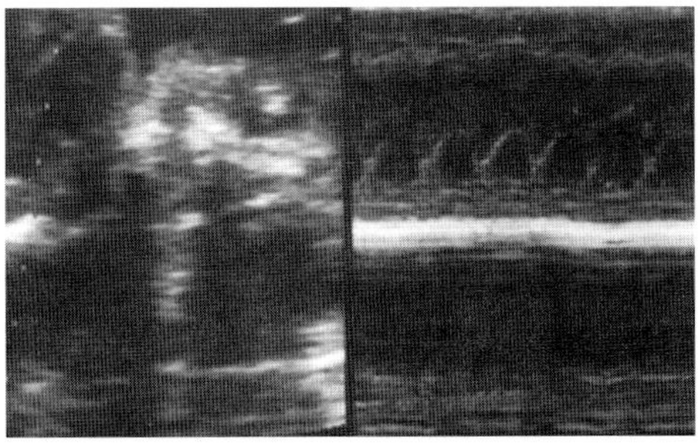

PARAMETER	METHOD	US APPEARANCE
CROWN RUMP LENGTH (CRL) -useful from 6.5 to 12 weeks -after 12 weeks accuracy becomes variable due to flexion and extension movements of fetus -most accurate method of measuring fetus in 1st trimester Accuracy within +/- 4 days -most accurate sonographic dating method	-measure top of head to rump (exclude limbs and yolk sac) -several attempts should be made to ensure longest measurement gestational age (weeks) = CRL < 1.0 cm = CRL (cm) + 6 CRL > 1.0 cm = CRL (cm) + 6.5	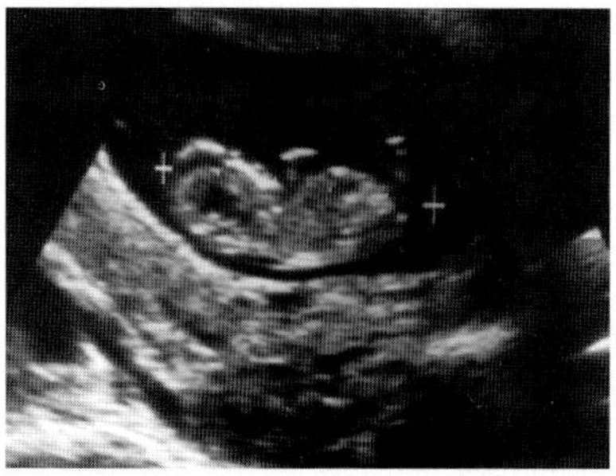
FEMUR LENGTH -easiest and most reliable long bone for measurement -major role in evaluation of fetal weight and body proportions -not affected as much as other parameters in IUGR -some tendency to underestimate length -below 2 standard deviations suggest skeletal dysplasia	-whole length of femur seen with both ends sharp (not tapered) and with good acoustic shadow -measure only diaphysis of femur (femoral neck to distal end of femoral condyles) -exclude distal femoral epiphysis -severe bowing of femur could be from tangential scan planes (try different angle) or from congenital bone abnormalities	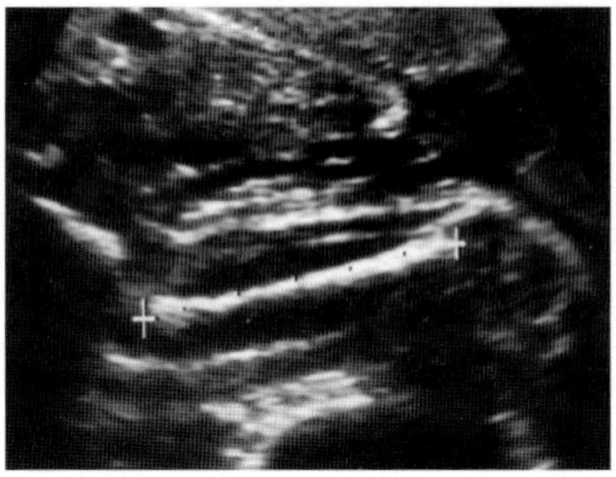

SECOND AND THIRD TRIMESTER

HEAD AND NECK

PARAMETER	METHOD	US APPEARANCE
BIPARIETAL DIAMETER (BPD) -largest transverse diameter of head which is perpendicular to midline echo -used from 12 weeks to term -most accurate from 14–20 weeks -most accurate parameter for assigning dates in second trimester If fetal skull low in pelvis try: -Trendelenburg position -gentle manual upward pressure on head -distend maternal urinary bladder	-transaxial, image of head, measuring from outer surface of skull table (nearest transducer) to the inner margin of opposite skull table at widest plane -accuracy depends on ideal ovoid head shape -use cephalic index if head is abnormal <u>Scan plane landmarks</u>: 1. falx (midline echo) 2. thalamus 3. choriod plexus in atria of lateral ventricles 4. cavum septi pelucidi 5. 3rd ventricle Arrows indicate placement of calipers in head perimeter measurement 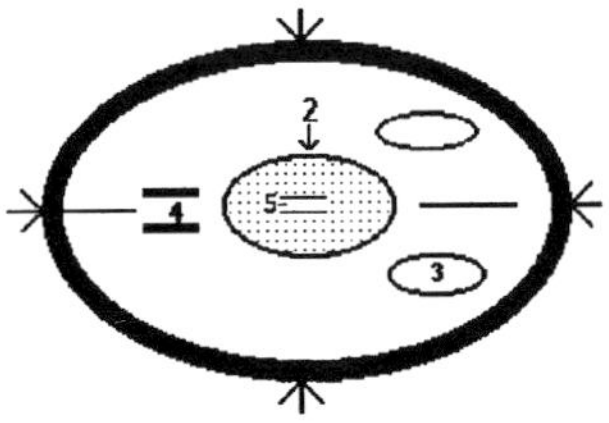	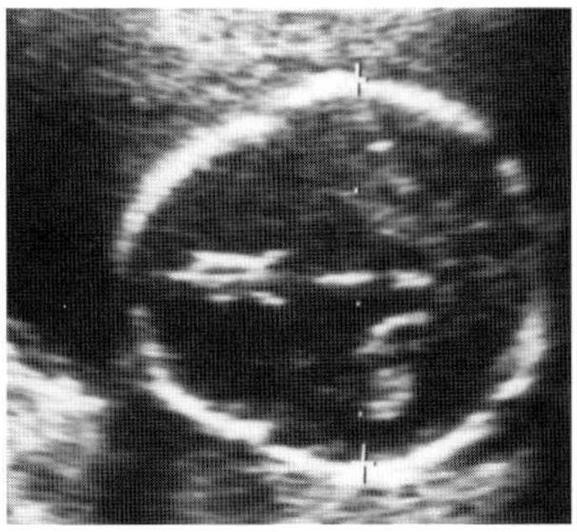 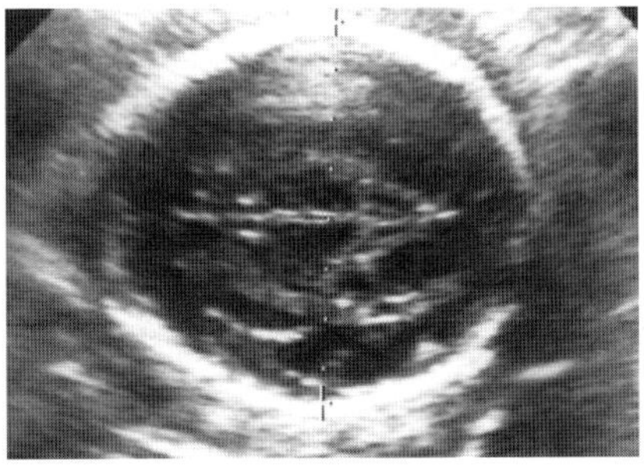

CORRECTED BPD:

-calculation used when cephalic index indicates that the BPD will be misleading

= square root of [(biparietal diameter x fronto occipital diameter) / 1.265]

CEPHALIC INDEX (CI):

-ratio of biparietal diameter to occipitofrontal diameter and is an indication of head shape

-dimensions should be measured from outer-to-outer aspects when calculating cephalic index

$$CI\ \% = \frac{\text{BPD (biparietal diameter)}}{\text{OFD (occipital-frontal diameter)}} \times 100$$

NORMAL CEPHALIC INDEX RANGE = 70–85%

LOW CI= dolichocephaly HIGH CI= brachycephaly

HEAD PERIMETER (HP) / HEAD CIRCUMFERENCE (HC) -not as reproducible as BPD, but used when cephalic index indicates flattened or rounded head shape -same plane as for BPD	3 methods: 1. directly traced on screen with light pen or joy stick 2. traced by digitizer and circumference calculated 3. outer-to-outer occipitofrontal diameter (OFD) and biparietal diameter and calculated: HC=[(BPD + OFD)/2] x 3.14 or =(BPD + OFD) x 1.57	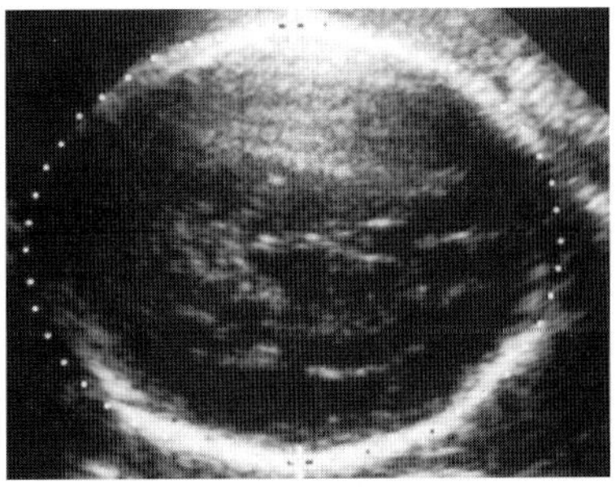

PARAMETER	METHOD	US APPEARANCE
CEREBELLAR HEMISPHERES & CISTERNA MAGNA -transverse measurements across hemispheres can be used in confirming gestational age as well as ruling out CNS anomalies -cisterna magna lies between cerebellum and cranium	-slight posterior/inferior rotation of the probe from the BPD plane angled through posterior fossa and cisterna magna Measure: 1. bilobar diameter of cerebellum 2. anterior–posterior depth of cisterna magna (Normal <1 cm)	measurement of cisterna magna (arrows) 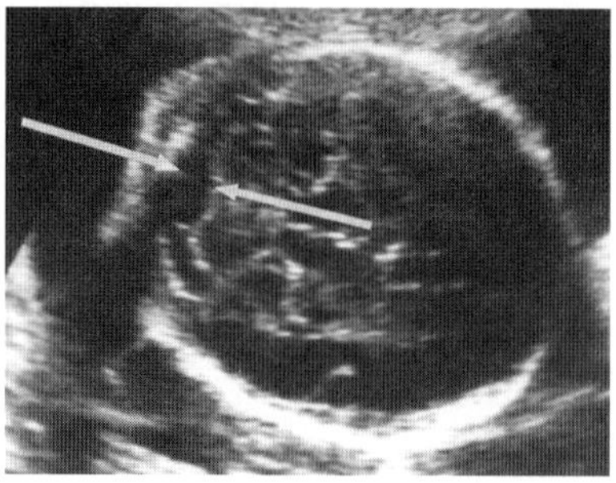 measurement of cerebellum (between arrows) 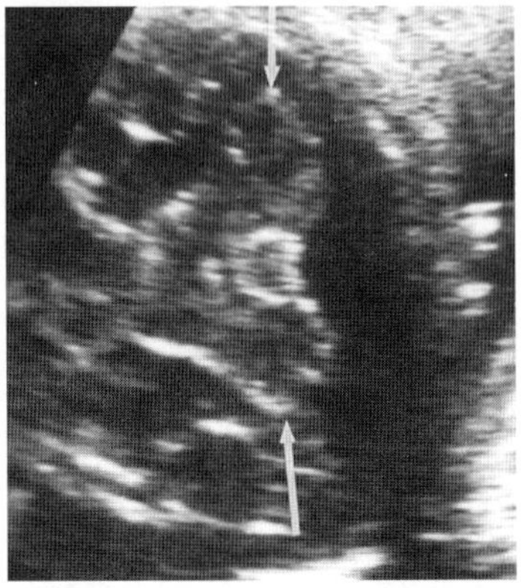
VENTRICLES -important indicator of normal internal anatomy Atrium Diameter -transverse diameter of the ventricular atrium at the level of the glomus of the choroid plexus -from 16 weeks to term Lateral Ventricular Ratio -ratio of lateral ventricle to its hemisphere's width -helpful after 24 weeks	Atrium Diameter -transverse axial scan plane, just superior to BPD scan plane -measure width lateral ventricle normal < 10 mm Lateral Ventricular Ratio= $\frac{\text{lateral ventricular width}}{\text{hemispheric width}}$ abnormal >50%	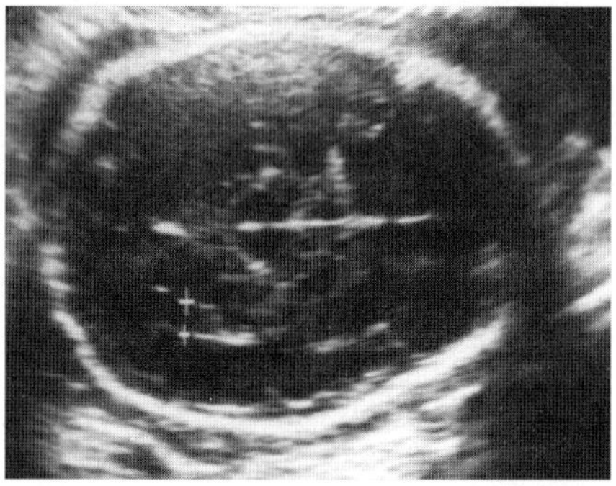

PARAMETER	METHOD	US APPEARANCE
ORBITAL DISTANCE Biocular -distance from lateral aspect of one eye to lateral aspect of other eye Ocular -width of one eye Interocular -width between eyes <u>Hypotelerorism</u> -eyes too close together <u>Hyperteleroism</u> -eyes too far apart	Biocular: -measure outer-to-outer margins of the eyes -start at same plane as BPD and angle transducer caudally until orbits are visualized	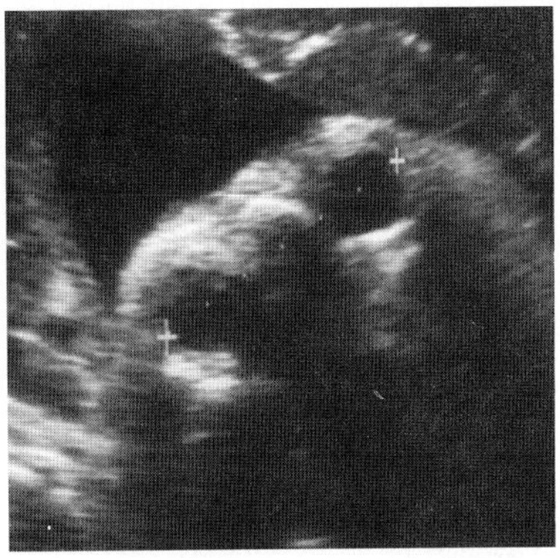 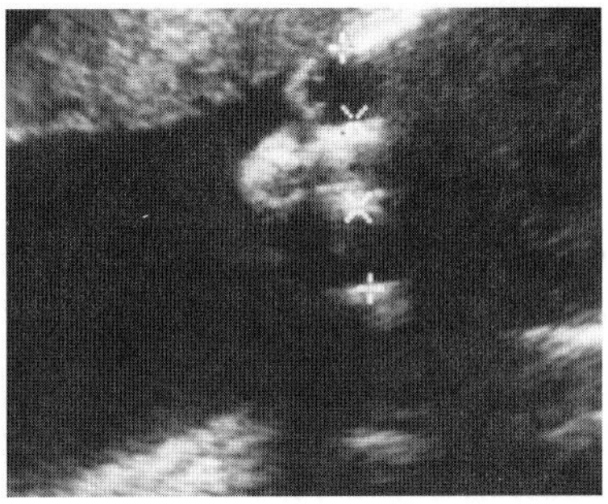
NUCAL SKIN FOLD -measurement of the skin at the back of the neck -measured between 15 and 21 weeks gestation -thickened nucal fold associated with Trisomy 21	-measure from outer skull table to outer skin surface on transcerebellar view of cranium in 2nd trimester -abnormal > 6 mm -appropriate scan plane landmarks: 1. cavum septa pellucidi 2. cerebellar hemispheres 3. cerebral peduncles 4. cisterna magna	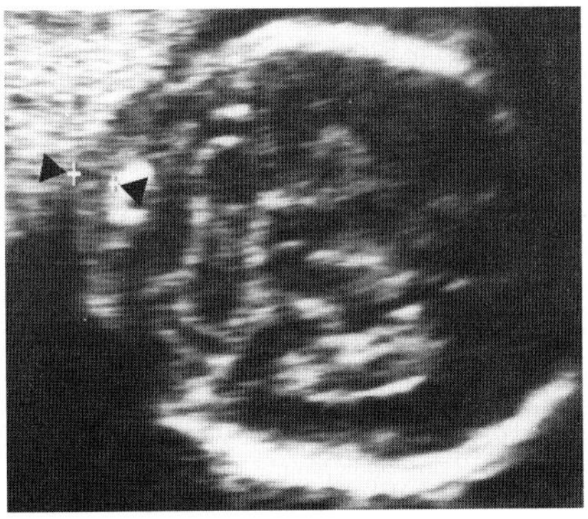

BODY		
PARAMETER	**METHOD**	**US APPEARANCE**
ABDOMINAL CIRCUMFERENCE (AC) / ABDOMINAL PERIMETER (AP) -used in estimation of fetal weight and diagnosis of macrosomia and IUGR -reflects liver size, amount of fatty tissue -has greatest interobserver and intraobserver variability of all fetal measurements TECHNICAL HINTS: -excessive transducer pressure can distort abdomen circumference -to avoid using oblique scan plane, fetal spine should line up across from portal vein	<u>Scan Plane Landmarks:</u> 1. umbilical part of left portal vein enters liver (gall bladder on right may be mistaken for umbilical vein) 2. stomach 3. 3 ossification centers of spine (adrenals can be in scan plane but scan plane must be below heart and above kidneys) 3 methods of calculation: 1. directly traced on screen with light pen or joy stick 2. traced by digitizer and circumference calculated 3. outer lateral diameter (D1) + outer AP diameter (D2) AC= (D1+D2) x 1.57	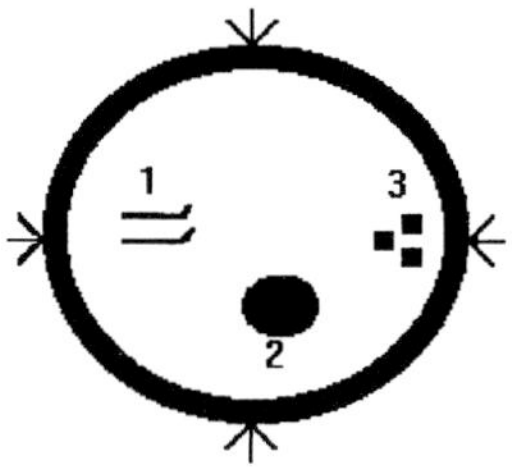 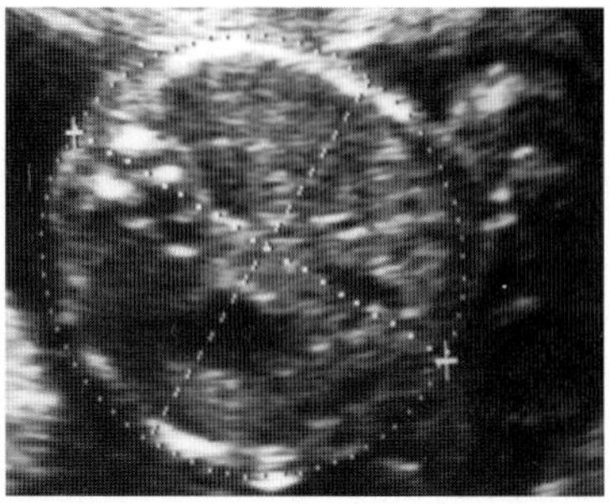
KIDNEYS -significant deviation enables antenatal detection of renal enlargement -small kidneys maybe more difficult to measure because of ill-defined renal outline	-an approximate calculation of normal kidney size for gestation age Gestational age (weeks) = length (mm) = 2 x AP diameter (mm)	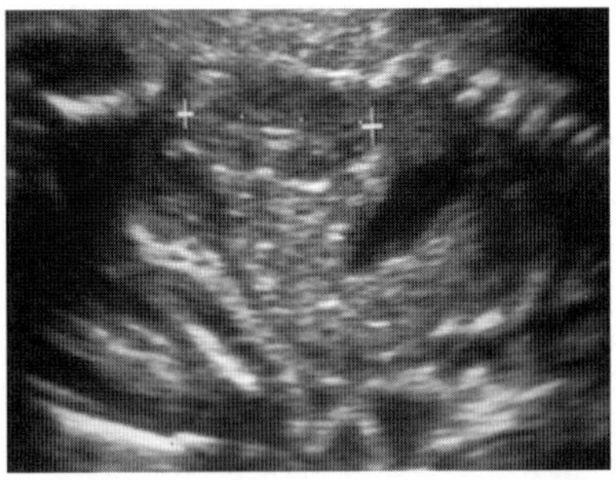
THORACIC CIRCUMFERENCE -useful in detecting fetal anomalies such as dwarfism	-transverse diameter (mm) + AP diameter (mm) x 1.57 -obtained in transverse scan plane at level of the four-chamber view of the heart	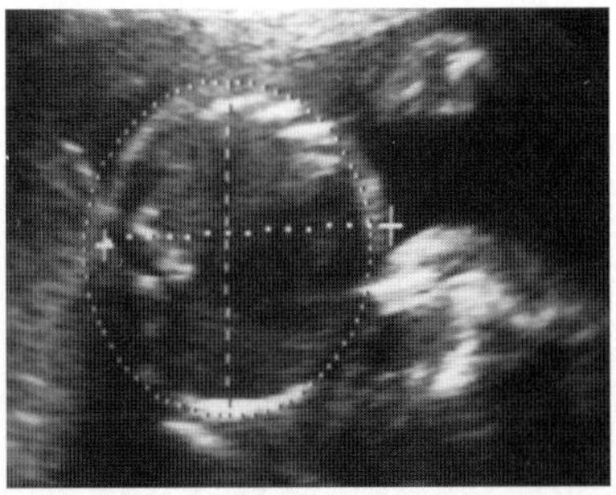

FETAL WEIGHT

-indications: suspected IUGR, macrosomia, twins, breech prior to trial labor, threatened pre-term labor
-accuracy in estimating birth weights using abdominal circumference depends on weight of fetus (the smaller the fetus, the greater the accuracy)

weight difference in twins =

$$\frac{\text{EFW (large)} - \text{EFW (small)}}{\text{EFW (large)}} \times 100$$

-calculated by combining multiple fetal parameters
-most accepted method uses BPD, FL and AC
-corrected BPD should be used if CI is abnormal
-if BPD not available, FL alone is used

FETAL BODY RATIOS

- used to detect fetal asymmetry and fetal growth patterns in cases such as IUGR, ascites, macrosomia, dwarfism

HEAD TO ABDOMEN CIRCUMFERENCE RATIO (HC/AC)
FEMUR LENGTH TO BPD RATIO (FL/BPD)
FEMUR LENGTH TO ABDOMEN (FL/AC)

FETAL PRESENTATION

-described in relation to presenting part

CEPHALIC	COMPLETE/ FULL BREECH	FRANK BREECH	FOOTLING BREECH
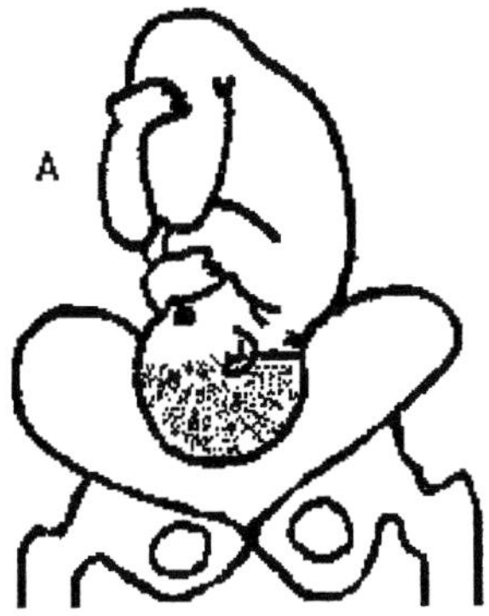	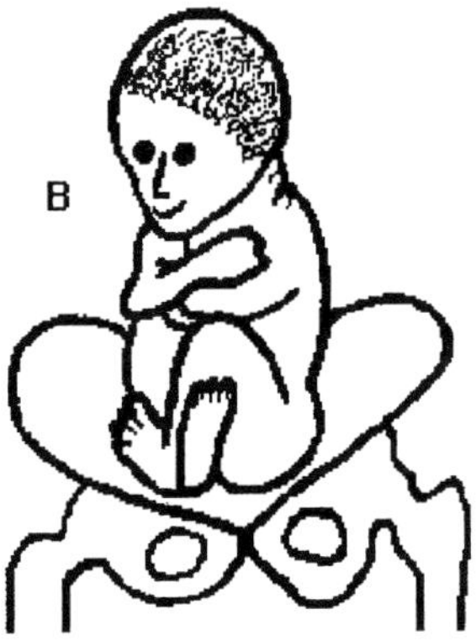	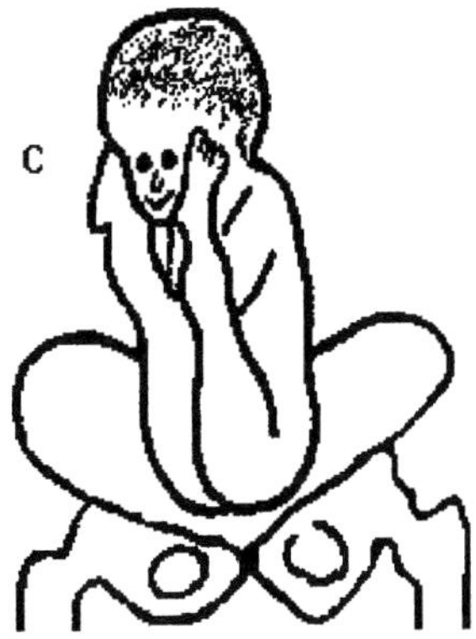	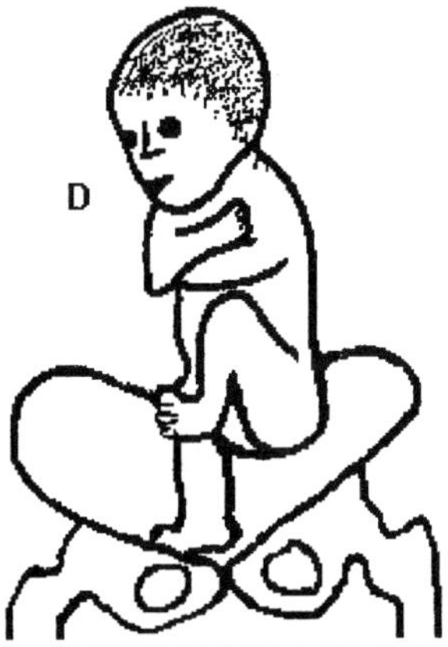

transabdominal sagittal midline scan of cephalic presentation; head directly over os (arrow)

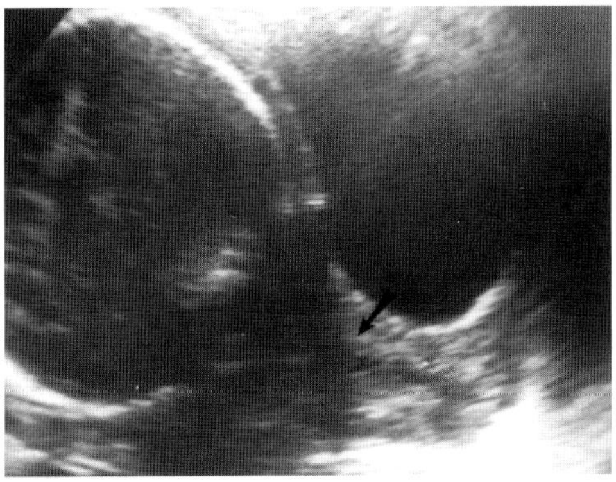

transabdominal sagittal midline scan of breech presentation; fetal lower limbs directly over os (arrow)

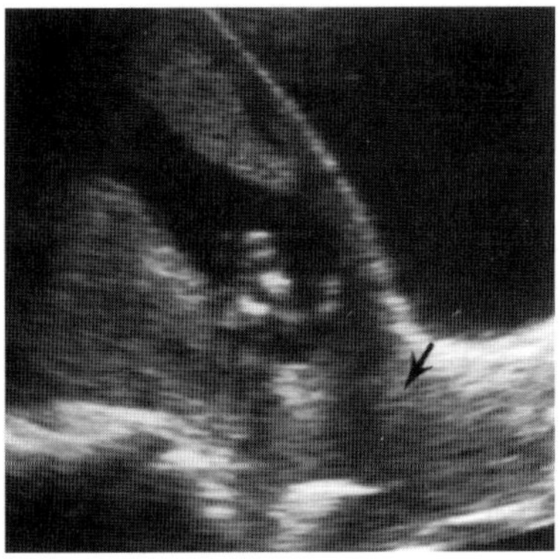

INTRAUTERINE GROWTH RETARDATION - IUGR

DEFINITION: most commonly defined as a fetus who measures below the 10th percentile of weight for gestational age or a term fetus that is less than 2500 grams

-a fetus that has not reached its genetic growth potential because of pathologic restrictions

SGA - small for gestational age: 3 types

1. genetically small babies: are NOT IUGR, and are not at increased risk for perinatal morbidity and mortality
2. intrinsic causative factors
3. extrinsic causative factors

LBW - low birth weight: 2 types

1. infants whose birth weight is low because they were born early but whose weights are above the 10th percentile for gestational age
2. infants who are below the 10th percentile for gestational age

CLINICAL SIGNS	CLINICAL SIGNIFICANCE
-small symphysis fundal height -decrease in maternal weight -decrease in symphysis-fundal height (SFH) Risks -previous history of IUGR -mother < 17 or > 35 years old	Fetus: death, premature delivery, in utero starvation, asphyxia at delivery, muscle wasting, thermal instability Newborn: increased association with perinatal mortality acidosis, meconium aspiration, cerebral hemorrhage, convulsions, hypoglycemia, hypocalcaemia,, Long-term: increased risk for neurologic and intellectual impairment

TYPES: not absolute concepts as growth-retarded fetuses display a wide spectrum of body proportions

SYMMETRICAL - PRIMARY	ASYMMETRICAL - SECONDARY
-least common (25-35%) -proportionate reduction of all fetal measurements -prior to 26 weeks persisting until delivery -unknown dates can lead to IUGR not being recognized	-most common (65-75% of IUGR) -decrease in body size (abdominal circumference and soft tissue growth) -head sparring: placental blood flow compromise (blood shunted to brain at expense of liver and body) -in severe cases, the head sparing is compromised and fetus is more symmetrically growth retarded -occurs after 30 weeks
CAUSES: Intrinsic causes DECREASED GROWTH POTENTIAL OF FETUS 1. chromosomal abnormality (eg. trisomies 13,18,21) 2. major congenital abnormality (eg. bone dysplasia) 3. early environmental insult (eg. TORCH)	CAUSES: Extrinsic causes DECREASE IN NUTRIENTS AND OXYGEN TO FETUS Maternal—malnutrition, significant hypertension, anemia, substance abuse, smoking, overt diabetes, uterine anomaly Placenta—premature aging, hemangiomas, infarcts, circumvellate, abruptio, subchorionic hematoma

SONOGRAPHIC FINDINGS: to identify "at risk" fetuses

1. SMALL SIZE FOR DATES: must have reliable LMP or early scan

a) head size - BPD, HC -symmetrical: frequently compromised early
-asymmetrical: normal until late pregnancy

b) abdominal circumference < 10th percentile
-most sensitive single indicator of IUGR and nutritional status of fetus

c) femur length -degree of compromise is less well established
-used primarily in evaluating fetal weight and body proportionality

d) estimated fetal weights < 10th percentile (fetal gender specific weight charts should be used)

2. SLOW GROWTH: serial scans with 2-week intervals are indicated once diagnosis of IUGR suspected
abdominal circumference - should average growth of 1 cm/week in 3rd trimester
growth in estimated fetal weight should be documented

3. EVIDENCE OF ASYMMETRY
HC/AC ratio -normal values change with time, therefore, menstrual age is required to diagnose IUGR
FL/AC ratio -constant after 24 weeks, therefore, could be used as age independent indicator

4. OLIGOHYDRAMNIOS

5. GRADE 3 PLACENTA BEFORE 36 WEEKS

6. DELAYED APPEARANCE OF DISTAL FEMORAL EPIPHYSEAL OSSIFICATION CENTER

7. DOPPLER ULTRASOUND UMBILICAL ARTERY

-if resistance to blood flow is abnormally elevated, there is a decrease in nutrients and oxygen exchange which can limit fetal growth and cause hypoxia

-abnormal uterine arterial doppler suggest IUGR

-absent or reversed end-diastolic flow in fetal umbilical arteries can indicate fetal compromise and poor outcome

-not every pregnancy with abnormal Doppler findings has a poor outcome and, therefore, must be used in conjunction with maternal history, fetal biometry, intrauterine observations

MACROSOMIA

-most commonly defined as a fetus who measures over the 90th percentile of weight for gestation age or a term fetus that weighs over 4000 grams
LGA - large for gestational age - macrosomia, > 90 %tile, > 4000 grams
-poorly defined group
1. large normal babies
2. fetuses of diabetic mothers

CLINICAL SIGNS:	CLINICAL SIGNIFICANCE:
-large for dates -maternal gestational diabetes	-increased perinatal mortality (birth trauma, hemorrhage, meconium aspiration) -stillbirth if associated with diabetes

ETIOLOGICAL FACTORS IN DEVELOPMENT OF MACROSOMIA:

1. PROLONGED GESTATION
2. MATERNAL - obesity, previous history, glucose intolerance, diabetes mellitus, multiparity, age over 35

SONOGRAPHIC FINDINGS:

1. LARGE FOR DATES
   -abdominal circumference- most sensitive indicator of macrosomia (AC >3SD for gestational age)
   -high fetal weight
2. ACCELERATED GROWTH
   -serial measures of AC at 2-week intervals above the 90th percentile for growth
3. EVIDENCE OF ASYMMETRY
   -HC/AC or FL:AC ratio low
4. OTHER
   -thick subcutaneous fat line seen about head, abdomen and thigh

transverse scan of fetal abdomen; skin 1 cm. thick which is an indication of macrosomia

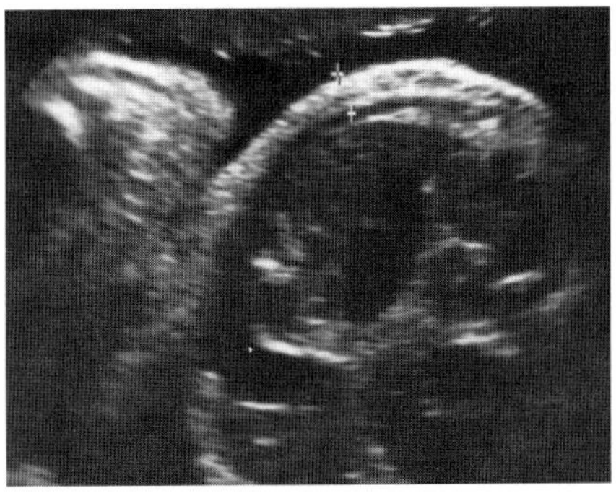

PITFALL don't confuse hair or bone for thickened skin
-hair (H), skin (S), bone (B)

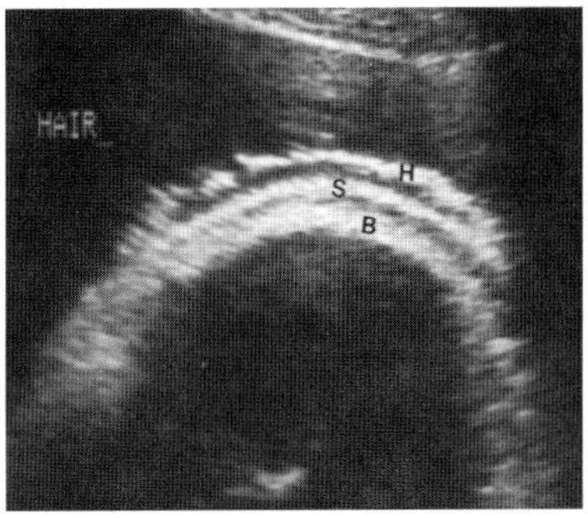

DIFFERENTIAL DIAGNOSIS FOR CLINICAL EXAMINATION

SMALL FOR DATES	LARGE FOR DATES
-incorrect dates	-incorrect dates
-missed abortion	-multiple gestation
-fetal death	-hydatidiform mole
-IUGR	-fetal macrosomia
-oligohydramnios	-maternal gestational diabetes
-premature rupture of membranes	-uterine fibroids
	-polyhydramnios

CHAPTER 15 - EVALUATING FETAL FUNCTION AND WELL-BEING

BIOPHYSICAL PROFILE

-antepartum fetal risk assessment based on dynamic ultrasound survey of biophysical variables in 30 minutes of continuous observation

Score: 8-10 = fetal well being-normal infant, low risk for chronic asphyxia
4-6 = repeat in 24 hours- suspect chronic asphyxia
0-2 = strong suspicion of chronic asphyxia-extend testing time to 120 minutes and a persistent score of < 4 is an indication for delivery

-two types of scoring in literature:
1) more commonly accepted method scores each variable either as normal (score 2) or abnormal (score 0)
2) each variable including placenta grading receives a score of 0, 1 or 2

Factors affecting score: hypoxemia, drugs, fetal sleep cycles

BIOPHYSICAL VARIABLE	NORMAL - 2 POINTS	ABNORMAL - 0 POINTS
<u>REACTIVE FETAL HEART RATE</u> Non stress Test -external system to monitor fetal movement, uterine contractions and fetal heart rate	-normal baseline heart rate (110-160) -presence of at least 2 accelerations of 15 bpm for 15 seconds in 30 minutes	-baseline rate < 100 bpm -unexplained persistent baseline tachycardia >160 bpm -less than 2 episodes of acceleration
<u>AMNIOTIC FLUID VOLUME</u> -largest pocket of fluid free of umbilical cord	-pocket of 2 cm in two perpendicular planes -Normal Amniotic Fluid Index (90%< Normal >10% percentile	-no pockets OR -pocket < 2 cm in two perpendicular planes OR -AFI < 10th percentile
<u>GROSS BODY MOVEMENTS</u> -single or clusters of activity involving limbs and/or body	-three separate fetal/limb movements within 30 minutes	-two or fewer episodes of body/limb movement
<u>FETAL TONE</u> -extension movement with return to flexion	-at least 1 episode of active flexion-extension movements of limbs or trunk	-slow extension with return to partial flexion or movement or no fetal movement
<u>FETAL BREATHING MOVEMENTS</u> -inward movement of thorax with descent of diaphragm and abdominal contents	-30 -60 second episode in 30 minutes	-absent or no episode of > 30 second duration in 30 minutes

DEATH IN UTERO

-fetal death is defined as death over 20 weeks, with fetus weighing more than 500 grams
-before 20 weeks is termed abortion

<u>Specific Signs:</u>
-absent cardiac motion with doppler, M-mode or with real-time sonography

<u>Nonspecific Signs (seen 48 hours after death):</u>
-development of dolichocephaly -- "spalding sign": overlapping fetal skull bones
-distorted fetal anatomy: difficult to distinguish structures, gas and /or thrombis in vascular system
-loss of falx cerebri
-diffuse skin edema
-echogenic foci in amniotic fluid-decrease in size of uterus
-polyhydramnios or oligohydramnios

<u>Clinical & Laboratory Signs:</u>
-2 negative pregnancy tests
-failure of uterus to grow
-no fetal movement
-no heart sounds with auscultation
-red or brown amniotic fluid

-transverse scan of fetal heart showing large clot (arrow) within heart

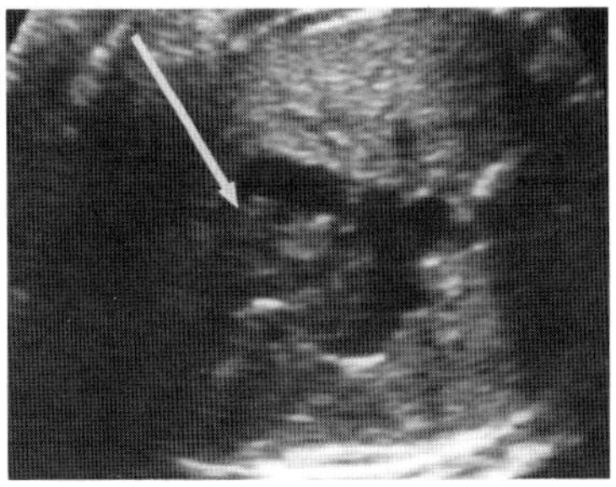

-fetal death with large placental hematoma(arrows)

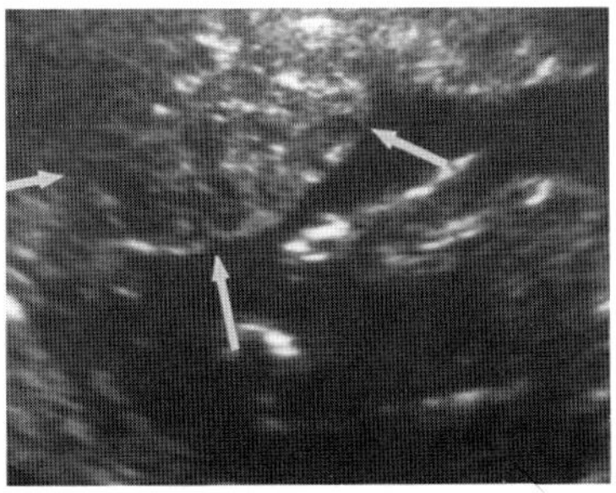

DOPPLER

The placenta and fetus circulations are normally of low resistance, which enables large volumes of blood to be involved in gas and substrate exchange. There have been many Doppler studies on various fetal vasculature: Umbilical artery and vein, aorta, cerebral and renal vessels. When Doppler is used to evaluate a selected high-risk population such as IUGR fetuses, abnormal waveforms seem to be associated with adverse outcomes. Whether Doppler gives superior information compared to other fetal tests remains unclear. An abnormal waveform does not always indicate immediate delivery but does suggest an at-risk pregnancy. The potential value is still being evaluated and using Doppler as a screening test remains uncertain.

Normal Umbilical Artery Doppler

R.I. = 4.7
P.I. = 0.82
S/D = 2.5 (gradually declines during pregnancy)
-waveform characteristics change during pregnancy
-factors such as fetal breathing, heart rate accelerations and activity can produce changes in waveform

Abnormal Umbilical Doppler

1. Absent End Diastolic:
-due to very high umbilical outflow resistance so that there is little or no flow during diastole
2. Reverse Diastolic:
-due to extremely high outflow resistance causing vascular recoil with retrograde blood flow at end of cardiac cycle
3. Elevated Systolic:Diastolic Ratio
-indicating increased vascular resistance

Normal Cerebral Doppler

-normally shows typical low resistance patterns
-factors such as cigarette smoking, patient position and duration of pregnancy produce marked changes in cerebral Doppler waveforms

Abnormal Cerebral Doppler

1. Increased Diastolic Flow:
-caused by vasodilatation or brain hyperfusion compensation due to hypoxia
2. Decreased Diastolic Flow:
-caused by cerebral vascular resistance due to acidosis

ABNORMAL DOPPLER SONOGRAPHIC APPEARANCE

appearance of umbilical artery reversal of flow in diastole (white arrow)

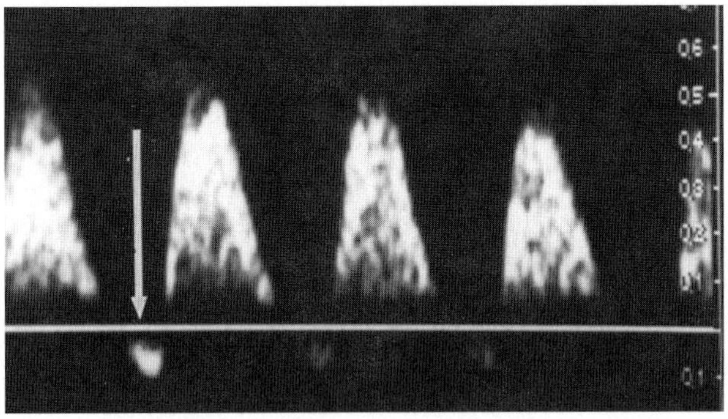

appearance of absent diastolic flow in umbilical artery

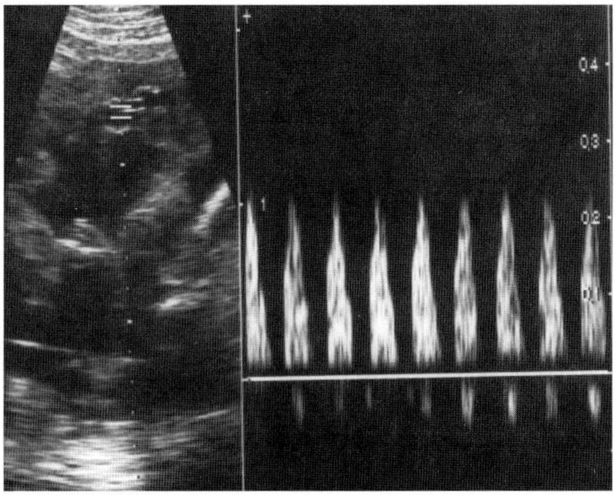

FETAL BLOOD TREATMENTS

CORDOCENTESIS - PERCUTANEOUS UMBILICAL BLOOD SAMPLING (PUBS)

-similar to amniocentesis procedure.
-involves cord insertion site localization and puncture of cord for blood sample.
-indications for fetal blood sampling include: confirm chromosomal mosaicism found on amniocentesis, rapid karyotyping, evaluation of isoimmunization, fetal blood grouping, assessment of fetal anemia, blood transfusion

INTRAUTERINE TRANSFUSIONS

Indications:
-erythroblastosis fetalis: when fetus too immature for early delivery and the bilirubin level in the amniotic fluid is dangerously high
Method:
-under sonographic guidance, a needle is inserted into fetal peritoneum and group O Rh -ve blood is injected
-the fetus absorbs intact transfused red blood cells from the peritoneum to the bloodstream via the lymphatic system
-these red cells which are compatible with the maternal antibody, lessen the risk of anoxia and cardiac failure and the fetus is able to mature sufficiently to survive early delivery
-repeated as necessary during pregnancy

MATERNAL SERUM SCREENING (TESTING) MSS

-involves measuring markers in the maternal serum
1. Alpha-Fetoprotein (AFP)
2. Estriol (uE3)
3. Human Gondotrophin (hCG)

-allows for improved detection of Down syndrome, trisomy 18 and neural tube defects
-fetal age must be known prior to testing and usually a dating ultrasound scan is performed for this
-some degree of false positive and false negative results
-test performed at approximately 16 weeks gestation

MSS RESULTS	POSSIBLE ULTRASOUND FINDINGS
↑ hCG ↓ AFP ↓ ESTRIOL	**TRISOMY 21 - DOWN SYNDROME** -heart: VSD, ASD, AV canal -GI: duodenal atresia, esophageal atresia, omphalocele -GU: pyelectasis -skeletal: short femur, humerus, clinodactyl 5th finger, widely spaced 1st & 2nd toes
↓ hCG ↓ AFP ↓ ESTRIOL	**TRISOMY 18 - EDWARD SYNDROME** -heart: ASD, VSD -GI: esophageal atresia, omphalocele -GU: hydronephrosis, horseshoe kidney -skeletal: overlapping fingers, clenched fist, club foot -CSN: large cisterna magna, myelomeningocele, choroid plexus chsts -OTHER: IUGR, polyhydramnios, single umbilical artery
↑↑ AFP	**-OPEN NEURAL TUBE DEFECTS** -encephaly, encephalocele, spina bifida **-ABDOMINAL WALL DEFECTS** -omphalocele, gastroschisis **-CYSTIC HYGROMA** **-CNS ANOMALY** -Dandy-Walker syndrome, hydrocephalus

PRENATAL CYTOGENETIC STUDIES

INDICATIONS	ULTRASOUND ROLE
1. Abnormal Biochemical markers a) maternal serum alpha fetoprotein b) maternal serum unconjugated estriol c) maternal human chorionic gonadotropin 2. Family History a) previous pregnancy with abnormality b) parental translocation c) relatives (other than offspring) with trisomies d) genetic disorders with chromosome marker or abnormality 3. Advanced Maternal Age 4. Abnormal Ultrasound Scan 5. Parental Anxiety	1. detect multiple gestation 2. document fetal viability before and after procedure, detect obvious fetal malformations, molar pregnancies 3. confirm gestation age 4. localize placenta, fetal position 5. amnios: locate the most accessible pocket of fluid CVS: locate the trophoblast 6. monitor the needle tip/catheter with continuous scanning during procedure

	AMNIOCENTESIS	**CHORIONIC VILLUS SAMPLING (CVS)**
DEFINE	-insertion of a needle through the abdominal wall into the amniotic fluid that surrounds the fetus; a small amount of fluid is removed and the cells contained in the fluid are cultured for study; ultrasound is used to safely guide the needle to ensure that it avoids the fetus, umbilical cord and placenta; in multiple gestations, separate amniocentesis of each is necessary; each amniotic sac may be identified by injecting a dye after aspiration of first fluid sample but before withdrawal of needle	-because genetic material found in chorionic villus is identical to the developing fetus, studies can be made of that tissue instead of culturing amniotic fluid; a narrow plastic tube (catheter) is guided through the vagina into the trophoblast (chorion) under ultrasound guidance; a small sample of villi is removed by suction.
WHEN	-chromosomal analysis is performed at about 16 weeks (although centers are now testing the safety and accuracy of doing amniocentesis at 11–12 weeks) -fetal lung maturity in 3rd trimester: usually between 34 and 37 weeks, when there is a varying degree of lung maturity	-from 8–12 weeks
WHAT	-some amniotic fluid tests include: bilirubin, blood, lecithin/sphingomyelin ratio-L/S (fetal lung maturity), genetic analysis, AFP levels	-genetic analysis
ADVANTAGES	-lower risk of miscarriage than chorionic villus sampling. -fetal lung maturity can be accurately assessed by biochemical analysis of amniotic fluid obtained by amniocentesis	-earlier and faster diagnosis than amniocentesis -termination of an abnormal pregnancy may be made much earlier
DISADVANTAGES	-performed later in pregnancy usually around 16 weeks, requiring about 2 weeks to obtain the results, therefore, fetal diagnosis can rarely be established prior to 18 weeks -if termination is selected, it is performed well into second trimester -requires additional time for tissue culturing except for L/S ratios that can be done the same day	-higher risk of miscarriage than amniocentesis
POTENTIAL COMPLICATIONS	-premature separation of placenta, premature rupture of membranes, premature labor, fetal or maternal bleeding, fetal death -serious maternal risks are almost nonexistent	-bleeding, infection, spontaneous abortion

amniocentesis: length of needle in fluid (bright echogenic line)

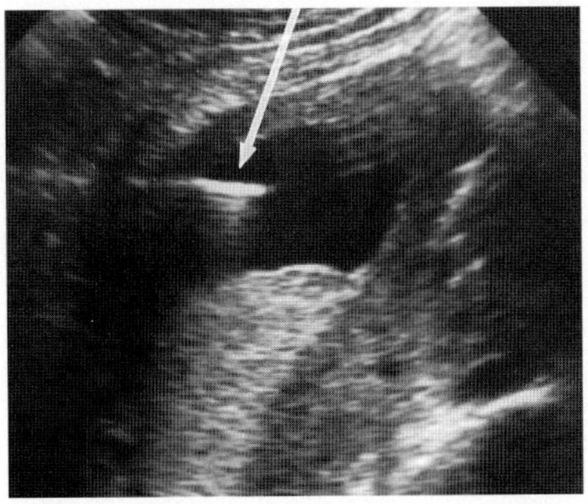

amniocentesis: cross section needle in fluid (arrow)

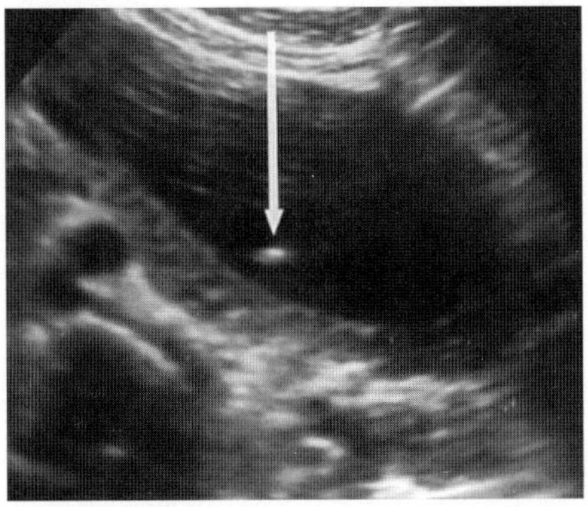

CHAPTER 16 - SONOGRAPHIC EVALUATION OF MATERNAL DISORDERS OF PREGNANCY

DIABETES MELLITUS

-disorder of carbohydrate metabolism from inadequate production or utilization of insulin
-symptoms include: elevated blood sugar (hyperglycemia), sugar in urine (glycosuira), polyuria, excessive thirst, increase food intake, loss of weight
-accurate estimation of gestation age is critical due to increased possibility of growth abnormalities
-patient education about diabetes; how it is managed and controlled, diet, insulin dosage is important for successful pregnancy

	GESTATIONAL (TYPE A,B,C)	IDDM-OVERT (TYPES D,F,H,R,T)
DEFINE TYPES	-can appear suddenly in pregnant women who have never exhibited any signs of high blood glucose -hormonal changes of pregnancy stress the woman's system and in some cases, the pancreas is unable to produce sufficient insulin treatment: ranges from diet management, exercise to insulin therapy	-mother who has chronic insulin dependent diabetes mellitus -for women with diabetes, a glycosylated hemoglobin test can measure the quality of blood sugar control over the last 6–8 weeks which assesses if the diabetes control is adequate to start a pregnancy
EFFECTS OF DIABETES ON PREGNANCY	-higher risk of miscarriage in early stages of pregnancy and birth defects, especially for women in poor diabetic control or with other complications -toxemia: increased blood pressure, protein in urine, swelling of hands and feet -well-controlled diabetes has little harmful effects on the fetus and the danger seems to arise from repeated high blood sugar levels and persistent ketones associated with poor control -chance of baby having diabetes at birth is small	
CLINICAL SIGNS	-large for dates	-small for dates
CLINICAL SIGNIFICANCE	-usually disappears after the birth of baby -30–40% develop Type I (or non-insulin dependent) diabetes within 5 to 10 years -associated with increased perinatal mortality	-increase incidence of intrauterine sudden death at 35–36 weeks -increased risk for development of preeclampsia
SONOGRAPHIC FINDINGS	Macrosomic Fetus: -asymmetric macrosomia head & femur vary in size, but usually are below 90th %tile while abdominal circumference and thigh diameter are significantly larger than normal indicating abundance of soft tissue mass Placenta: -thick placenta > 4 cm Other: -polyhydramnios	Microsomic Fetus: -IUGR due to vascular insufficiency Placenta: -small placenta Associated Finding: -congenital anomalies due to hyperglycemia at organogenesis ie. neural tube defects, cardiovascular, GI tract, renal, skeletal: caudal regression

FETAL HYDROPS

	NONIMMUNE HYDROPS (NIH)	IMMUNE HYDROPS ERYTHROBLASOSIS FETALIS HEMOLYTIC DISEASE OF THE NEWBORN (HDN) ISOIMMUNIZATION
DEFINE TYPES	-excess of total body water evident as extracellular accumulation of fluid in tissues and serous spaces without antibodies against RBC -outcome usually fatal	-lysis of fetal RBCs by maternal IgG antibodies -Rh(+) father and Rh(-) mother carrying Rh(+) fetus. Mother may become isoimmunized if exposed to Rh(+) blood. Maternal Rh(+) antibodies develop which can cross placenta attacking fetus's blood cells causing hemolytic disease or <u>ERYTHROBLASTOSIS FETALIS.</u> treatment: intrauterine transfusions if fetus too immature for early delivery prevention: in subsequent pregnancies Rh immune globulin (Rhogam) is given to Rh -ve women
CAUSE	1. Fetal -cardiac anomalies, hematologic causes, idiopathic, twin-to-twin transfusion, chromosomal abnormalities, skeletal dysplasias, renal disease, TORCH, chest and abdominal masses 2. Maternal -gestational diabetes, hypertension 3. Placental -chorioangioma, thrombosis, AV shunts	-feto-maternal transplacental hemorrhage in 3rd stage labour, miscarriage, abortion -usually doesn't manifest itself until 2nd or 3rd pregnancy

SONOGRAPHIC FINDINGS

1. Fetal Change
-fetal skin thickening (>5 mm), hepato/splenomegally, ascites, pleural and/or pericardial effusion
2. Placental enlargement > 4 cm thickness
3. Polyhydramnios

sagittal scan of fetus showing skin thickening

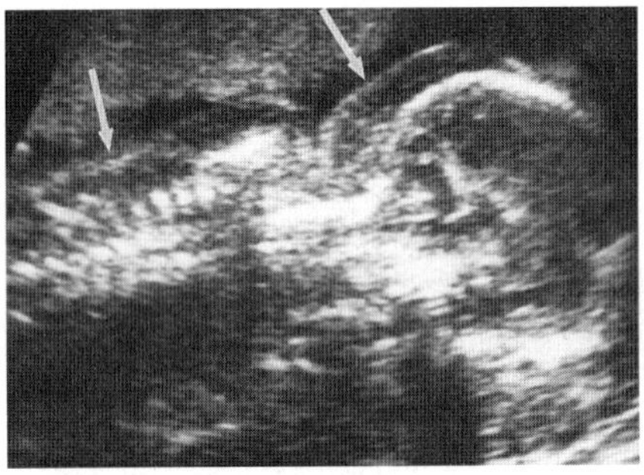

transverse scan of fetal abdomen with thickened (9 mm) skin marked by calipers

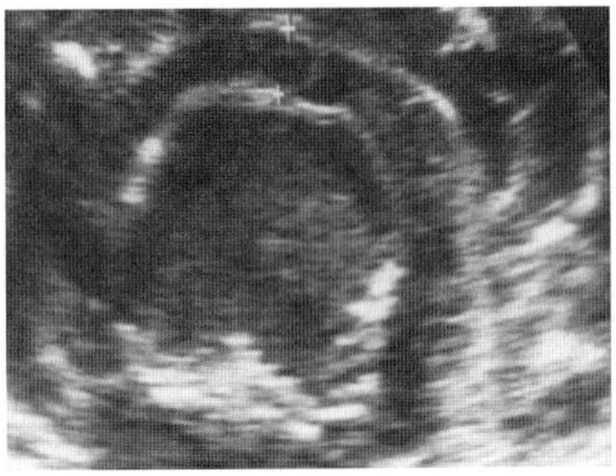

massive amount of fetal ascites with nonimmune hydrops

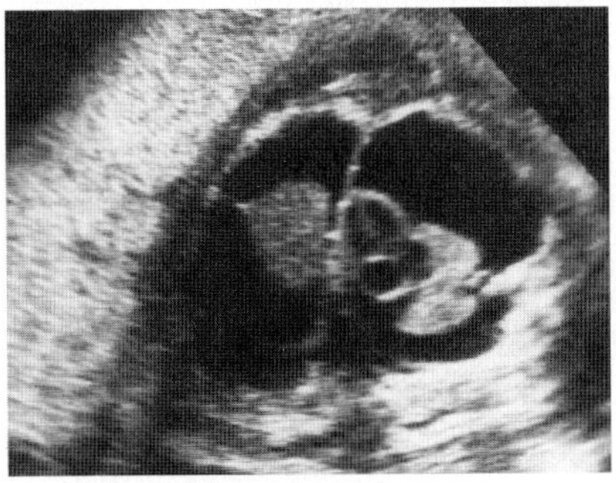

massive amount of pleural and abdominal ascites in a fetus with nonimmune hydrops

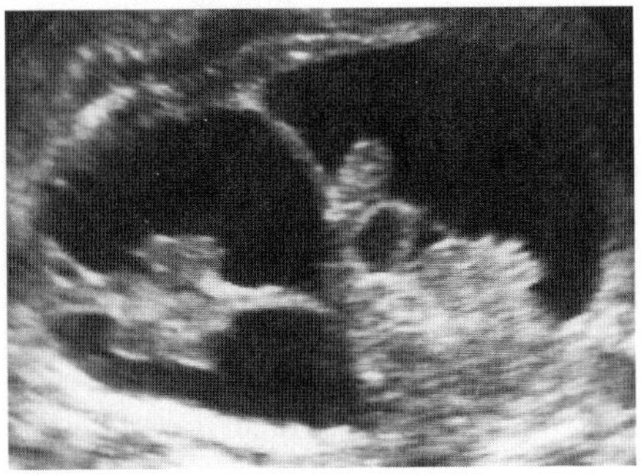

HYPEREMESIS GRAVIDARUM (MORNING SICKNESS)

-nausea and vomiting associated with pregnancy
causes:
-exact cause is unknown
-possibly due to high levels of human chorionic gonadotropin (HCG) secreted by the placenta
-associated with trophoblastic disease

INFERTILITY

PRIMARY - pregnancy does not result after one year of attempting to conceive
SECONDARY - conception is possible but aborts repeatedly

	FEMALE	MALE
FACTORS	1. Mechanical (eg. fibroids, tube damage) 2. Genetic (eg. Turners Syndrome) 3. Developmental (eg. congenital anomalies) 4. Iatrogenic (eg. removal of reproductive organs) 5. Vascular (eg. poor perfusion) 6. Endocrine (eg. PCO, ovulatory failure)	-oliogospermia -azoospermia -impaired motility of sperm -abnormal formation of sperm
TREATMENTS	1. Surgery 2. Pharmacological treatment to improve mucous consistency 3. Hormone Induced Ovulation (clomid, pergonal) 4. In Vitro Fertilization (IVF) -patients have normal ovarian function and normal uterus, but have tubal pathology or dysfunction causing infertility -ultrasound used to follow development of stimulated follicles and to guide in egg aspiration -embryo replacement into uterus can also be guided by ultrasound Complications: ovarian hyperstimulation syndrome, multiple gestations	-androgens -interventional therapy (varicocele repair)

MATERNAL HYDRONEPHROSIS

-maternal kidneys often seen with mild to severe hydronephrosis
-more severe usually on right due to cushioning effects of sigmoid colon
-renal failure is an uncommon, extreme complication and if left untreated it can compromise the fetus
-etiology unknown, although an increase in progesterone causes ureters to relax

sagittal scan of maternal kidney showing mild to moderate hydronephrosis

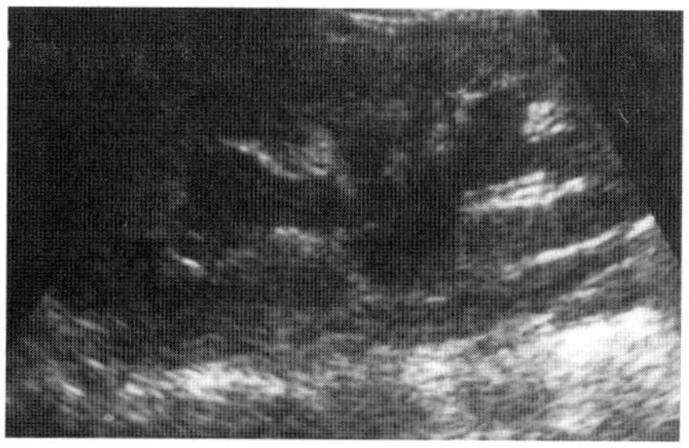

POSTPARTUM COMPLICATIONS

BLADDER FLAT HEMATOMA

-hematoma from cesarean section incision site

US

-inhomogenous convexity on the anterior surface of uterus

-this complex anechoic mass must measure greater than 2 cm to be considered a bladderflap hematoma

sagittal scan of uterus with small complex mass (calipers) which is a small bladder flap hematoma at anterior aspect of uterus

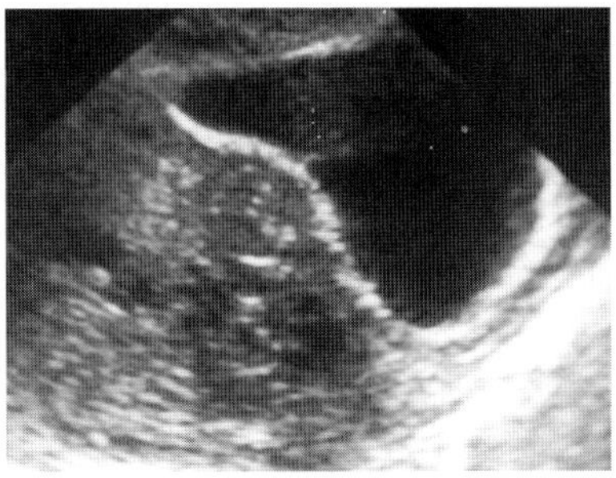

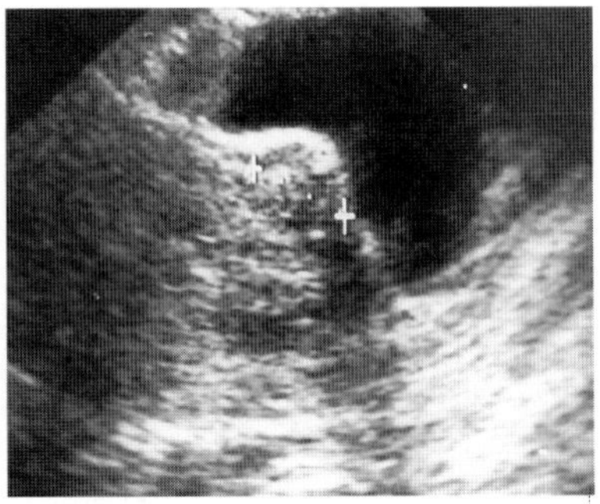

RETAINED PRODUCTS OF CONCEPTION

-echogenic material and fluid within endometrial canal can represent retained blood, clot or placental tissue

-placental-type blood flow is detected in most instances of retained products

-may cause secondary postpartum hemorrhage and infection

US

-thickened, echogenic endometrium which occasionally contains placental tissue

-can also have the appearance of a complex echogenic mass in the endometrium

transvaginal sagittal scan of uterus with hyperechoic tissue within the endometrial cavity

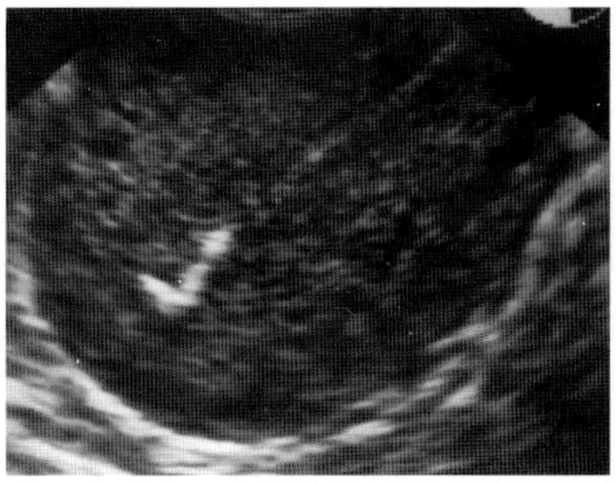

PREGNANCY INDUCED HYPERTENSION - PIH /TOXEMIA		
	PRE-ECLAMPSIA	**ECLAMPSIA**
DEFINE	1. hypertension > 20-week pregnancy Mild : BP: 140/90 or Systolic ↑ 30 mmHg or diastolic ↑ 15 mm Hg over baseline values observed twice, 6 hours apart after 20-week pregnancy Severe: BP: Systolic >160 mm Hg or diastolic >110 mm Hg observed twice, 6 hours apart on bedrest 2. maternal edema 3. proteinuria	-end stage, untreated preeclampsia -preeclampsia plus seizures and/or coma -can lead to death -not common due to advanced detection of pre-eclampsia
PATIENTS AT RISK	-chronic vascular disease -older primigravidas -multiple gestation -trophoblastic disease	
CLINICAL FINDINGS	-hypertension -rapid weight gain -lower extremity edema -progresses to cerebral/visual disturbances, lung edema -oligouria, proteinuria	
SONOGRAPHIC FINDINGS	-oligohydramnios -IUGR -placental abruption -advanced grade 3 placenta, small infarcts -abnormal umbilical artery waveform: high systolic:diastolic ratios	

SUPINE HYPOTENSION SYNDROME

-occurs when a pregnant patient lies supine and becomes faint, nauseous
-due to pressure of gravid uterus on the inferior vena cava causing a drop in blood pressure
-when it occurs, turn patient immediately on her side to a lateral decubitus position
-patient will feel better very quickly after being turned

BIBLIOGRAPHY

NAME	AUTHORS/EDITORS	PUBLISHER	DATE, LOCATION
DIAGNOSTIC ULTRASOUND VOLUMES 1 & 2	RUMACK, CAROL WILSON, STEPHANIE CHARBONEAU, J.WM.	MOSBY	
THE PRINCIPLES AND PRACTICE OF ULTRASONOGRAPHY IN OBSTETRICS AND GYNECOLOGY	FLISCHER, ARTHUR ROMERO, ROBERTO MANNING, FRANK A. JEANTY, PHILLIPPE JAMES, A. EVERETTE JR.	APPLETON & LANGE	1991
PRENATAL ULTRASOUND	SPIRT, BEVERLY GORDON, LAWRENCE OLIPHANT, MICHAEL	CHURCHILL LIVINGSTON	1987, NY
RADIOGRAPHICS (PERIODICAL) SEPT 1993, VOLUME 13 N#5 PAGE 969	ENDOVAGINAL SONOGRAPHY OF THE NONGRAVID UTERUS MOGAVERO, GERALINE GERALDINE, SHEILA ULRIKE, M. HANPER		
ROBBINS PATHOLOGIC BASIS OF DISEASE 4TH EDITION	COTRAN, RAMZI KUMAN, VINAY ROBBINS, STANLEY	WB SAUNDERS CO	1989 PHILADELPHIA
SEMINARS IN US, CT, & MRI EDITORS RAYMOND, HOWARD W. ZWIEBEL, WM. HARNSBERGER, H.R.	VOL. 11 NO. 1 FEB. 90 TV SONOGRAPHY MENDELSON, ELLEN	WB SAUNDERS COMP	
RADIOLOGY OF SYNDROMES	TAYBI, HOOSHANG	YEAR BOOK MEDICAL PUBLISHERS	1975
GYNECOLOGY ILLUSTRATED 4TH EDITION	GOVAN, A.D.T. HART, D. MCKAY CALLANDER, ROBIN	CHURCHILL LIVINGSTON	1993
LANGMAN'S MEDICAL EMBRYOLOGY 5TH EDITION	SADLER, T.W.	WILLIAMS & WILKINS	1985
A PRACTICAL GUIDE TO ULTRASOUND IN OBSTETRICS AND GYNECOLOGY	SAUERBREI, ERIC E. NGUYEN, KHANH T. NOLAN, ROBERT L.	RAVEN PRESS	1987
A PRACTICAL GUIDE TO ULTRASOUND OF FETAL ANOMALIES	HEGGE, FREDERICK N.	RAVEN PRESS	1992
CORE TEXTBOOK OF ANATOMY	THOMPSON, JS.S.	J.B. LIPPINCOTT COMPANY	1977
APPLETON & LANGE'S REVIEW FOR THE ULTRASONOGRAPHY EXAMINATION 2ND EDITION	ODWIN, CHARLES S. DUBINSKY, TRUDY FLEISCHER, ARTHUR	APPLETON & LANGE	1993

SYLLABUS: SPECIAL COURSE ULTRASOUND 1991-PRESENTED AT THE 77TH SCIENTIFIC ASSEMBLY OF THE RSNA	EDITOR : RIFKIN, MATTHEW CO-EDITORS: CHARBONEAU, J. WM. LAING, FAYE C.	RSNA PUBLICATIONS	1991
TABERS CYCLOPEDIC MEDICAL DICTIONARY 17TH EDITION	THOMAS, CLAYTON	F.A. DAVIS COMPANY	1993 PHILADELPHIA
OVARIAN MALIGNANCIES	PIVER, M. STEVEN	CHURCHILL LIVINGSTON	1983
ESSENTIALS OF HUMAN EMBRYOLOGY	MOORE, KEITH	B.C. DECKER INC	1988
PRINCIPLES OF ANATOMY AND PHYSIOLOGY 5TH EDITION	TORTORA, GERALD ANAGNOSTAKOS, NICHOLAS	HARPER & ROW	1987
ENDOVAGINAL ULTRASOUND 2ND EDITION	GOLDSTEIN, STEVEN R.	WILEY-LISS	
RADIOLOGY REVIEW MANUAL	DAHNER, WOLFGANG,	WILLIAMS & WILKINS	1990
ULTRASONOGRAPHY IN OBSTETRICS AND GYNECOLOGY 3RD EDITION	CALLEN, PETER	W.B. SAUNDERS	
FUNDAMENTALS OF OBSTETRICS AND GYNECOLOGY 6TH EDITION	LLEWELLYN-JONES, DEREK	MOSBY	1994
DOPPLER ULTRASOUND IN OBSTETRICS ABD GYNECOLOGY	COPEL, JOSHUA A. REED, KATHRYN L.	RAVEN	1995
ATLAS OF ULTRASOUND MEASUREMENTS	GOLDBERG, BARRY KURTZ, ALFRED	YEAR BOOK MEDICAL PUBLISHERS	1990, CHICAGO
BASIC IMAGING AND CONGENITAL HEART DISEASE 3RD EDITION	SWISCHUK, LEONARD E. SAPIRE, DAVID W.	WILLIAMS & WILKINS	1986

SUBJECT INDEX